Epidemiology and the Delivery of Health Care Services

T0203058

Denise M. Oleske

Epidemiology and the Delivery of Health Care Services

Methods and Applications

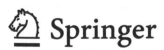 Springer

Denise M. Oleske
Chicago, IL
USA

ISBN: 978-1-4899-8343-5   ISBN: 978-1-4419-0164-4 (eBook)
DOI 10.1007/978-1-4419-0164-4
Springer New York Dordrecht Heidelberg London

Springer is part of Springer Science+Business Media (www.springer.com)

Preface

As the obesity epidemic widens to all age groups and nations, chronic conditions increase in frequency, and populations grow in number, the costs of treatment will exhaust future health care resources. The only alternative is population-based management emphasizing prevention, health promotion, and environmental modifications. Dissemination of information on risk factors derived from epidemiologic studies to evoke individual, community, and policy change is a strategy in supporting this approach. Complementing this needs to be health care services based upon the knowledge and application of epidemiologic concepts and methods to achieve control of existing and emerging health problems given resource constraints and ethical considerations. While some of these health problems and their consequences are predictable and generally addressed by health systems, health care services need to address unpredictable exposures and events as well. Epidemiology also provides a framework for planning health services for unpredictable events such as natural and man-made disasters.

This text focuses on the unique application of epidemiology to health care management practice, regardless of the setting of that practice. This emerging discipline termed is "managerial epidemiology." Managerial epidemiology draws from the traditional disciplines of public health, epidemiology, and health care management for improving the health of populations, be those in communities or served by health plans or systems. Competencies from each of these traditional disciplines which are fundamental to managerial epidemiology are emphasized throughout this text, starting from the basic core domains which focus on the conceptual orientation of management epidemiology and the basic skills and to the competencies needed for assessment and prioritization in chapters under Part I. This is followed by competencies required for specialization of the ever-changing fields of infectious disease, environmental, health care quality, and patient safety concerns are illustrated in chapters under Part II. And finally, managerial epidemiology requires competencies which span health care settings requiring leadership, systems thinking, and professionalism which are emphasized in chapters under Part III covering policy and ethics in managerial epidemiology.

Finally, this updated text overviews aspects of the five core areas of public health (biostatistics, environmental health, epidemiology, health policy, and social and behavioral health factors) and the interdisciplinary domains of communication and informatics, diversity and culture, professionalism, program planning, and systems thinking. Practice examples throughout illustrate the integration of core competencies and interdisciplinary domains. Discussion questions are presented at the end of each chapter to promote critical thinking in deriving creative solutions using epidemiologic methods to real-life problem situations to promote the health, safety, and quality of life of populations.

Chicago, IL

Denise M. Oleske

Contents

Part I
Foundations of Managerial Epidemiology

Chapter 1
An Epidemiologic Framework for the Delivery of Health Care Services

Learning Outcomes

After completing this chapter, you will be able to:

1. Estimate population health care needs from a demographic profile of the population served.
2. Ascertain factors that are potential barriers to utilization of health care services in a population subgroup.
3. Identify the factors that are determinates of health in a community.

Keyterms Epidemiologic model of health care delivery • Epidemiology • Health • Health care needs • Population pyramid

Increasingly, health care management has shifted from a focus upon organizing care around individuals to strategizing the delivery of health care regardless of setting for populations. This has been largely driven by worldwide problems related to population growth, aging populations, decreasing resources (nursing shortage, lower reimbursement, etc.), and increasing costs. Although the use and introduction of new technology has been identified as a major factor for increasing costs, a small number of medical conditions, or treated prevalence in epidemiologic terms, account for the marked rise in cost and use of resources (Thorpe, 2006). This further prompts the shift to a population-based viewpoint in all aspects of health care management. It also prompts an increasing focus on prevention and reliance upon various indicators, particularly safety and quality indicators, to make informed decisions and inform providers, insurers, policy-makers, and consumers regarding how the care planned, delivered, and monitored. The value of any indicator is only as good as the quality of the information upon which it was based. To represent the application of epidemiology in the new era of the delivery of health care services, the following definitional orientation is offered:

D.M. Oleske (ed.), *Epidemiology and the Delivery of Health Care Services: Methods and Applications,*
DOI 10.1007/978-1-4419-0164-4_1, © Springer Science+Business Media, LLC 2009

Epidemiology is the study of the distribution of health needs, including disease, impairments, disability, injuries, and other health problems in human populations and the factor contributing to their emergence, severity, and consequences. The ultimate goal of epidemiology is to identify the causal factors that could be eliminated or modified to prevent or control adverse health outcomes and apply the knowledge of these to improve the health of populations.

An epidemiologic model is essential to understand how health care delivery can affect population health. A model that represents this orientation is displayed in Fig. 1. This conceptual model is the focus of this chapter and provides the orientation for the remainder of the volume. First, each component of the model is discussed. An explanation of how the model provides a framework the health care management practice follows.

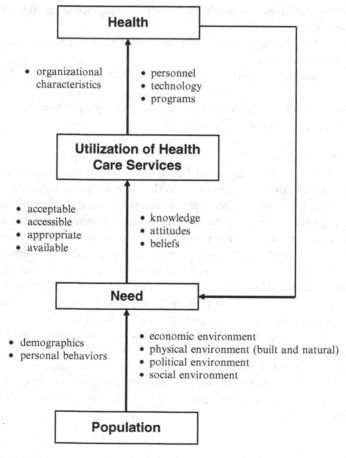

Fig. 1 Epidemiological model of the delivery of health care services

The Population

Defining the population and understanding its characteristics are fundamental to the epidemiology model of health services delivery. Population characteristics form the basis for the type of health care needs it requires. Populations targeted may be defined in terms of geopolitical boundaries, as users of health services (e.g., hospital, physician group practice, public clinic, etc.), as potential users (e.g., members of a health insurance plan, Health Maintenance Organization [HMO]), by institutional membership (e.g., school children, prisoners, orphanages, etc.), because of a special group membership (e.g., military personnel), or some combination thereof. The demographic features of a population, its size, and growth trends are the fundamental determinants of the types of health problems likely to emerge in a geographic area and concomitantly what types of health services would be required.

Factors affecting population size are: birth rate, fertility rate, migration, and mortality rate. The greatest amount of natural change in a population over the short term is usually attributable to the difference between the birth rate and the death rate. However, over time or because of natural disasters or civil strife, migration contributes a major influence to population change in terms of numbers and composition. With the exception of Europe, the global population is expected to increase despite decreased fertility levels in many countries, the widespread devastation of HIV/AIDS, and the emergence of new transmissible diseases (United Nations [UN], 2007). A global population which is estimated to increase by 77.8% between 2007 and 2050 will present a health care challenge unto itself with increasing units of resources for prevention to treatment care needing to be garnered to provide the services (Table 1). It will be particularly challenging to maintain a healthy world given that most of the population growth anticipated is in countries classified by the UN as developing.

Table 1 Population of the world, major development groups and major areas, 1950, 1975, 2007, and 2050 according to different growth projection variants

Major area	Population (millions)			Population in 2050 (millions)			
	1950	1975	2007	Low	Medium	High	Constant
World	2,535	4,076	6,671	7,792	9,191	10,756	11,858
More developed regions	814	1,048	1,223	1,065	1,245	1,451	1,218
Less developed regions	1,722	3,028	5,448	6,727	7,946	9,306	10,639
Least developed countries	200	358	804	1,496	1,742	2,002	2,794
Other less developed countries	1,521	2,670	4,644	5,231	6,204	7,304	7,845
Africa	224	416	965	1,718	1,998	2,302	3,251
Asia	1,411	2,394	4,030	4,444	5,266	6,189	6,525
Europe	548	676	731	566	664	777	626
Latin America and the Caribbean	168	325	572	641	769	914	939
Northern America	172	243	339	382	445	517	460
Oceania	13	21	34	42	49	56	57

(Source: United Nations, 2007)

With respect to demographic and social characteristics, attributes of a population highly correlated with health events include age, gender, race, ethnicity, education, employment, and income, with age being the strongest and most consistent predictor of health needs in a population (Norris et al., 2003). A population pyramid is a graphical representation of age group by gender, ordered with the youngest age group at the base. The population pyramid can be constructed to represent the proportion of the population in the age group of the gender or as a frequency distribution with the latter being more frequently used. Figure 2 displays the projected age distribution

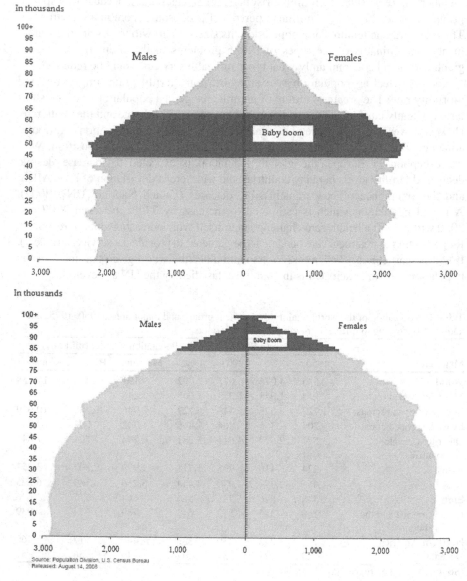

Fig. 2 (**a**) Population Pyramid, United States, 2010. (**b**) Population pyramid, United States, 2050

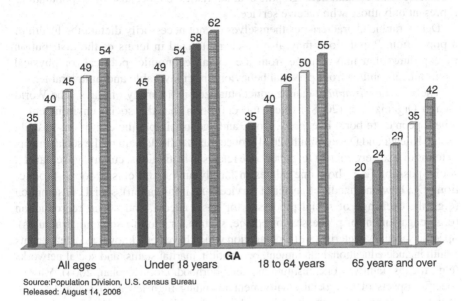

Source:Population Division, U.S. census Bureau
Released: August 14, 2008

Fig. 3 Projected percent minority by age group, 2010–2050, United States

changes in the USA. Notably, the proportion of the population that is 65+ years will continue to grow. The proportion of minorities will also grow such that by 2050 54% of the entire population will be compromised of minorities and in every age group except for those 65+ years, the minorities will comprise the majority of the population (Fig. 3).

As of July 1, 2007, the US population was 301.6 million, with Hispanics, the single largest minority group at 45.5 million (15.1% of the total population). Blacks are the second largest minority group at 40.7 million, followed by Asians, who totaled 15.2 million; American Indians and Alaska Natives, who totaled 4.5 million; and Native Hawaiians and Other Pacific Islanders, with one million. The population of whites (single race and not of Hispanic origin) totaled 199.1 million. Hispanics were the fastest-growing minority group, with a 3.3% increase between July 1, 2006 and July 1, 2007 followed by Asians, who were the second fastest-growing minority group.

The population data referred to above are from the decennial. The census provides the basic information on demographic and other characteristics of population residing in a community. A census is a count of everyone (citizens and non-citizens). The US Census counts everyone as of April 1 living in the USA, Puerto Rico, and the Island Areas. The US Census was mandated by the US Constitution (Article I, Section 2). It was first conducted in 1790 and since then every 10 years with next census occurring in 2010. Federal law protects the personal information shared during the census. Other sources of population demographic characteristics can be obtained from birth certificates and death certificates. Health care claims data (hospital discharge abstracts, physician bills) and health insurance beneficiary files

(Medicare) also contain demographic characteristics, but because these populations represent only those who receive services.

Demographic characteristics themselves do not necessarily dictate the health of a population. Populations may also be characterized in terms of the distribution of exposures that may emerge from the social, economic, political, or physical environments and/or from personal behaviors, both favorable and unfavorable.

The *social environment* can be conceptualized in a variety of ways. The World Health Organization (2008a) offers the definition that the social environment is where people are born, live, grow, work, and age, or simply the conditions of daily living. Krieger and Davey-Smith (2004) conceptualize the domain of the social factors in terms of a society context (e.g., how one relates to institutions, culture, governance), social position (e.g., how one relates in family and social class), social production (e.g., how one handles transfer of services and information), social consumption (e.g., the exchange of social processes for basic needs), and social reproduction (e.g., engagement of processes to replace, sustain, or modify societal structures). Specific social characteristics of a population which have been known as determinants health include educational attainment, occupation, marital status, and social networks (e.g., friends, family, work, institutions, neighborhood, etc.) (Kaplan, 2004). Various specific aspects of the social environment including high levels of social support, social integration, and diversity of social roles have been reported in a number of studies to reduce morbidity and mortality for a variety of conditions, particularly in the elderly (Barefoot et al., 2005; Ertel et al., 2008; Lett et al., 2007; Mortimore et al., 2008). The WHO (2008a) reports data that social gradients, such as differences in educational attainment, in turn give rise to health gradients such as higher mortality in groups with lower educational attainment. The slope of the gradients for these factors may vary among different countries, but the phenomena are universal. The major *economic environmental* factors impacting health are largely those derived from the census and include: household wealth, unemployment rate, proportion of heads of households in lower social class occupation, proportion living in overcrowded housing, and proportion without access to a car. Wealthier societies have different health problems than poorer ones. Downturns in the economy and involuntary unemployment are also associated with mortality (Kim et al., 2004; Steenland and Pinkerton, 2008). *Political environmental* factors, such as public policies, direct to whom health care resources are distributed and how much is allocated. Political environmental forces act largely in terms of their distributive properties regarding laws, representation in government, and governmental budget distribution that could influence health. The *physical environment*, its natural as well as built features, is known to impact health. Favorable environments include access to safe recreational areas, healthy food, and safe drinking water (Cubbin et al., 2008). Climate variation and extremes also affect the emergence of health problems. High ambient temperatures are associated with mortality and tropical climates and warmer seasons are linked to more frequently occurring infectious diseases particularly gastroenteritis (Basu and Ostro, 2008). Colder climates can give rise to cases of frostbite and fall injuries from icing conditions. On a more micro physical environmental level, lead paint, dust, mold, and pest infestation can influence health in unfavorable ways (Cubbin et al., 2008).

Lastly, personal behaviors of the population effect exposures which may result in health problems. These behaviors include: tobacco use, physical activity, dietary habits, alcohol and illicit drug use, and violence.

Epidemiologic studies aid in determining which demographic and other exposures are risk factors. A risk factor is an attribute or an exposure that is statistically associated with a health-related condition. It is, thus, important to know the demographic characteristics of a population as well as the distribution of exposures and risk factors in a population. A risk factor may be immutable (e.g., age) or potentially modifiable (e.g., safe pedestrian walkways), with the latter targeted to improve the health of a population.

Need for Health Care

A health care "need" is a perceived or real deviation from a societal norm of health or health problem that is antecedent and is the impetus for the potential entry into the health care or public health system. Population demographic and economic characteristics are determinates that are needed for health care. An individual's perception of the degree of need is influenced by past experiences with a situation, health information, health education, or a changing socioeconomic situation (e.g., inability to perform work tasks). The need can be also identified by a health care provider and is similarly influenced by education (e.g., educational tract of practitioner, physician versus. chiropractor), health information (dissemination of guidelines regarding a specific practice, e.g., requesting mammography in high-risk younger women), a changing economic situation (e.g., financial incentives by an insurer to avoid hospitalization), and past experiences. The degree of deficit perceived or identified regarding the health need influences when and how much health care services are utilized to produce the desired level of health. Perceived need can also be determined by public authorities in circumstances, such as interventions to prevent a suicide. Different populations, given the same measure of need, can also exhibit highly variable levels of need. For example, the incidence rate of tuberculosis in the US general population is 5.2 per 100,000 persons, but may be as high as 110.3 among homeless persons (Miller et al., 2006).

Health care needs can be measured through a variety of methods including vital records, surveys, and medical care claims data. Need at the community level can be measured through the use of vital records, such as the birth certificate, which provides information on prenatal care and age of the mother. Lower levels of prenatal care relative to published recommended levels of prenatal care (AAP/ACOG, 2007) among pregnant teens may suggest the need for special adolescent health services in the community. A second approach is to measure health care needs through surveys of individuals for self-reported health, adverse exposures, signs (e.g., breast lump) and symptoms (e.g., pain) of disease, overt disease, injuries, impairments, and degree of disability (see chapter 2). An increasing depression score and increasing menopausal symptoms score have been found to be independent predictors of hospitalization in women with breast cancer controlling for age at diagnosis, disease stage, and time since diagnosis (Oleske et al., 2004). Individuals with self-reported chronic conditions are more likely to have a coexisting major depression, the combination of which is associated with significant increases in both emergency department visits and ambulatory visits (Egede, 2007). A third measure of need is withdrawal behavior, such as absentee rates, lost work days, and days confined to bed for illness or injury. High rates of withdrawal behaviors, such as a high rate of lost work days, could suggest high exposure to work-related stressors, such as ergonomic hazards from repeated motion jobs (e.g., nurses and lifting, admissions clerks, and frequent key strokes). A fourth approach is to assess the use of nonmedical services such as nonprescription medications. A fifth method is utilization of formal health care services, a proxy measure, with the assumption that the utilization rates reflect a level of need not met by preventive care or adequate primary care. An example of this is the measurement of avoidable hospitalization rates as measure of need. High rates of selected hospitalizations for certain conditions, termed "ambulatory care sensitive conditions" or "potentially avoidable hospitalizations" such as for asthma, diabetes, and pneumonia, indicate that if adequate primary care were available for control and management of these conditions, hospitalization would not be necessary (see Table 2) (Cloutier-Fisher et al., 2006). Disparities in avoidable hospitalization rates

Table 2 Ambulatory sensitive conditions

Condition	ICD-9 code
Angina	411.1, 411.8, 413 (excludes cases with Procedure Codes 01-86.99)
Asthma	493
Bacterial pneumonia	481 482.1, 482.3, 482.9, 483, 485–486 (excludes patients aged < 2 months and cases with secondary diagnosis of Sickle cell 282.6)
Bronchitis	466.0 only if secondary diagnosis is 491, 492, 494, or 496
Cellulitis	681, 682, 683, 686 (excludes cases with any procedure codes except 860 where it is the only procedure)
Congenital syphilis	090 (secondary diagnosis for newborn only)
Congestive heart failure	428, 402.01, 402.11, 402.91, 518.4
Chronic obstructive pulmonary disease	491, 492, 494, 496,
Dehydration/volume depletion	276.5
Dental conditions	521–523, 525, 528
Diabetes	250.0, 250.1, 250.2, 250.3, 250.8, 250.9
Failure to thrive	783.4
Gastroenteritis	558.9
Grand mal and other epileptic convulsive disorders	345, 780.3
Hypertension	401.0, 401.9, 402.00, 402.10, 402.90 (excludes cases with procedure codes 36.01, 36.02, 36.05, 36.1, 37.5, 37.7)
Hypoglycemia	251.2

(continued)

Table 2 (continued)

Condition	ICD-9 code
Immunization preventable conditions (1 <= age <= 5 years)	033, 037, 045, 320.0, 320.2, 390, 391
Iron deficiency anemia (age <5 years)	280.1, 280.8, 280.9
Kidney and urinary tract infection	590, 599.0, 599.9
Nutritional deficiencies	260–262, 268.0–268.1
Pelvic inflammatory disease (women only)	614 (cases with surgical procedure of hysterectomy 683 688 excluded)
Pneumonia	481, 482.2, 482.3, 482.9, 483, 485, 480
Ruptured appendix	540.0–540.1
Severe ear, nose, throat infection	382 (excludes cases with procedure code 2001), 462, 463, 465, 472.1
Skin graft with cellulitis	DRG 263, 264 (excludes admission from skilled nursing facility or intermediate care facility)
Tuberculosis	011–018

(Adopted from Bindman et al., 2005 and DeLia, 2003)

reflect unmet or unequal levels of responses to the needs of population subgroups. Alternatively, low levels of utilization can represent lack of adequate (e.g., low rates of breast conserving surgery for breast cancer) or lack of access to care (e.g., low mammography utilization rates). Lastly, a sixth approach for quantifying need is through clinical or anthropomorphic measurements such as body mass index (BMI, weight in kilogram per square meters), physical function, blood pressure, cognitive impairment, or cholesterol level. The high proportion of obesity among certain age, race, and gender population sub-groups indicates the need for weight reduction interventions, namely for Mexican American and Black females. Where possible, physical measurements of needs are desirable as reported symptoms may be over-looked, ignored or under-reported, or vary by gender or ethnic/racial group. This point is illustrated by the emerging findings of the variability in symptom reporting related to heart attack symptoms by women who are significantly less likely to relate chest pain or discomfort symptoms as compared with men (Canto et al., 2007).

The selection of a measure of need depends upon what type of health service utilization is anticipated. A population survey of the blood pressure level in a community is a means of determining both the need for preventive services (e.g., education on factors associated with high blood pressure) as well as treatment services (e.g., identifying individuals with asymptomatic high blood pressure). Prevention of depression in a community with a high prevalence of this disorder may be more effectively managed by an educational program aimed at primary care providers to improve their ability to identify depression-related symptoms that left untreated could become disabling. The concept of defining need is most difficult for mental disorders where the spectrum can range from "diseases of the brain" to "problems of everyday living" (Mechanic, 2003). This is because some health services for mental disorders may be more appropriately delivered as behavioral interventions when the disorder (such as a chemical dependency) affects social role capabilities than an intervention for a bipolar disorder managed by medication.

Utilization of Health Care Services

The utilization of health care services reflects the entry into formal health care or the public health system resulting from a need for health services determined by a health care professional, health agency, community, or an individual or family. Ultimately and optimally, utilization of health services is intended to improve health. Health services utilization can be conceptualized as informal or formal. Informal health services are those derived from personal family care, self-help sources (e.g., Internet health care sites). Formal health care services are commonly organized around the health-disease continuum as primary prevention, secondary prevention, and tertiary prevention (see Table 3). Primary prevention services are those activities or initiatives designed to reduce the likelihood of a health problem or to prevent its onset in healthy persons. Secondary prevention services are those activities or initiatives designed at reducing the morbidity or morbidity from a health problem due to early identification of a health problem before its signs and symptoms occur and to alter its natural history through effective early intervention (see also chapter 5). Tertiary prevention services are those activities, interventions, or initiatives aimed at reducing morbidity, mortality, disease progression, and complications among individuals who have an existing health problem. Ideally, health care services when efficacious and delivered in a timely, safe, patient-centered, efficient, and equitable manner result in improved health for individuals and populations (IOM, 2001). Health services utilization markedly increases with age (Fig. 4) and thus, as an increasing number and proportion of the US population ages, the demands for both ambulatory and hospital services will continue to increase.

Table 3 Level of prevention and examples of health services

Level of prevention	Health services
Primary	Meals-on-wheels for seniors
	Immunization programs
	WIC (Women's, Infants, and Children's) Program (*supplemental foods, health care referrals, and nutrition education for low-income pregnant, breastfeeding, and non-breastfeeding postpartum women, and to infants and children up to age five who are found to be at nutritional risk*)
Secondary	Screening mammography
	Blood pressure screening
	Body mass index assessment to identify obesity (*weight in kilograms/height in m^2, a measurement standard to determine obesity [BMI $\geq$ 30]*)
Tertiary	Postoperative physical therapy after joint replacement surgery
	Aspirin therapy to prevent secondary acute myocardial infarction
	Administration of tissue plasminogen activator (tPD) within 3 hours of ischemic stroke onset to minimize damage and prevent stroke recurrence
	Hypertension control to prevent stroke
	Cholesterol reduction by diet and/or use of cholesterol-lowering drugs in persons with coronary heart disease

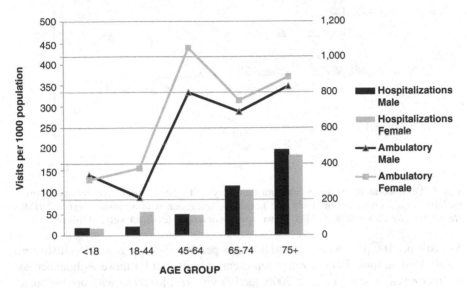

Fig. 4 Ambulatory visits and hospitalization rates by age group and gender (Source: National Center for Health Statistics, 2007)

Health care utilization is influenced by the level and degree of perceived health care need realized through behaviors stimulated knowledge, attitudes, and beliefs. Knowledge of the condition, either by the individual, most common interpretation, or by the provider is required as well as the attitude by both that utilization can favorably influence health. Belief, is defined according to the Health Belief Model requiring that perceived susceptibility, severity, benefits, barriers, cues to action, and self-efficacy which comprise the basis of action for utilization (Glanz et al., 2002). Health care utilization also varies with need, regardless of the measure of need. Figure 5 illustrates this concept with self-rated health resulting in varying frequency of hospitalization and visit to physician. Utilization was directly correlated with lower levels of self-rated health as well as higher mortality.

Other factors affecting utilization include demographics, household income, relation between zip code residence and choice of care, type of service, type of provider, type of organization, cultural competence of provider, payment source for health care, cost of care, and an individual's beliefs, knowledge, and attitudes regarding the efficacy of health services, the curability of their condition, and self-help seeking behaviors. Important ambulatory care utilization patterns discerned from sociodemographic factors occurring between 1996 and 2006 are: an increase in the number of ambulatory care visits by 26% to a rate of 381.9 visits per 100 persons annually; 29% increase in the annual visit rate to medical specialty offices with a significant increase noted for white patients but not black patients; 32% increase in the number of ED visits to a rate of 40.5 per 100 persons annually; adjusted rate of annual visits to EDs increased among blacks by about 40%, from

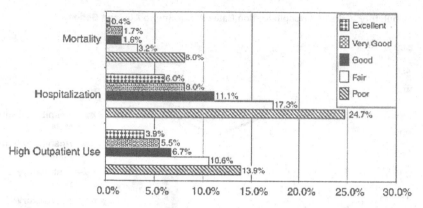

Fig. 5 Distribution of mortality and utilization by self-reported health (Reproduced from DeSalvo, et al., Predicting mortality and healthcare utilization with a single question," *HSR: Health Serv. Res.* 2005;40(4):1234–1246 with permission of Wiley-Blackwell Publishing)

58 visits per 100 persons in 1996 to 81 visits per 100 (Schappert and Rechtsteiner, 2008). High hospital ED utilization represents a safety net for those without access to other types of health care. In 2006, the ED visit rate for those with no insurance was nearly twice the rate of persons with any form of private insurance (47.4 visits per 100 persons versus. 24.9 visits per 100 persons) (Schappert and Rechtsteiner, 2008). The disparity in the utilization of EDs by race (whites, 36.1 per 100 persons versus blacks, 79.9 per 100 persons in 2006) further suggests lack of access to primary care in communities with high concentrations of blacks.

The features of a health care organization can affect health, including its technology, personnel, and types of programmatic efforts. Organizations can be characterized in a variety of dimensions, commonly ownership (public, private, etc.), form, decision-making, system membership, personnel, and technology. Gillies et al. (2006) report differential impacts based upon health plan configuration which impact clinical performance indicators. Schmittdiel et al. (2006) in studying physician organizations found presence of an electronic standardized problem list improved chronic care. Personnel refers to the number, type, credentials, experience, training, and continued training, Technology refers to inputs into the utilization of the organization's services from drugs, devices, machines, bureaucratic procedures, management strategies (e.g., case management). Programmatic efforts represent what services are provided, how these are organized, the means that they are delivered, and how the results of the programs are utilized and reported. Examples of programs include lactation services and a "Rapid Response Team," a multi disciplinary group clinicians who bring critical care expertise to the bedside or wherever it's needed.

Utilization of formal health care services, even with optimal organizational structure, personnel, technology, and programs, cannot occur unless there are health care resources in a community that are accessible, acceptable, and available. Accessibility, as defined from an epidemiological point of view, is the proportion or number of a population that use a service or facility as a function of physical (e.g., distance, wheel chair access), economic (e.g., copayment amount), cultural factors (e.g., translation services), or other aspects of the health care system (e.g., time to appointment, policies on referral to specialist). Optimally, the resources that need to be accessible are primary and specialty providers, mid-level providers (physician assistants, nurse practitioners, etc.), acute care (hospitals, emergency services, outpatient care), home health care services, mental health care, long-term care, oral health care, and rehabilitation services. The resources must also be in sufficient ratio. An alternative to a ratio measurement of access is geographic access in terms of time or distance. The use of geographic information systems (GIS) allows for assessing accessibility from a spatial perspective. These systems allow for modeling access to care in consideration interactions between patients and providers across administrative borders, including competition among providers and demand for services (Yang et al., 2006). Access may also be a subjective consideration. Perceptions of lack of access may also influence utilization. GIS systems may also be used to model the impact of perception of lack of access by also including spatial parameters (line distance to health care for an individual) (Fone et al., 2006). Acceptability is the perception of the consumer or patient that the service(s) provided are consistent with and reflect sensitivity to the norms, culture, aesthetics, and spiritual values of the population or population subgroup served. The race/ethnic composition ratio of the providers to the population facilitates acceptability by the community in addition to the linguistic/cultural competence of the organization. Availability is the ratio between the population of an administrative or geographic unit and the health facilities, personnel, and technology to support the delivery of health care. Higher utilization occurs with greater availability of resources.

Lastly, utilization of health services may not necessarily facilitate the achievement of optimal health unless they are appropriate. Lavis and Anderson (1996) propose two distinct types of appropriateness: appropriateness of a service and appropriateness of the setting in which care is provided. The appropriateness of a service is the effectiveness and potential benefit of that service for a condition exceeds harm, given a consideration of signs and symptoms, results of diagnostic test and patient or consumer preferences for the service. The appropriateness of a setting (e.g., inpatient, outpatient, specialty center, center of excellence) extends this definition to consider the cost. Additionally, given the current health care environment alternative settings now also needs to consider patient safety before appropriateness can be established. Not all utilization of health care is viewed as appropriate. Wennberg (1996) found marked variation in the delivery of health care across different regions of the US that is not explained by patient characteristics or preferences, medical conditions, or recommendations of evidence-based medicine. Instead, variations in physician practice styles and intensity in the use of medical resources and technology exist by systems of care and geographic areas independent of patient demographics and clinical conditions (viz., health care needs). Studies of this variation have included chronically ill, end-of-life care, mammography rates, prostate biopsy rates, and several other surgical procedures. The conclusion from these studies of variability in utilization that more is not necessarily better. Consequences of inappropriate utilization, in addition to increased costs, include the potential for adverse events, such as surgical complications, health–care acquired infections, and medication errors. Increasingly, evidence-based practice is the management strategy for determining appropriate utilization of any type of health care service. Evidencebased practice reports, data, and consensus guidelines on the appropriateness of various health care services from the Agency for Health Care Research and Quality (http://www.ahrq.gov), the Centers for Medicare and Medicaid Services, the National Registry of Evidence-based Programs and Practices (a searchable database of interventions for the prevention and treatment of mental and substance use disorders, http://nrepp.samhsa.gov), the Cochrane Reviews (http://www.cochrane.org), and among others provide guidance in determining the appropriateness of any health service, be it primary prevention or tertiary services.

The Health of Populations

There are a myriad of definitions and approaches for determining the health of a population. The World Health Organization in its 1948 Constitution offered a definition of health as "the state of complete physical, mental and social well-being," a definition that still has relevance today. The measure selected for assessing the health depends upon the target population (geographically defined, members of a health plan, etc.), the goal of the assessment (overall health, specific aspect of health), and the scope of the assessment (e.g., local, national, international). Historically, for geographically defined populations, health has been quantified with the proxy measure, mortality, because of its universality of recording of deaths, and because of the widespread availability and general comparability of these records across geographic areas, even across nations (see chapter 3 for sample death certificate).

More recently, additional global indicators of health are now commonly used as more nations are recording them because of their public health importance. Thus, the indicators used by the World Health Organization (2008b) to compare health of populations have now expanded to include the following:

- Infant mortality rate (the number of deaths under 1 year of age per 1,000 live births)
- Maternal mortality ratio (number of deaths of mothers attributable to childbirth per 100,000 live births)
- Life expectancy at birth (average number of years of life than an individual is expected to live from birth assuming the current mortality rates prevail)
- Healthy life expectancy at birth (average number of years that a person can expect to live in "full health" by taking into account years lived in less than full health due to disease and/or injury as estimated from incidence, prevalence, duration and years lived with disability for 135 major causes determined from self-reports for a set of core health domains which includes a health state valuation module for assessing the severity of reported health states relative to a life table calculated from mortality data)
- Neonatal mortality rate per 1,000 live births
- Under-5 mortality rate (probability of dying by age 5 per 1,000 live births)

- Adult mortality rate (probability of dying between 15 and 60 years per 1,000 population)
- Cause-specific mortality rate (per 100,000 population) (separately for HIV/AIDS, TB/HIV+, TB/HIV-)
- Age-standardized mortality rates by cause (per 100,000 population) (separately for noncommunicable, cardiovascular, cancer, and injuries)
- Prevalence of tuberculosis (per 100,000 population)
- Incidence of tuberculosis (per 100,000 population)
- Prevalence of HIV among ≥15 years (per 100,000 population)
- Number of confirmed cases of poliomyelitis

The above measures are also useful for both cross-national comparisons of health and the health of population subgroups (see also chapter 3 on computing rates). Health can also be determined by a health care provider or can be self-reported by an individual (see also chapter 2). Survey formats are used to evaluate health in populations, but the logistics may be challenging. The use of Internet-based and surveys along with other technologies may facilitate the use of self-ratings of health in large populations.

Health assessed in reference to a specific intervention is referred to as a "health outcome." Health outcomes commonly represent the end results of therapeutic interventions and can include self-rated health, quality of life, functional ability, and mental status. Examples of therapeutic population interventions include internet-based smoking cessation programs and programs aimed at improving the health of arthritics (Lorig et al., 2008; Strecher et al., 2008). The concept of health in this context is becoming increasingly important and continuing to evolve as some therapeutic interventions are targeted at populations as a strategy for improving health. Managed care plans and insurers are particularly keen on population-based interventions in support of promoting health.

Regardless of the measure of health used, better health should be the overall goal of any health care provider, organization, or system with focus on resolving the health care needs and promoting health in populations served and those in the surrounding communities.

Other Models of Epidemiology

Other models of epidemiology related to understanding causation here are presented for sake of completeness and in appreciation of the origins of the discipline of epidemiology as oriented to the identification of risk factors and control of disease in the context of public health.

The simplest model of epidemiology is the agent–host–environment triangular model. This model conceptualizes that a health problem can be prevented by severing any one side of the triangle (Fig. 6). This model also acknowledges that health problems are not necessarily caused by one factor, but the interaction of agent-host

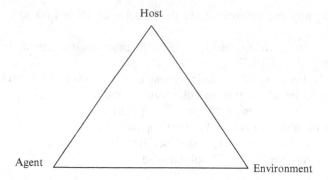

Fig. 6   The triangular theory of epidemiology

and the environment. This model can be applied to infectious, chronic disease, and even behavioral health problems. For example, the epidemic of obesity in youth may be diminished by increasing physical activity (host modification) but also providing a safe neighborhood (environment) in which to play. Additional examples are provided in Hogue (2008).

Web of causation model posits that a health condition may have multiple links, even some quite distant as possible etiologic factors. The web strands more proximate to the health problem represent factors with known immediate impact or "causative" factors. The web strands more distal represent "pathway" factors that are important to the genesis of the health problem but give rise to or mitigate more proximate and more precisely defined causative risk factors. This model represents the theory that when more links are broken within the "web" of potential factors, the chances of controlling the problem increases. This model is more useful in conceptualizing health problems with multi factorial etiologies such as diabetes mellitus. For example, a new potential risk factor for diabetes, neighborhood of residence, may be a distant variable in the "web" representing either a toxic environment giving rise to diabetes or a variable representing an access to care barrier to care for possible underlying causes of diabetes such as obesity (Grant, 2007). The limitations of the web-of-causation model are that latency periods or interactions among variables are not conceptually represented.

Rothman (1995) presents a causal model of epidemiologic utilizing statistical concepts into understanding the etiology of illness. Rothman characterizes the pathway to illness in terms of types of causes. According to Rothman, a cause is "an act or event or state of nature which initiates or permits, alone or in conjunction other causes." He further states that causes are influenced by confounding ("a distortion in the effect measure introduced by an extraneous variate"), effect modification (different values of the variable at different levels of the variable). This is a useful model for interpreting the statistical results of studies because it recognizes that the pathway to illness cause is not necessarily linear, nor independent of other causes but actually may emerge because of the strength of a specific causative factor or synergy (or interaction) among factors. The reader should consult Greenland and

Brumback (2002) for more complex models of causality which consider assumptions about exposure quantitatively modeled including a potential-outcome (counterfactual) model that examines exposure other than what occurred.

Applying Epidemiology in Health Care Management Practice

From this conceptual orientation, it should be clear that a basic knowledge of epidemiological methods and their applications is essential for all health care managers. Specifically, the health care manager must continuously monitor in the populations served: (1) the service population size, (2) the distribution of health needs, (3) the genesis and consequences of health care problems, (4) how the health care system and organizational characteristics impact health, (5) the appropriates of the structure and performance of the health system, organization, and/or program with epidemiological techniques, (6) the impacts of a changing environment, and (7) response to public policy affecting health care delivery. These tasks comprise the practice of management epidemiology. Questions providing the framework for the practice and the description of the tasks below are listed in Table 4.

Table 4 Questions to answer when managing health systems from an epidemiologic framework

1. Who is the population served?
    a. How is the population defined?
    b. What are the size, demographic composition, and trends of this population?
    c. What social, political, physical, and environmental factors affect the population?
2. What are the population's health care needs?
    a. How can those needs be measured?
    b. What is the prevalence of exposure risk factors for adverse health?
    c. What are the most common diseases, disability, injuries, and other health problems?
3. Where are health services in relationship to the population? Are they available, accessible, acceptable, and appropriate for addressing the population's health care needs?
    a. What are barriers the population can experience when attempting to access health care services?
    b. What distances do individuals have to travel to receive health care?
    c. What are the capabilities of services relative to the size and needs of the population (organization, personnel, technology)?
    d. How do the services of the local health system link to local and national goals or initiatives?
    e. What environmental influences affect health services delivery (market competition, trends affecting delivery model/setting)?
4. How can the health of the population be promoted?
    a. How will health be measured at the present and over time?
    b. Is the population becoming healthier?
    c. Are there inequalities in the health of population subgroups relative to the larger population?
    d. Will variations in health affect health needs such that different health services are required for different population subgroups?

Monitoring Service Population Size

The primary role of the health care manager is to align resources with the goals of the organization to improve the health of populations served. This function requires an understanding of the boundaries and definition of the population, its size, and factors affecting the size of the population. Typically, the health care manager is responsible for populations who are defined as potential users from a community (who are within the "market area"), eligible beneficiaries (i.e., of a managed care plan), or a service population of current users (e.g., hospitalized patients). The major factors affecting population size relative to the need for and/or utilization of health services are:

- Birth rate
- Fertility rate
- Mortality rate
- Migration/immigration
- Health care facility closures
- Changes in the service offerings of health care facilities (e.g., elimination of emergency or obstetrics services)
- Horizontal integration of organizations (e.g., affiliations, joint ventures, partnerships)
- Vertical integration of organizations or services (e.g., addition of palliative care unit in a hospital)

As mentioned previously, the health care manager should plan for, in general, a population which is increasing in diversity, size, and age regardless of the definition or boundaries of the population.

Distribution of Health Needs in a Population

Epidemiological measures enable the distribution of health needs in a population to be characterized in terms of, "Who is affected? When are they affected? Where are population affected?" An estimate of the distribution and frequency of health needs in a population enables the projection of the amount of resources that would be required. For example, a health plan should consider screening for diabetes in a population known to be a high risk for the condition, to determine the number of persons affected with the anticipation that early identification and glycemic control of the condition would reduce the likelihood of hospitalization through preventing potential complications of this disease such as diabetic retinopathy and foot complications (Knight et al., 2005).

Understanding the Genesis and Consequences of Health Problems

Risk factors are attributes or exposures that influence the chance of the occurrence (or genesis) of a health outcome or health problem, favorably or unfavorably.

Prognostic factors, are exposures or clinical conditions, which influence the course of a disease favorably or unfavorably (consequences). Knowing the distribution of risk factors and prognostic factors associated with the health problems common in the population served can aid in developing more effective health services. For example, fractures, particularly of the hip, are a major health problem of the elderly in community-dwelling as well as for hospitalized populations. Risk factors for the condition include psychotropic drug use, impaired vision, confusion, assisted ambulation, low weight, history of falls, and hospitalization (Myers et al., 1991; Gardner et al., 2008; Lichtenstein et al., 1994). High mortality and morbidity are associated with fractures in the elderly, but can be greater diminished with the use of immediate rehabilitation intervention. The health care management implications are that the introduction of preventive services (e.g., communitybased physical activity programs and medication management education, fall risk assessment of newly admitted hospitalized patients), secondary prevention (e.g., screening elderly at high risk because of gait problems), and tertiary prevention (e.g., ensuring hospital-based and community rehabilitation services) when offered through community partnerships (hospital-primary care-public health agency) can improve the health of the elderly population in the service area.

Understanding the Relationship Between Health System Characteristics and the Health of Populations Served

The body of literature indicating that features of a health system, its organization, its personnel, its available technology, and programmatic efforts have been linked to changes in the health of population served, even when considering its demographics and presence of clinical conditions. In drawing an analogy to classic epidemiology, these organizational features may be characterized as "exposure factors." An organization is commonly characterized by its ownership (e.g., government, for profit, not-for-profit, membership in a system, patient volume, and accreditations).

Personnel considerations of an organization primarily refer to the number of staff, number in relationship to persons served, their credentials, experience, training, and other factors such as turnover. The composition of personnel or staff mix can have substantial impact upon the health of populations served, both in the inpatient as well as ambulatory settings. Higher educational level of nursing and higher proportion of RN staff to patients has been observed to be associated with lower hospital mortality, adjusting for patient and organizational characteristics (Aiken et al., 2006). Alternatively, in certain circumstances, different types of providers may have comparable effects on population health. Mundinger et al. (2000) demonstrated that it was possible to achieve similar patient outcomes at least when comparing nurse practitioners and physicians in an ambulatory setting. Other features, such as high provider turnover can decrease the likelihood that preventive services are delivered in managed care settings (Plomondon et al., 2007).

The application of technology is intended to improve the health of populations served. The introductions of neonatal intensive care units and surfactant therapies are examples of therapies for premature babies. However, the health care manager must keep mindful that technologies may produce risk, be associated with high cost, yield false negative or false positive results when applied as a screening or diagnostic test (see chapter 3), or even adverse effects if the technology is intended for treatment.

Monitoring Health Care Systems, Organizations, and Program Performance

The increased necessity for continuous monitoring the health care system, organization, and program performance is another reason for the use of epidemiology in management practice. The impetus for monitoring performance has been stimulated by the continuous quality improvement movement, the patient safety movement, and the pay for performance initiatives by insurers. Monitoring is also formalized as part of various specialty accreditation standards, of facilities, as well as of programs. The Commission on Cancer American College of Surgeons, for example, as part of one standard for designation as a Cancer Program, requires the compilation and monitoring of survival statistics of populations treated (http://www.facs.org/cancerprogram/home.html).

Modifying Structure and Processes to Respond to Environmental Change

The environment, as described in the epidemiological model of health services delivery, is continuously changing and evolving. Climates are changing the global environment. Governments change and so do their policies. Social environments change when displacement from war and civil conflicts emerges. Among the most universal change in health care management practice embracing epidemiologic principles is the modification of service delivery in response to potential disasters, both manmade and natural (see chapter "Health Risk from the Environment: Challenges to Health Services Delivery"). New conditions, such as post-traumatic stress disorders and new threats of greater magnitude (e.g., mass physical trauma from terrorist attacks) require new facilities (e.g., decontamination sites), manpower training, and re-organization of services. For example, according to the Joint Commission for Accreditation of Healthcare Organizations (http://www.jointcommission.org) requires "that health care organizations that offer emergency services or are designated as disaster receiving stations must have an emergency management plan that addresses both external and internal disasters." Epidemiologic data provide the information to the health care manager on the types of disasters likely to be encountered by an organization such that the appropriate emergency management program plans could be developed.

Response to Public Policy Affecting the Delivery of Health Care Services

Epidemiological data and methods are critical for the development and assessment of public policy affect the delivery of health care services. Health care managers have the opportunity to participate in public policy development, but more commonly, are required to develop systems in response to public policies. An example of a change in public policy that health care managers should initiate immediate response to in terms of organizational structure and policies is The Deficit Reduction Act (DRA) of 2005. The DRA required that for certain conditions that are not present upon admission, hospitals will not receive additional payment. Section 5001(c) provides that the Centers for Medicare and Medicaid Services (CMS) can revise the list of conditions from time to time, as long as it contains at least two conditions. There are 10 categories of conditions designated by CMS (2008):

1. Foreign Object Retained After Surgery
2. Air Embolism
3. Blood Incompatibility
4. Stage III and IV Pressure Ulcers
5. Falls and Trauma
   - Fractures
   - Dislocations
   - Intracranial Injuries
   - Crushing Injuries
   - Burns
   - Electric Shock
6. Manifestations of Poor Glycemic Control
   - Diabetic Ketoacidosis
   - Nonketotic Hyperosmolar Coma
   - Hypoglycemic Coma
   - Secondary Diabetes with Ketoacidosis
   - Secondary Diabetes with Hyperosmolarity
7. Catheter-Associated Urinary Tract Infection (UTI)
8. Vascular Catheter-Associated Infection
9. Surgical Site Infection Following:
   - Coronary Artery Bypass Graft (CABG) - Mediastinitis
   - Bariatric Surgery
     - Laparoscopic Gastric Bypass
     - Gastroenterostomy
     - Laparoscopic Gastric Restrictive Surgery
   - Orthopedic Procedures
     - Spine
     - Neck
     - Shoulder
     - Elbow

10. Deep Vein Thrombosis (DVT)/Pulmonary Embolism (PE)
   *   Total Knee Replacement
   *   Hip Replacement

Policy documents referencing epidemiologic data such as *Healthy People 2010*, those from the CMS (2008) and state agencies (Weinick, 2007) aid in benchmarking organizational performance relative to national and state standards (see also chapter, "Delivering Health Care with Quality: Epidemiologic Considerations"). As new national policies are introduced, epidemiological methods also can be used to determine if organizational restructuring will be required to meet the health needs of the populations targeted for service and whether the reconfiguration will favorably affect the health of the population served.

Summary

The population characteristics of the United States as well as globally will continue to increase, increase in aging and increase in diversity, particularly among those who are most likely to be in need of health care. One crucial step for all health care providers is to be aware of this forthcoming global transition and to recognize that any inequalities in the distribution of risk factors for adverse exposures and health services will influence population health. Data systems must be continuously enhanced to monitor trends. But, so too should efforts to ensure that the distribution of these services are handled equitably across population subgroups to not lose ground on maintaining overall health in communities and nations.

Discussion Questions

Q.1. You have been appointed the new vice president for community and external affairs at an academic medical center which is located in an urban area serving a population according to the 2000 U.S. Census is 82.2% Black, has 32.8% of families below the poverty level, and 26.3% with a long-standing disability. According to a recent survey conducted by the academic medical center, many people in this community go to its emergency room even when they have conditions and symptoms that can be treated and managed through regular visits with a primary care provider. Develop a plan based upon the epidemiologic model of health services delivery to build community partnerships with health care services to efficiently connect patients with appropriate primary care sources in the community (Boxed Example 1).

**Boxed Example 1.1 Demographic Changes Change the Way Health
Care Is Delivered**

Problem: The foreign born population living in the US increased by 44%
between 1990 and 2000, comprising 12.5% of the total US population, the
highest since 1930. Over 24 million or 8.7% of the population speak English
less than very well (U.S. Census Bureau, 2000). Disparities may continue to
exist and grow because health care services cannot be patient-centered, safe,
timely, or equitable if language serves as a barrier to their delivery.

Data and Results: Hasnain-Wynia et al. (2006), (http://www.ama-assn.org/
ama1/pub/upload/mm/433/hasnain-wynia_oct07.pdf) obtained the following
results from their survey for the Commission to End Health Care Disparities
of the American Medical Association: 63% of hospitals encountered limited
English proficiency (LEP) patients daily or weekly; 54% of general internal
physicians treat LEP patients at least once a day or a few times a week; 84%
of federally qualified health centers see at least one LEP patient a day.

Managerial Epidemiology Interpretation: Data on race, ethnicity, and
primary language spoken are important to collect upon enrollment or admission regardless of health care setting. These data can be linked to quality
measures or for quality improvement activities to ensure that disparities in
care do not emerge in a health service delivery setting because of language,
race, or ethnicity. The collection of accurate and timely information requires
training of staff in how to collect the information and in cultural competency
training. Health care managers can utilize strategies suggested by Hasnain-
Wynia and Baker (2006) for guidance in developing the implementation of
a systematic collection of race, ethnicity, and primary language data from
patients. The collection of data will guide in the selection of and scheduling
appropriate interpreters, and appropriately identified, developed, and translated patient information (e.g., consent forms) and education materials. The
data will also aid the organization in assessing the diversity of its patient
population and form its practices upon the National Standards on Culturally
and Linguistically Appropriate Services (CLAS) (USDHHS, Office of
Minority Health 2001). CLAS contain the principles and activities of culturally and linguistically appropriate services should be integrated throughout
an organization and undertaken in partnership with the communities being
served. Further, it contains mandates that are current Federal requirements
for all recipients of Federal funds. These mandates are as follows:

Boxed Example 1.1 (continued)

Standard 4: Health care organizations must offer and provide language assistance services, including bilingual staff and interpreter services, at no cost to each patient/consumer with limited English proficiency at all points of contact, in a timely manner during all hours of operation.

Standard 5: Health care organizations must provide to patients/consumers in their preferred language both verbal offers and written notices informing them of their right to receive language assistance services.

Standard 6: Health care organizations must assure the competence of language assistance provided to limited English proficient patients/consumers by interpreters and bilingual staff. Family and friends should not be used to provide interpretation services (except on request by the patient/consumer).

Standard 7: Health care organizations must make available easily understood patient-related materials and post signage in the languages of the commonly encountered groups and/or groups represented in the service area.

The health care manager must understand the changing demographics of the populations served as well as their needs. The increasing diversity of a population signals an increasing diversity of needs. This trend will prompt policy makers to change laws, rules, and regulations which affect the delivery of health care. Compliance with these and other new standards and mandates will not only ensure on-going federal funding for an organization, but also improve the health outcomes of diverse populations treated and then ultimately the health of the community's population.

Q.2. As part of its planning efforts, a local health department examined the patterns of deaths from diabetes found marked variation in diabetes mortality according to geographic area (town and township) within the county served. Identify the social determinants of health which could explain these differences and propose actions to reduce disparities.

Q.3. Select another community area from the Health Resources Administration Geospatial Data Warehouse. Compare your selected community area's need for health care services with the Managerial Epidemiology Interpretation for the community area evaluated in Boxed Example 2.

Boxed Example 1.2 Determining the Need for Health Care Services

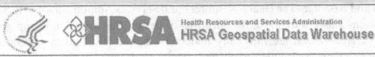

Health Resources and Services Administration
HRSA Geospatial Data Warehouse

Community Fact Sheet
Cook County, Illinois, HHS Region V

Collection	Characteristic	Population	% of Pop.	Hispanic or Latino Population	% of Pop.
Population	Total	5,288,655	---	1,200,957	22.71 %
(U.S. Census 2006)					
Race / Ethnicity	White	3,519,844	66.55 %	1,143,522	21.62 %
(U.S. Census 2006)	Black or African American	1,390,689	26.30 %	26,765	0.51 %
	Asian	295,735	5.59 %	5,096	0.10 %
	American Indian or Alaskan Native	20,239	0.38 %	12,708	0.24 %
	Native Hawaiian or Other Pacific Islander	5,400	0.10 %	3,451	0.07 %
	One Race	5,231,907	98.93 %	1,191,542	22.53 %
	Two or More Races	56,748	1.07 %	9,415	0.18 %
Income in Relation	Statistical Total	5,376,741	---		
to U.S. Federal	Known Poverty Status Total	5,285,159	---		
Poverty Level	Below 100%	713,040	13.49 %		
Note: % is relative to	Between 100% and 199%	845,740	16.00 %		
known poverty status.	200% and Above	3,726,379	70.51 %		
(U.S. Census 2000)	Unknown	91,582	---		

Living Below	Under 5 Years of Age	75,855	Median Household		$48,919
U.S. Federal Poverty	Age 5 Years	16,183	Income		
Level (USFPL) by Age	6 to 11 Years of Age	95,383	Estimate Living Below USFPL		
(U.S. Census 2000)	12 to 17 Years of Age	76,766	Ages 5-17		191,551
	18 to 64 Years of Age	386,830	Under Age 18		289,146
	65 to 74 Years of Age	31,646	All Ages		780,189
	75 Years of Age and Greater	30,377	(U.S. Census 2005)		

Health Care	Uninsured	852,932
Payment Source	Medicare (Elderly)	577,235
(2005)	Medicare (Disabled)	89,487

Health Providers	Primary Care Physicians per 100,000 Population	137.17
(2005)	Dentists per 100,000 Population	67.39

Employment	Unemployed	167,659
(2005)	No High School Diploma	767,904

Births and Infant	Statistic	Total	Black	White	Other
Deaths	Live Births	417,862	121,478	272,788	23,596
(1999-2003)	Low Birth Weight	37,646	17,593	18,029	2,024
	Low Birth Weight Rate Per 1,000 Births	90.09	144.82	66.00	85.78
	Infant Deaths	3,886	2,048	1,725	113
	Infant Death Rate Per 1,000 Births	9.30	16.86	6.32	4.79
(2001-2003)	Teenage Pregnancy (Mothers < 18) as Percentage of All Births	4.40 %	---	---	---

Problem: Many urban areas face the dual challenge of a high proportion of the population being in poverty and at the same time limited city budgets to provide for health services at any level.

Boxed Example 1.2 (continued)

Data and Results: The Health Resources and Services Administration (HRSA) maintains a data warehouse for purposes of monitoring and identifying geographic areas which are medically underserved. The HRSA data warehouse focuses on uninsured, underserved, and special needs populations. Additionally, the database provides information on Health Professional Shortage Areas (HPSA) by address and locates Medically Underserved Areas and Population (MUA/P) groups by area and address. Displayed herein is a Community Fact Sheet from the HRSA data warehouse for Cook County, Illinois, USA. Data from the census, vital data, and information from insurance payors are summarized and can be used to quickly estimate health needs of a population and project the types of health services to promote population health.

Managerial Epidemiology Interpretation: Since nearly a third of the population is either at less than 200% of the poverty level or uninsured, and nearly 300,000 children living below the federal poverty level, hospital managers should partner with community groups, health department, and other nonprofit organizations to coordinate, in particular preventive services which could include nutrition and immunization campaigns, important health needs of childhood.

References

Aiken, L.H., Clarke, S.P., Cheung, R.B., Sloane, D.M., and Silber, J.H., 2006, Educational levels of hospital nurses and surgical patient mortality, *J.A.M.A.* **290**:1617–1623.

American Academy of Pediatrics/American College of Obstetrics and Gynecology (AAP/ACOG), 2007, *Guidelines for Prenatal Care*, 6th ed., American Academy of Pediatrics, Elk Grove Village, IL.

Barefoot, J.C., Gronbaek, M., Jensen, G., Schnohr, P., and Prescott, E., 2005, Social network diversity and risks of ischemic heart disease and total mortality: findings from the Copenhagen City Heart Study, *Am. J. Epidemiol.* **161**:960–967.

Basu, R., and Ostro, B.D., 2008, A multicounty analysis identifying the populations vulnerable to mortality associated with high ambient temperature in California, *Am. J. Epidemiol.* **168**: 632–637.

Bindman, A.B., Chattopadhyay, A., Osmond, D.H., Huen, W., and Bacchetti, P., 2005, The impact of Medicaid managed care on hospitalizations for ambulatory care sensitive conditions, *HSR: Health Services Res.* **40**:19–38.

Canto, J.G., Goldberg, R.J., Hand, M.M., Bonow, R.O., Sopko, G., Pepine, C.J., and Long, T., 2007, Symptom presentation of women with acute coronary syndromes – myth vs. reality, *Arch. Intern. Med.* **167**:2405–2413.

Centers for Medicare and Medicaid Services, 2008, *Hospital Acquired Conditions* (July 5, 2009) http://www.cms.hhs.gov/HospitalAcqCond/06_Hospital-Acquired_Conditions.asp.

Cloutier-Fisher, D., Penning, M.J., Zheng, C., and Druyts, E.F., 2006, The devil is in the details: trends in avoidable hospitalization rates by geography in British Columbia, 1990–2000, *BMC Health Serv. Res.* **6**:104 (December 29, 2008), http://www.biomedcentral.com/1472–6963/6/104.

Cubbin, C., Pedregon, V., Egerter, S., and Braveman, P., 2008, Where we live matters for our health: neighborhoods and health, Issue Brief 3: *Neighborhoods and Health*, Robert Wood Johnson Foundation, http://www.commissiononhealth.org.

DeLia, D., 2003, Distributional issues in the analysis of preventable hospitalizations, *HSR: Health Serv. Res.* **38**:1761–1779.

DeSalvo, K.B., Fan, V.S., McDonell, M.B., and Fihn, S.D., 2005, Predicting mortality and healthcare utilization with a single question, *HSR: Health Serv. Res.* **40**:1234–1246.

Egede, L.E., 2007, Major depression in individuals with chronic medical disorders: prevalence, correlates and association with health resource utilization, lost productivity and functional disability, *Gen. Hosp. Psychiatry* **29**:409–416.

Ertel, K.A., Glymour, M.M., and Berkman, L.F., 2008, Effects of social integration on preserving memory function in a nationally representative US elderly population, *Am. J. Pub. Health* **98**:1215–1220.

Fone, D.L., Christie, S., and Lester, N., 2006, Comparison of perceived and modelled geographical access to accident and emergency departments: a cross-sectional analysis from the Caerphilly Health and Social Needs Study, *Int. J. Health Geogr.* **5**:16.

Gardner R.L., Harris, F., Vittinghoff, E., and Cummings, S.R., 2008, The risk of fracture following hospitalization in older women and men, *Arch. Intern. Med.* **168**:1671–1677.

Gillies, R.R., Chenok, K.E., Shortell, S.M., Pawlson, G., and Wimbush, J.J., 2006, The impact of health plan delivery system organization on clinical quality and patient satisfaction, *HSR: Health Serv. Res.* **41**:1181–1199.

Glanz, K., Rimer, B.K., and Lewis, F.M, 2002, *Health Behavior and Health Education*, Jossey-Bass, San Francisco, CA.

Grant, R.W., 2007, Invited commentary: untangling the web of diabetes causality in African Americans, *Am. J. Epidemiol.* **166**:388–390.

Greenland, S., and Brumback, B., 2002, An overview of relations among causal modeling methods, *Int. J. Epidemiol.* **31**:1030–1037.

Hasnain-Wynia, R., and Baker, D.W., 2006, Obtaining data on patient race, ethnicity, and primary language in health care organizations: current challenges and proposed solutions, *HSR: Health Services Research* **41**:1501–1518.

Hogue, C.J., 2008, The triangular future of epidemiology, *Ann. Epidemiol.* **18**:862–863.

Institute of Medicine (IOM), 2001, *Crossing the Quality Chasm: A New Health System for the 21st Century*, National Academy Press, Washington, DC.

Kaplan, G.A., 2004, What's wrong with social epidemiology, and how can we make it better? *Epidemiol. Rev.* **26**:124–135.

Kim, H., Song, Y.J., Yi, J.J., Chung, W.J., and Nam, C.M., 2004, Changes in mortality after the recent economic crisis in South Korea, *Ann. Epidemiol.* **14**:442–446.

Knight, K., Badamgarav, E., Henning, J.M., Hasselblad, V., Gano, A.D., Ofman, J.J., and Weingarten, S.R., 2005, A systematic review of diabetes disease management programs, *Am. J. Manag. Care* **11**:242–250.

Krieger, N., and Smith, G.D., 2004, "Bodies count," and body counts: social epidemiology and embodying inequality, *Epidemiol. Rev.* **26**:92–103.

Lavis, J.N., and Anderson, G.M., 1996, Appropriateness in health care delivery: definitions, measurement and policy implications, *Can. Med. Assoc. J.* **154**:321–328.

Lett, H.S., Blumenthal, J.A., Babyak, M.A., Catellier, D.J., Carney, R.M., Berkman, L.F., Burg, M.M., Mitchell, P., Jaffe, A.S., and Schneiderman, N., 2007, Social support and prognosis in patients at increased psychosocial risk recovering from myocardial infarction, *Health Psychol.* **26**:418–427.

Lichtenstein, M.J., Griffin, M.R., Cornell, J.E., Malcolm, E. and Ray, W.A., 1994, Risk Factors for hip fractures occurring in the hospital, *Am. J. Epidemiol.* **140**:830–838.

Lorig, K.R., Ritter, P.L., Laurent, D.D., and Plantv, K., 2008, The internet-based arthritis self-management program: A one-year randomized trial for patients with arthritis or fibromyalgia, *Arthritis Rheum.* **59**:1009–17.

Mechanic, D., 2003, Is the prevalence of mental disorders a good measure of the need for services? *Health Affairs* **22**:8–27.

Miller, T.L., Hilsenrath, P., Lykens, K., McNabb, S.J.N., Moonan, P.K., and Weis, S.E., 2006, Using cost and health impacts to prioritize the targeted testing of tuberculosis in the United States, *Ann. Epidemiol.* **16**:305–312.

Mortimore, E., Haselow, D., Dolan, M., Hawkes, W.G., Langenberg, P., Zimmerman, S., Magaziner, J., 2008, Amount of social contact and hip fracture mortality, *J. Am. Geriatrics Soc.* **56**:1069–1074.

Mundinger, M., Kane, R.L., Lenz, E.R., Totten, A.M., Tsai, W., Cleary, P.D., Friedewald, W.T., Siu, A.L., and Shelanski, M.L., 2000, Primary care outcomes in patients treated by nurse practitioners or physicians: a randomized trial, *J.A.M.A.* **283**:58–68.

Myers, A.H., Robinson, E.G., Van Natta, M.L., Michelson, J.D., Collins, K., and Baker, S.P., 1991, Hip fractures among the elderly: factors associated with in-hospital mortality, *Am. J. Epidemiol.* **134**:1128–1137.

Norris, J.C., van der Laan, M.J., Lane, S., Anderson, J.N., and Block, G., 2003, Nonlinearity in demographic and behavioral determinants of morbidity, *HSR: Health Serv. Res.* **38**:1791–1818.

Oleske, D.M., Cobleigh, M.A., Phillips, M., and Nachman, K.L., 2004, Determination of factors associated with hospitalization in breast cancer survivors, *Oncol. Nurs. Forum.* **31**:1081–1088.

Plomondon, M.E., Magid, D.J., Steiner, J.F., MaWhinney, S., Gifford, B.D., Shih, S.C., Grunwald, G.K., Rumsfeld, J.S., 2007, Primary care provider turnover and quality in managed care organizations, *Am. J. Managed Care* **13**:465–472.

Rothman, K.J., 1995, Causes, *Am. J. Epidemiol.* **141**:90–95.

Schappert, S.M., and Rechtsteiner, E.A., 2008, Ambulatory medical care utilization estimates for 2006. *National Health Statistics Reports*; no 8, National Center for Health Statistics, Hyattsville, MD.

Schmittdiel, J.A., Shortell, S.M., Rundall, T.G., Bodenheimer, T., and Selby, J.V., 2006, Effect of primary health care orientation on chronic care management, *Ann. Fam. Med.* **4**:117–123.

Steenland, K., and Pinkerton, L.E., 2008, Mortality patterns following downsizing at Pan American World Airways, *Am. J. Epidemiol.* **167**:1–6.

Strecher, V., McClure, J., Alexander, G., Chakraborty, B., Nair, V., Konkel, J., Greene, S., Collins, L., Carlier, C., and Wiese, C., 2008, Web-based smoking-cessation programs: results of a randomized trial, *Am. J. Prev. Med.* **34**:373–381.

Thorpe, K.E., 2006, Factors accounting for the rise in health-care spending in the United States: the role of rising disease prevalence and treatment intensity, *Public Health* **120**:1002–1007.

United Nations, Department of Economic and Social Affairs, Population Division, 2007, *World Population Prospects: The 2006 Revision, Highlights*, Working Paper No. ESA/P/WP.202, United Nations, New York, NY.

U.S. Census Bureau, 2000, *Census 2000 Gateway* (July 5, 2009) http://www.census.gov/main/www/cen2000.html.

U.S. Department of Health and Human Services, Office of Minority Health, 2001, *National Standards for Culturally and Linguistically Appropriate Services in Health Care*, (http://www.omhrc.gov), Rockville, MD.

Weinick, R.M. 2007, *Pay-for-Performance to Reduce Racial and Ethnic Disparities in Health Care in the Massachusetts Medicaid Program* Institute for Health Policy, Massachusetts General Hospital, Boston, MA (http://www.cms.hhs.gov/MedicaidSCHIPQualPrac/Downloads/disp4p.pdf).

Wennberg, J.E. (ed.), 1996, The Dartmouth Atlas of Health Care in the United States, American Hospital Publishing, Inc., Chicago, IL.

World Health Organization (WHO), 2008a, *Closing the Gap in a Generation: Health Equity through Action on the Social Determinants of Health*, WHO Press, Geneva, Switzerland.

World Health Organization (WHO), 2008b, *World Health Statistics 2008*, WHO Press, Geneva, Switzerland.

Yang, D.H., Goerge, R., and Mullner, R., 2006, Comparing GIS-based methods of measuring spatial accessibility to health services, *J. Med. Syst.* **30**:23–32.

Chapter 2
Measurement Issues in the Use of Epidemiologic Data

Learning Outcomes

After completing this chapter, you will be able to:

1. Construct a self-administered survey form to measure a community's health.
2. Interpret a survey form's reliability and validity in measuring health, disability, or quality of life.
3. Outline steps to represent the logistics of administering a survey form to assess the health of a community.
4. Devise a plan for controlling measurement error when using a survey form.

Keyterms Error • Health Primary data • Reliability • Secondary data • Sensitivity • Specificity • Validity • Variable

Introduction

There are many different types of health care services. It is the health care manager's responsibility to employ epidemiologic strategies to continuously monitor the services provided to determine if they are achieving the health goals of a community. Fundamental to monitoring is determining what to measure and if it could or should be measured. Accurate measurement of exposure in the community to risk factors, use of health care services, and the hypothesized health outcomes associated with the services is essential in determining the impact of health services delivery and optimizing the allocation of services as needed. Health care managers must decide what data should be collected for monitoring, how frequently it should be collected, and what measurement is most appropriate for the particular service(s) delivered. This chapter discussed the major issues pertinent to the measurement of exposure to risk factors and of the health outcomes of health services delivery, including the methods and logistics of measurement, reliability and validity, classification systems, and reduction of measurement error.

D.M. Oleske (ed.), *Epidemiology and the Delivery of Health Care Services: Methods and Applications,*
DOI 10.1007/978-1-4419-0164-4_2, © Springer Science+Business Media, LLC 2009

Measurement

To determine what should be measured, one must first specify or conceptualize the relationship among variables and their hypothesized direction of influence, this is called a conceptual model. A variable is an element or entity in a model that takes on different values represented as attributes of a variable. Variables can represent any quantitative or qualitative values. For example, the variable consumer relations (Fig. 1) can be represented through two or more attributes (e.g., Present/absent or 1 = high degree, 2 = medium degree, 3 = low degree). Latent variables represent the category of the variables, but they themselves are not directly observed or measured. Sechrest (2005) argues that blood pressure is a latent variable for this reason as it indirectly measures the pressure in the blood vessel. Also, because it is comprised of two concepts, systolic and diastolic blood pressure, the latter of which requires a judgment of when the audible sound changes to reflect the artery is no longer constricted and hence representing the diastolic pressure. Observed variables represent the variable of the unit upon which the measurement is performed. In Fig. 1, the latent variables are consumer relations, hospital relations, physician relations, quality of care, and quality of work life for physicians. The "x's" represent the observed variables. The relationship among latent variables specifying the indicators that are observed (or measured) is called the measurement model. Instrumental variables are intended to control for confounding and measurement

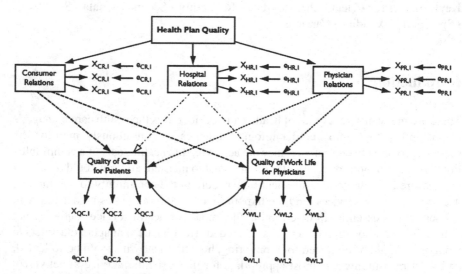

Fig. 1 Diagram of conceptual model and measurement model. *X* indicates observed variables; e, random errors; labels (CR [consumer relations], HR [hospital relations], PR [physician relations], QC [quality of care for patients], WL [quality of work life for physicians]), latent variables; →, causal arrow. Reproduced from Wholey, D.R. et al. (2003) with permission from the *American Journal of Managed Care: The Forum For Peer-Reviewed Literature on Healthcare Outcomes* Medical Publishing Division

error, particularly in observational studies (Greenland, 2000). An example of an instrumental variable would be a variable that influences a level of a hospital's patient safety activity, but does not directly affect patient safety. Instrumental variables in this example could be presence of an electronic health record system or board monitoring of patient safety initiatives. Figure 1 displays a conceptual model of the inter-relationship of health plan to the variables of quality of care for patients and quality of work life for physicians through the variables of consumer relations, hospital relations and physician relations. Embedded within the conceptual model is a measurement model. Although all relationships are specified in a conceptual model when examining the causal pathway of a health service delivery problem, typically only one component is studied and analyzed.

Methods of Measurement

Numerous methods exist for measuring exposure variables, health, and other variables which could mitigate the relationship between exposure and health. These include survey forms, laboratory tests, imaging techniques, and physical measurements. Physical measurements include direct measurement such as obtaining blood pressure, height, weight, or ambient air concentrations, or indirect physical measurement such as observation of gait.

The survey form is the most widely used method for obtaining information about exposure factors, health outcomes, and covariates. Survey forms may be designed to collect information using one of three modes: a data abstractor, interviewer, or self-administrated. The types of surveys include: data abstraction, personal interview, telephone interview, or self-administered. The media for collecting survey information include: paper and pencil, computer, web-based, or through some other technology or device. The advantages and disadvantages of the various modes of survey data collection are contrasted in Table 1. Audio-assisted self-interviewing has been proposed as a means of addressing problems related to literacy and questions about risk or sensitive behaviors (Edwards et al., 2007).

A survey form, regardless of the mode of administration, type, or media for data collection, consists of the following elements: (1) an introduction (2) the body of the survey form containing the questions or items themselves, and (3) a conclusion. The *introduction* contains the title and purpose of survey, special instructions to the respondent (or abstractor). Studies with a longitudinal component would ascertain here information about informants (relatives, etc.) who could be contacted in the event of relocation of the respondent. The *body* of the survey contains questions or items grouped into meaningful categories in a logical sequence and their associated responses including how to respond if an item does not apply. The body of the survey form may contain both items pertaining to exposure as well as outcome information, depending upon the study design. Exposure measurement should include: the source, periods or exposure, intensity, frequency, and duration. Outcome measurement (e.g., onset of an acute myocardial infarction) should include: the date of onset of symptoms, date

Table 1 Advantages and disadvantages of various survey methods

Survey method	Advantages	Disadvantages
Data abstraction	Reduces nonresponse error Can quickly obtain information. Eliminates possibility of recall error when abstracting from primary sources (e.g., medical records) or recording information each day	Unable to determine if missing information represents a positive or negative exposure
Telephone (mostly random-digit-dial)	Less likely to have interviewer response bias Yields information similar to in-person interviews using memory aids	Cannot reach households without telephones Higher likelihood of missing height and weight information
Self-administered paper and pencil[a]	Provides access to cell-phone only households, households without telephones Useful for collecting sensitive behavioral data Response rate 33.9% to mail survey	May not be able to clarify instructions Participant response may be affected by physical abilities (inability to read, lack of corrective lenses, etc.)
Self-administered web-based or computer-based[a]	Response rate 50% Item completion rate 98.3% Useful for collecting sensitive behavioral data. Ease of use and high acceptance reported	Provides more complete contact information including email addresses Responders more likely to be obese, smoke, and report occupational exposures Lower educational level and infrequent computer use have usability trouble
In-person interviews	May be conducive to lengthier surveys. Allows probing of responses	May not provide complete information on sensitive behavioral data. May respond differently to different features of interviewer. Interviewer body language may affect participant response

[a]Includes questionnaire and diary formats

sought care for the condition, and the name of the physician/hospital where care was received. Cues (either verbal or pictorial, also known as memory aids) and definitions within the body of the form may be used in the item or question to stimulate recall and/ or provide more accurate responses (Cook et al., 2003). Table 2 displays an example of pictorial cues for accurate recall of portions for dietary surveys. Cues in data abstraction survey forms commonly refer the abstractor to the location in the source document where the data elements can be found. The *conclusion* contains verbiage that no more responses are required, and when and where the completed form should be sent (or submitted if faxed or web-based). Figures 2 and 3 display a sample telephone interview survey form and a data abstraction form, respectively.

Throughout the survey form, attention should be given to the level of measurement desired for each response item, nominal, ordinal, interval, or ratio. Regardless of the level of measurement, each item or type questions should have a highlighted time referent for the respondent (e.g., within the last 24 h, in your lifetime, etc.) as in the examples below.

Table 2 Using everyday objects as cues to estimate serving sizes in food surveys

1 cup of cereal = a fist

1/2 cup of cooked rice, pasta, or potato = 1/2 baseball

1 baked potato = a fist

1 medium fruit = a baseball

1/2 cup of fresh fruit = 1/2 baseball

1 1/2 ounces of low-fat or fat-free cheese = 4 stacked dice

1/2 cup of ice cream = 1/2 baseball

2 tablespoons of peanut butter = a ping-pong ball

Source: Available from: http://win.niddk.nih.gov/publications/just_enough.htm (2006)

A *nominal* measurement categorizes information into two or more levels of mutually exclusive categories, illustrating a survey question pertaining to cancer screening:

Q. A Prostate-Specific Antigen test, also called a PSA test, is a blood test to check men for prostate cancer. Have you *ever* had a PSA test?

1	Yes
2	No
7	Don't know/not sure
8	Not applicable
9	Refused

An *ordinal* measurement categorizes information into levels which have meaning to the ordering, with the ordered responses typically assigned the most conventional options. Two common ways of capturing ordinal information are through Likert-type scales or visual analog scales (VAS). The Likert-type scale uses a number in association with the rating of a response to an item. Because

Q. In the past <u>seven days</u>, how bothersome has your low back pain been?

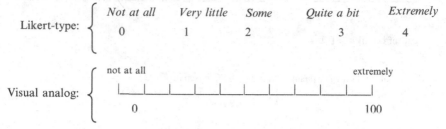

Likert-type:

Not at all	*Very little*	*Some*	*Quite a bit*	*Extremely*
0	1	2	3	4

Visual analog:

not at all   extremely

0   100

Interviewer's Script

HELLO, I am calling for the **(health department).** My name is **(name).** We are gathering information about the health of **(state)** residents. This project is conducted by the health department with assistance from the Centers for Disease Control and Prevention. Your telephone number has been chosen randomly, and I would like to ask some questions about health and health practices.

I will not ask for your name, address, or other personal information that can identify you. You do not have to answer any question you do not want to, and you can end the interview at any time. Any information you give me will be confidential. If you have any questions about this survey, please call **(give appropriate state telephone number).**

Module 3: Healthy Days (Symptoms)

The next few questions are about health-related problems or symptoms.

1. During the past 30 days, for about how many days did pain make it hard for you to do your usual activities, such as self-care, work, or recreation?

　　_ _　　Number of days
　　8 8　　None
　　7 7　　Don't know / Not sure
　　9 9　　Refused

2. During the past 30 days, for about how many days have you felt sad, blue, or depressed?

　　_ _　　Number of days
　　8 8　　None
　　7 7　　Don't know / Not sure
　　9 9　　Refused

3. During the past 30 days, for about how many days have you felt worried, tense, or anxious?

　　_ _　　Number of days
　　8 8　　None
　　7 7　　Don't know / Not sure
　　9 9　　Refused

4. During the past 30 days, for about how many days have you felt very healthy and full of energy?

　　_ _　　Number of days
　　8 8　　None
　　7 7　　Don't know / Not sure
　　9 9　　Refused

Fig. 2 Selected sections of Behavioral Risk Factor Surveillance Survey form (From Centers for Disease Control and Prevention, 2008)

Resident _____　　　Numeric Identifier _____

MINIMUM DATA SET (MDS) — *VERSION 2.0*
FOR NURSING HOME RESIDENT ASSESSMENT AND CARE SCREENING

BACKGROUND (FACE SHEET) INFORMATION AT ADMISSION

SECTION AB. DEMOGRAPHIC INFORMATION

1.	DATE OF ENTRY	Date the stay began. Note — Does not include readmission if record was closed at time of temporary discharge to hospital, etc. In such cases, use prior admission date
		☐☐ – ☐☐ – ☐☐☐☐ Month Day Year
2.	ADMITTED FROM (AT ENTRY)	1. Private home/apt. with no home health services 2. Private home/apt. with home health services 3. Board and care/assisted living/group home 4. Nursing home 5. Acute care hospital 6. Psychiatric hospital, MR/DD facility 7. Rehabilitation hospital 8. Other
3.	LIVED ALONE (PRIOR TO ENTRY)	0. No 1. Yes 2. In other facility
4.	ZIP CODE OF PRIOR PRIMARY RESIDENCE	☐☐☐☐☐
5.	RESIDENTIAL HISTORY 5 YEARS PRIOR TO ENTRY	(Check all settings resident lived in during 5 years prior to date of entry given in item AB1 above) Prior stay at this nursing home — a. Stay in other nursing home — b. Other residential facility—board and care home, assisted living, group home — c. MH/psychiatric setting — d. MR/DD setting — e. NONE OF ABOVE — f.
6.	LIFETIME OCCUPATION(S) [Put "/" between two occupations]	☐☐☐☐☐☐☐☐☐☐☐☐☐☐☐☐
7.	EDUCATION (Highest Level Completed)	1. No schooling　　5. Technical or trade school 2. 8th grade/less　6. Some college 3. 9-11 grades　　7. Bachelor's degree 4. High school　　8. Graduate degree
8.	LANGUAGE	(Code for correct response) a. Primary Language 0. English　1. Spanish　2. French　3. Other b. If other, specify
9.	MENTAL HEALTH HISTORY	Does resident's RECORD indicate any history of mental retardation, mental illness, or developmental disability problem? 0. No　　1. Yes
10.	CONDITIONS RELATED TO MR/DD STATUS	(Check all conditions that are related to MR/DD status that were manifested before age 22, and are likely to continue indefinitely) Not applicable—no MR/DD (Skip to AB11) — a. MR/DD with organic condition Down's syndrome — b. Autism — c. Epilepsy — d. Other organic condition related to MR/DD — e. MR/DD with no organic condition — f.
11.	DATE BACKGROUND INFORMATION COMPLETED	☐☐ – ☐☐ – ☐☐☐☐ Month Day Year

SECTION AC. CUSTOMARY ROUTINE

1. CUSTOMARY ROUTINE	(Check all that apply. If all information UNKNOWN, check last box only.)	
(In year prior to DATE OF ENTRY to this nursing home, or year last in community if now being admitted from another nursing home)	**CYCLE OF DAILY EVENTS**	
	Stays up late at night (e.g., after 9 pm)	a.
	Naps regularly during day (at least 1 hour)	b.
	Goes out 1+ days a week	c.
	Stays busy with hobbies, reading, or fixed daily routine	d.
	Spends most of time alone or watching TV	e.
	Moves independently indoors (with appliances, if used)	f.
	Use of tobacco products at least daily	g.
	NONE OF ABOVE	h.
	EATING PATTERNS	
	Distinct food preferences	i.
	Eats between meals all or most days	j.
	Use of alcoholic beverage(s) at least weekly	k.
	NONE OF ABOVE	l.
	ADL PATTERNS	
	In bedclothes much of day	m.
	Wakens to toilet all or most nights	n.
	Has irregular bowel movement pattern	o.
	Showers for bathing	p.
	Bathing in PM	q.
	NONE OF ABOVE	r.
	INVOLVEMENT PATTERNS	
	Daily contact with relatives/close friends	s.
	Usually attends church, temple, synagogue (etc.)	t.
	Finds strength in faith	u.
	Daily animal companion/presence	v.
	Involved in group activities	w.
	NONE OF ABOVE	x.
	UNKNOWN—Resident/family unable to provide information	y.

SECTION AD. FACE SHEET SIGNATURES

SIGNATURES OF PERSONS COMPLETING FACE SHEET:

a. Signature of RN Assessment Coordinator　　　　　　Date

I certify that the accompanying information accurately reflects resident assessment or tracking information for this resident and that I collected or coordinated collection of this information on the dates specified. To the best of my knowledge, this information was collected in accordance with applicable Medicare and Medicaid requirements. I understand that this information is used as a basis for ensuring that residents receive appropriate and quality care, and as a basis for payment from federal funds. I further understand that payment of such federal funds and continued participation in the government-funded health care programs is conditioned on the accuracy and truthfulness of this information, and that I may be personally subject to or may subject my organization to substantial criminal, civil, and/or administrative penalties for submitting false information. I also certify that I am authorized to submit this information by this facility on its behalf.

Signature and Title	Sections	Date
b.		
c.		
d.		
e.		
f.		
g.		

☐ = When box blank, must enter number or letter　☐a. = When letter in box, check if condition applies　　　　MDS 2.0 September, 2000

Fig. 3 Minimum Data Set (MDS) for Nursing Home Resident Assessment and Care selected page from form, face sheet (Source: Centers for Medicare and Medicaid Services, 2000)

bias inherent in the value of the rating may occur such that an individual may misinterpret the rating (e.g., 1 = excellent, but the respondent perceives the low numeric value to be a low rating) or does not feel the score represents the condition accurately, the VAS is a method that may be used as alternative measure. The magnitude of the perception is scored on a straight line, usually 100 mm, with either a horizontal or vertical orientation. At each end of the line, the extreme values are anchored (e.g., no pain, extreme pain). There are different types of VAS scales including simple (no scale marks), middle marked, marked every 10 mm without numbers, marked every 10 mm with numbers, and a scale with numbers every 10 mm but no line. The VAS scales can be oriented either horizontally or vertically. The type of VAS used influences the percentage of zero ratings as well as low- and high-intensity ratings, so care needs to be taken (Paul-Dauphin et al., 1999). Examples of the two measurement types are below:

Q. In the past *7 days*, how bothersome has your low back pain been?

In *interval* measurement, the distance between data points has meaning such that the distance between 5 and 10 miles is the same as the distance between 25 and 30 miles. Ratio measurement is characterized by an absolute zero that has meaning. The number of cases of a disease is a ratio measurement, because having zero cases of the disease has meaning. Blood pressure is another example of ratio measurement. When recording values on a survey form to obtain interval or ratio measurements, the value, the units of measurement, and the maximum number of integers anticipated for the variable during the time interval queried should be indicated. For example:

Q. The next question asks about recent falls. By a fall, we mean when a person unintentionally comes to rest on the ground or another lower level. *In the past 3 months*, how many times have you fallen? (Write number or circle response.)

–	–	Number of times
8	8	None
7	7	Don't know/not sure
9	9	Refused

Coding conventions typically designate the use of "9" for items that a respondent refuses to answer.

The level of measurement guides in determining the type of statistical test that will be used to evaluate the relationship between exposure and outcome. Each item or question on the survey form may have a different level of measurement. The highest level of measurement should be obtained for an item where feasible as it yields the most information. Grouping responses to items or questions can occur during programming the data. Devising cut-points or grouping data from measurements should be determined by: (1) common convention (e.g., hospital bed groups); (2) clinical significance (e.g., LDL > 130); (3) database rules such as quartiles of a distribution; (4) plots of exposure vs. outcome (e.g., Q–Q plots, splines); or, statistical models (recursive partitioning analysis [tree-based models], multiple stepwise linear or logistic regression).

Validity, Reliability, and Responsiveness of a Measure

A measure should be valid, reliable, and responsive. This means a measure should truly capture a phenomenon (validity), repeatedly over time if it remains unchanged (reliability) and represent it accurately if it changes over time (responsiveness).

A measure should not be used unless these attributes are known in advance. The information can be obtained from prior studies of the use of the measure or at the very least initiate a pilot in the population intended for measurement. In evaluating a measure, typically a random sample from the pool of all eligible participants is selected to make the comparisons.

Validity

Validity represents the degree of precision to which the measure truly characterizes the phenomenon being studied. The process of establishing validity is influenced by the type of measurement device or form used, what population it is validated in, and how large is the sample obtained to validate the phenomenon. Additionally, the representativeness of the sample, the organizational structure and processes in the organization in which the population receives services may influence the determination of the validity of a measure (e.g., measure validated in persons from a Veterans Administration health system vs. those in a federally qualified health center) (Morgan et al., 2005). Devices and technical instruments require calibration against a known entity to assure validity. Measurements obtained through survey forms also require proper validation. The validation process can be complicated if proxies or external raters are involved (Snow et al., 2005). In its simplest form, survey forms evaluated for validity require proper formatting and then must be subject to a validation process using some a priori defined "gold standard." The validation process described herein emphasizes the validation process for survey forms.

Formatting Survey Forms

The structure of survey forms should follow the principles outlined in Table 3. The proper formatting to capture the appropriate measurement level in a survey form was previously discussed. Other considerations of formatting, regardless of the media, consider the physical appearance of qualitative aspects of the form, such as the colors used or any designs on the form. Surveys formatted for web-based data collection have the advantage of preventing multiple responses to single response questions. Survey data collected electronically can also promote clarity in free-text responses and ease response involving respondents skipping items that do not apply. Although characteristics of responders relative to survey format have been reported, completeness of information relative to type of question and response fatigue have been reported to be comparable between paper and pencil and web-based survey formats (Smith et al., 2007).

Common Types of Validation Processes

The validation process is built upon the degree of knowledge about the concept being measured. The method chosen depends upon the level of measurement of the test

Table 3 Principles for structuring survey forms

1. Formatting
    a. Header: Display title of project, purpose, instructions to participant/interviewer (voluntary, procedures for maintaining confidentiality) at beginning (top) of form
    b. Body of form:
        i. Be consistent with the manner in which it is administered (e.g., data abstraction, self-administered, web-based)
        ii. Determine logical sequence of items/questions; number items/items; clearly identify breaks between categories
        iii. Always use complete sentences for items/questions, not phrases, words, or incomplete sentences
        iv. Use consistent codes for responses (e.g., 1 always equals "yes")
        v. Take into consideration special needs of target population (e.g., larger font for older population)
        vi. Keep all items/questions pertaining to a set of instructions on the same page (hard copy or web page)
        vii. Provide clear instructions if skip patterns are used (e.g., *Skip to Q. 10, if you have never smoked cigarettes*)
    c. Concluding section:
        i. Place demographics last except in telephone survey forms where some demographic screening may be necessary to interact with appropriate individual or in data abstraction forms where it may be necessary to verify the correct case
        ii. Let the participant know the survey is complete; data abstraction forms should indicate the end of abstraction
        iii. Leave space for comments
        iv. Provide instructions on submitting the completed form (e.g., *Select "Submit" button when you have completed your survey*; *Return the completed survey in postage paid envelop*; *Fax your completed survey to the fax number xxx-xxx-xxxx.*)
        v. If submitting the form electronically, provide a statement/confirmation that submission was transmitted
        vi. Thank the participant
2. Clarity
    a. Provide instructions for individual items/questions as needed (e.g., "Check all that apply.")
    b. Provide referents as appropriate (e.g., events in the last 7 days vs. recent events; satisfaction with nursing care vs. satisfaction with service by hospital staff)
    c. Do not ask two questions and only provide one response
3. Balance
    a. Avoid providing more than 20 items/questions in a series with the same category of response
4. Length
    a. Keep each item/question as brief as possible
    b. Keep the total number of pages/screens as brief as possible

measure known to measure the concept or problem being measured. The most commonly used methods for evaluating validity are content validity (or face validity), criterion validity, and construct validity. In the validation process, the new or test measure is compared against measures which have known validity or professional opinions of validity.

Content validity is a first step in the validation process of a survey form when little is known about the concept being measured. Content validity is determined by an expert

Table 4 Assessing the criterion validity of a measure

Measure results	Disease		Total
	Present	Absent	
Positive	True positive (TP)	False positive (FP)	A + B
	A	B	
Negative	False negative (FN)	True negative (TN)	
	C	D	C + D
Total	A + C	B + D	A + B + C + D

Sensitivity[a] (those who have the disease and are so classified by the test) = A/(A + C) X 100% = TP/(TP + FN) × 100% = TP/(All those who have the disease)

Specificity[a] (those who do not have the disease and are so classified by the test) = D/(B + D) × 100% = TN/(TN + FP) × 100% = TN/All those without the disease

False negative rate[a] (those with the disease not identified by the test) = C/(A + C) × 100%

False positive rate[a] (those without the disease identified by the test) = B/(B + D) × 100%

Disease prevalence rate (proportion of those with the disease times a factor of 10) = (A + C)/ (A + B + C + D) × 100%

Positive predictive rate (the number with disease who test positive) = A/(A + B) × 100%

Negative predictive rate (the number without the disease who test negative) = D/(C + D) × 100%

Diagnostic accuracy rate (the total number of individuals correctly classified as having the disease or correctly classified as not having the disease from the total sample) = (A + D)/ (A + B + C + D) × 100% = (TP + TN)/All those evaluated

[a]Can also be expressed as a probability

panel, usually at least three, make a subjective determination that the measure accurately represents the full domain of the concept or condition. The panel typically consists of three to four members (who represent a "gold standard") including subject matter experts as well as those knowledgeable of measurement. Survey forms addressing cultural or behavioral practices (e.g., dietary patterns, drug usage) or health-related quality of life (HRQoL) may also be validated qualitatively using focus groups consisting of representatives of the population subgroups being measured such as patients and/or caregivers. In this way, familiar terminology, idioms, and phrases may be used to clarify the questions being and provide sensitivity to the ordering of the items on the form.

Criterion validity is the comparison of a test measurement against a known outcome or phenomenon. In epidemiological studies, the known outcome is typically a clinical laboratory measurement such as a blood test or results from a pathology examination. The test measures can be at any level of measurement. If the referent and test measures are nominal levels of measurement, present or absent (e.g., disease present or absent), an R × C table format is used to quantitatively assess the measure of level of validity. The validity is assessed through the computation of the sensitivity, specificity, and positive predictive values of the test measure (Table 4). The ideal measure of validity has 100% sensitivity, 100% specificity, and 100% positive predictive value. If the measures compared are interval or ratio, such as a plasma marker of carotenoid consumption vs. dietary self-report instruments obtained from all study participants, a linear regression can be performed with log transformation of the variables in the model to improve normality and stabilize variance (Natarajan et al., 2006).

Construct validity is the use of two or more measures yielding similar results to account for a phenomenon and as such represents a theoretical coherence. If many people do not believe in a construct, then it is futile to present evidence for a measure. Construct validity is used when multiple criteria are thought to measure a single concept, such as the quality of life or severity of illness. Thus, if one wanted to evaluate the validity of a new severity of illness scale, then that measure would be compared against mortality rates for that illness, medical resource consumption and other scale(s) with previously published correlation values. The degree of validity of a measure is statistically assessed as the degree of correlation across scales, using a correlation coefficient or R-squared from a linear regression model. High correlation among population subgroups (e.g., by age, gender, race) between the test (new) measure and the existing measure population subgroups provides even greater evidence for validity (Boxed Example 1).

Reliability and Responsiveness

A measure must be reliable in order for it to be valid. Reliability represents the extent to which a measure has consistency over time (stability or reproducibility), among various versions or applications (equivalence), within the measure itself (homogeneity) and the ability to detect valid changes in the phenomenon over time (responsiveness).

The statistical method used to assess reliability or responsiveness depends upon the level of measurement and aspect of reliability being assessed. Common test statistics used for evaluating reliability are the: correlation coefficient, the intraclass correlation coefficient (ICC), the kappa statistic, and the coefficient of variation (CV).

The *correlation coefficient* is used for evaluating the reliability of or correlation between two distinct variables from a measure. There are two types of correlation coefficients depending upon the level of measurement of the two variables compared. The product moment (Pearson) correlation coefficient (r) is used when both the independent and dependent variables are each continuous and have a normal distribution. The rank-difference correlation coefficient (r_s) (Spearman's *rho*) is used when either or both the independent and dependent variables are at least ordinal or when the total sample size is less than 30. The valid values for both correlation coefficients range from −1, a perfectly negative correlation, to +1, a perfectly positive correlation. The value "0" represents no correlation. The larger the value of the correlation coefficient (r or r_s), the greater the reliability of the measure; values of at least 0.70, either positively or negatively, represent a strong correlation.

When the reproducibility or reliability is assessed for two variables that cannot be distinguished from each other or replicate data from the same subject, such as comparing the mean cholesterol level from two samples from the same vial of blood, the *ICC* is computed. The ICC is the ratio of the between-person variance divided by the sum of the between-person and the within-person estimated from a one-way randomized effects ANOVA model variance. The valid values of the ICC range from 0 and 1. The reliability of the measure is determined both in terms of the point estimate of the ICC, with higher values indicating stronger agreement and the width of its associated confidence interval. A point estimate of ≥0.75 indicates excellent reproducibility (Rosner, 2006) and a narrow band bound of the 95% confidence

Boxed Example 1 Evaluation of the Validity of Self-Reported Endoscopies of the Large Bowel

Problem: One of the strongest predictors of protection against colorectal cancer is a history of endoscopy for large bowel screening. The validity of recall of this procedure is important in determining the extent of resources to be deployed for screening in a community or health plan.

Methods: Population-based case-control study validating all participants with a positive self-report and a random sample of 100 participants with a negative self-report of a previous endoscopy of the large bowel.

Data and Results

Gender*	Total (no.)	Self-report of colorectal endoscopy (no.)	No self-report of colorectal endoscopy (no.)	Sensitivity (%)	Specificity (%)	Chi-square test
Women	174	136	38	100	97	p = 0.85
Men	203	157	46	100	95	

Source: Hoffmeister et al., 2007

Yields the following data tables from which the results were computed:

Women	Yes on medical record	No on medical record	Total
Self-report Yes	135	1	136
Self-report No	0	38	38
Total	135	39	174

Men	Yes on medical record	No on medical record	Total
Self-report Yes	155	2	157
Self-report No	0	46	46
Total	155	48	203

Sensitivity$_{women}$ = No. True positive/total positives × 100% = 135/135 × 100% = 100%
Sensitivity$_{men}$ = No. True positive/total positives × 100% = 155/155 × 100% = 100%
Specificity$_{women}$ = No. True negative/total negatives × 100% = 38/39 × 100% = 97%
Specificity$_{men}$ = No. True negative/total negatives × 100% = 46/48 × 100% = 95%

Managerial Epidemiology Interpretation: The high sensitivity and specificity of self-reports of endoscopy, not significantly different between men and women, indicate that a well-constructed question on intake or a health survey form can aid a manager in accurately determining the timing of uses of resources for deploying endoscopies for screening the large bowel for cancer in communities or by a health plan.

Table 5 Calculating agreement of self-reports of colonoscopy with medical records among subjects with a previous colorectal endoscopy (Data from: Hoffmeister et al. (2007))

Self-report of procedure	Medical records documentation			
	Colonoscopy, n (p)	Sigmoidoscopy, n (p)	Rectoscopy, n (p)	Total n (p)
Colonoscopy	208[a] (0.8254)[b]	4	19	231 (0.9167)
Sigmoidoscopy	2	1 (0.0040)	0	3 (0.0119)
Rectoscopy	11	1	6 (0.0238)	18 (0.0714)
Total	221 (0.8770)	6 (0.0238)	15 (0.0992)	252 (1.0)

[a]Observed agreement (n) and [b]proportion (p) of total sample

interval would indicate a more narrow distribution of the point estimates and hence greater precision of the measure (Armstrong et al., 1992).

The *kappa statistic* (*k*) is used to assess reproducibility when the ratings from two measures, one measure with two or more raters, or one measure at two-time or more periods are compared and both are categorical levels of measurement. The components of this assessment are testing rater independence with a *k*-statistic. The null hypothesis is that agreement is no more than might what occur by chance alone given random sampling or that the level of agreement is 0. The *k*-statistic is computed as follows:

$$\bar{\bar{k}} = (P_o - P_e)/(1 - P_e)$$

where: $\bar{\bar{k}}$ = the overall kappa statistic

$P_o = \sum_{i=1}^{k} p_{ii}$ overall proportion of observations for which there is agreement.

$P_e = \sum_{i=1}^{k} p_1, p_1$. overall proportion of observations for which agreement is expected by chance alone.

Using the data from Table 5:

$$P_o = 0.8254 + .0040 + 0.0238 = 0.8532$$

$$P_e = 0.8770 \times 0.9167 + 0.0\ 238 \times 0.0119$$
$$+ 0.0992 \times 0.0714 = 0.8113$$

$$\bar{\bar{k}} = (0.8532 - 0.8113)/(1 - 0.8113) = 0.22$$

A scheme for assessing the degree of agreement of the *k*-statistic beyond chance supported by Fleiss et al. (2003) is: <0.40, poor; 0.40–0.75, fair to good; >0.75 excellent agreement. If the test measures evaluated are ordinal (i.e., as levels of agreement), a weighted *k*-statistic should be used (Fleiss et al., 2003). The example yields the interpretation that across the self-reported three specific types of colonoscopy with medical records, the agreement is poor, study subjects did not know the specific type of colonoscopy they had received. The significance of the *k*-statistic is computed and for this the reader is referred to Fleiss et al. (2003).

The *CV* is used when comparing interval level measures with respect to their dispersion or the variability or when comparing interval measures whose orders of magnitude of numeric values are very disparate. The CV is represented as:

$$CV = \text{s.d.} / \bar{x}$$

Where x_i = value for each observation; n = number of observations

$$\bar{x} = \left(\sum_{k=0}^{n} x^k \right) / n$$

s.d. = standard deviation of x_i observations

A CV over 50% indicates poor reliability and the use or purchase of the diagnostic material, technology or other measure is not advised (Boxed Example 2).

Boxed Example 2 Evaluation of the Reliability of a Health Assessment Survey Form

Problem: The validity and reliability of survey forms which measure health may vary among populations. It is necessary for the health care manager to use surveys which have been tested in the population targeted for survey or to develop a procedure for performing the test.

Methods: The Millennium Cohort study, a large, population-based military cohort, used a number of instruments standardized in other populations to gather health outcome information to assess the significant of various occupational and environmental exposures over time. Participants were asked to complete an additional survey within 6 months of their original submission. Kappa statistics were computed to measure the degree of nonrandom agreement over time between each of the items in the questionnaire.

Data and Results: Mean Kappa statistic scores between two surveys within 6 months

	Demographic	Exposure	Symptoms and conditions	Posttraumatic stress disorder checklist	Complementary and alternative medicine	Alcohol	Smoking
Male	0.85	0.62	0.43	0.55	0.54	0.55	0.82
Female	0.89	0.59	0.52	0.54	0.54	0.44	0.83

Source: Smith et al., 2007

Managerial Epidemiology Interpretation: Males and females had the same level of agreement over time except that women were more consistent in reporting symptoms and conditions than men. The highest level of agreement for both sexes was for demographic questions and smoking. Other kappa statistics revealed moderate level agreement for the items querried. The health care manager needs to be able to evaluate health outcomes in populations managed and be confident that the outcome values are accurately measured. High reliability of a survey form results suggests high validity in measuring the true health state even ones with low prevalences such as post-traumatic stress disorder. The more accurately a health problem can be classified, the more likely interventions can be targeted effectively and evaluated.

Logistics of Measurement

The logistics of measurement encompasses the: strategy of obtaining survey information, the feasibility of obtaining the information, addressing the barriers to obtaining information, training of the data collectors, administration and/or collection of the information and data processing (editing, coding, formatting of raw data for reports, and analyses), and strategy for handling refusals, nonresponders, and in the case of studies with a longitudinal component, dropouts, and withdrawals.

Strategies for Obtaining Survey Information

The first step in measurement is deciding how and what is the most appropriate method for obtaining the required information from the target population. As mentioned earlier, there are different survey methods for obtaining information from study participants regarding their exposures and diseases, health outcomes, or other factors related to health or illness (Table 1). Computer aided or web-based data collection can be well accepted and allow for the economical and accurate collection of data, particularly on sensitive topics Van Griensven et al. (2006) (Boxed Example 2).

Feasibility of Obtaining Survey Information

The feasibility of obtaining survey information requires knowledge of if and how the intended target audience can be reached and the acceptability of the measurement to

Table 6 Questions for evaluating the logistics of measurement

1. How is the measure administered (web, onsite abstraction, device, etc.)?
2. Has it been used in other similar situations and to what degree of success?
3. Will the sample (patients, records, specimens, community members) be accessible/available for measurement?
4. Should incentives be provided (e.g., transportation for in-person interviews for low socioeconomic status participants; monetary incentive for participation in phone interview)?
5. Is the measure understandable by the study sample? By those who administer it?
6. Are there any risks associated with its administration (e.g., security of website; risk to survey administrator, risk to participant due to sensitive nature of question)?
7. What are the potential restrictions of its use (e.g., format in paper and pencil only, cost, copyright, patent, proprietary software to calculate summary score)?
8. Are special training and equipment required?
9. What is the length of time involved in: Measuring each study subject? Or, abstracting each record? Entering the data from the form?
10. How is the measure scored? How are the data output from the measure?
11. Will the results of the measurement be available in a timely manner if sent out for scoring? How long does it take to compute summary scores from measure?
12. Are normative data and interpretation guidelines available? If so, what is the cost? Are normative data available for the population studied?

that target population. The questions in Table 6 must be addressed to determine whether the measurement process is feasible. Mail surveys are still an important strategy to reach households without telephones and cell phone only households (Link et al., 2006).

Addressing Barriers to Obtaining Measurements

A number of factors have affected responses to participation in measurement. Barriers to data obtained through surveys have been most thoroughly examined. These include: aggressive telemarketing, telecommunications technology allowing call screening, a decline in volunteerism, increased work hours, reduced number in the household to serve as informants, lengthy consents required by institutional review boards (which include HIPAA requirements, see also chapter "Ethics and Managerial Epidemiology Practice"), and lack of interest in science (Galea and Tracy, 2007). All of these affect the quality of the research study findings which is judged by the study's participation rate. A participation rate can have different definitions. A participation rate is defined as the number of interviews completed divided by the number of individuals who have been determined to be eligible after exclusion criteria are applied. Response rate is the most conservative measure of participation calculated as the number completing the survey divided by all possible contact including those with unknown eligibility. The refusal rate may not be an accurate measure of participation as the eligibility of a contacted individual may not be able to be ascertained or the respondent may decline further participation mid-stream during the contact to count its data is questioned.

The goal of obtaining survey information by practice is to obtain a 75% completion rate for all samples selected for interviews or self-administered methods and reduce error in measurement through the survey format. Because of the barriers listed above, some advocate a mixed-method approach to obtaining information by surveys (e.g., mailed questionnaire or introductory letter followed by an email for an Internet survey) to reduce nonresponse error (Galea and Tracy, 2007).

Classification Systems: Health, Disease, Disability, Injury, and Quality of Life

An essential component of the epidemiologic study is to ensure that the health problem under study is appropriately and accurately classified. The more precisely that the health problem can be classified, the more effective will be the design of interventions in promoting health, preventing illness, disease, disability, injury, or improving outcomes of health care. A *classification system* is a method for assigning individuals measured into one of *n*-number of mutually exclusively categories, aggregate indices, or single item questions using some form of measurement. Misclassification of information is error. The use of existing classification systems for health care conditions provides for a way of structuring information to reduce error. The more precisely a condition can be classified, the more likely that interventions can be effective as they are more precisely developed and targeted. Common classification systems used in epidemiology are described below.

Health

The 1946 Constitution of the World Health Organization (WHO) defines health as a "state of complete physical, mental and social well-being and not merely the absence of disease or infirmity." Further that Constitution acknowledges the role of health care services by stating, "the extension to all peoples of the benefits of medical, psychological and related knowledge is essential to the fullest attainment of health." The first common measure of health was the mortality rate (see chapter "Descriptive Epidemiological Methods") because of the universality of this measure among nations. Thus, a low mortality rate in a geographical area has general acceptance as an overall proxy measure of "good health"; a high mortality rate in a community is an indicator of poor health. Currently, one of the most robust, simple overall measures of health is ascertained through a response to a self-rated health (SRH) question:

Would you say that in general your health is – (or "How would you rate your health?)

1	Excellent
2	Very good
3	Good
4	Fair
5	Poor

This simple self-reported global measure of health has been validated in many US population subgroups as a predictor of both mortality risk, likelihood of morbidity and health services utilization, and even study participation (DeSalvo et al., 2005; Finch et al., 2002; Idler et al., 2000; Kennedy et al., 2001; Lee et al., 2007; Oleske et al., 2006, 2007). SRH has also been shown to be significantly related to both cohort and time changes, and thus, is an important measure for evaluating health interventions and planning demand for health care services (Chen et al., 2007).

Disease

Disease refers to a state of disruption of normal physiological processes manifest as signs, symptoms, and abnormal physical, behavioral, or social functioning. The most widely used schema for classifying disease is the *International Classification of Diseases* (ICDs). The ICD was originally developed with the intent of providing a uniform international classification of causes of death. Its codes can now also be used to classify symptoms, physical findings, drugs, pathological processes, procedures, external causes of injury (E-coding), and utilization of health care services.

The WHO owns the copyright to the ICD. The ICD continues to be revised and updated periodically with new scientific and medical information about diseases. Because of its continual revision, caution must be exercised in interpreting disease rates used with other than the current version of the ICD. The coding for a number of conditions has changed over time in particular for AIDS, pneumonias, and dementias. The ICD is currently in its tenth revision (ICD-10) as of January 1, 1999 and used throughout the world for coding mortality data. ICD-9 is still used in the USA to produce statistics and indices oriented toward costing medical care based upon severity (assembling individual ICD codes into Diagnostic Related Groups, DRG's for health care claims reimbursement). The major feature of ICD-10 is the

Table 7 Comparison of International Classification of Disease (ICD) major diagnoses codes and codes used to classify AIDS/HIV[a] and low back pain[b], ninth and tenth revisions

Revision	ICD diagnosis code	Label
Ninth		
	001–139	Infectious and parasitic diseases
	042–044 (1987)	AIDS
	140–239	Neoplasms
	240–279	Endocrine, nutritional and metabolic diseases, and immunity disorders
	279.19 (1986)	Other deficiency of cell-mediated immunity
	280–289	Diseases of the blood and blood-forming organs
	290–319	Mental disorders
	320–359	Diseases of the nervous system
	360–389	Diseases of the sense organs
	390–459	Diseases of the circulatory system
	460–519	Diseases of the respiratory system
	520–579	Diseases of the digestive system
	580–629	Diseases of the genitourinary system
	630–676	Complications of pregnancy, childbirth, and the puerperium
	680–709	Diseases of the skin and subcutaneous tissue
	710–739	Diseases of the musculoskeletal system and connective tissue
	724.2	Lumbago, low back pain, low back syndrome, lumbalgia
	724.5	Backache, unspecified
	740–759	Congenital anomalies
	760–779	Certain conditions originating in the perinatal period
	780–799	Symptoms, signs, and ill-defined conditions
	800–999	Injury and poisoning
	846.0–0.9	*Sprains and strains of sacroiliac region*
	847.2	Sprains and strains, lumbar
	847.3	Sprains and strains, sacrum
	847.4	Sprains and strains, coccyx
	E800–E999	External causes of injury and poisoning
	V01–V86	Supplementary classification of factors influencing health status and contact with health services

(continued)

Table 7 (continued)

Revision	ICD diagnosis code	Label
Tenth		
	A00–B99	Certain infectious and parasitic diseases
	B20–B24	*Human immunodeficiency virus (HIV) disease*
	C00–D48	Neoplasms
	D50–D89	Diseases of the blood and blood-forming organs and certain disorders involving the immune mechanism
	D80.8	*Other immunodeficiencies with predominantly antibody defects*
	E00–E90	Endocrine, nutritional, and metabolic diseases
	F00–F99	Mental and behavioral disorders
	G00–G99	Diseases of the nervous system
	H00–H59	Diseases of the eye and adnexa
	H60–H95	Diseases of the ear and mastoid process
	I00–I99	Diseases of the circulatory system
	J00–J99	Diseases of the respiratory system
	K00–K93	Diseases of the digestive system
	L00–L99	Diseases of the skin and subcutaneous tissue
	M00–M99	Diseases of the musculoskeletal system and connective tissue
	M54.3	*Sciatica*
	M54.4	Lumbago with sciatica
	M54.5	Low back pain
	N00–N99	Diseases of the genitourinary system
	O00–O99	Pregnancy, childbirth, and the puerperium
	P00–P96	Certain conditions originating in the perinatal period
	Q00–Q99	Congenital malformations, deformations, and chromosomal abnormalities
	R00–R99	Symptoms, signs, and abnormal clinical and laboratory findings, not elsewhere classified
	S00–T98	Injury, poisoning, and certain other consequences of external causes
	V01–Y98	External causes of morbidity and mortality
	Z00–Z99	Factors influencing health status and contact with health services
	U00–U99	Codes for special purposes

In bold italics codes for [a]*AIDS/HIV* or [b]*Low back pain*

reduction in the number of codes representing the same trait and increased precision in classifying disease for which there is more biological information. By global treaty, ICD-10 is currently used to code death certificates worldwide, including in the USA. For example, AIDS is no longer a single code, but now classified according to the immunological type (Table 7). Free searchable on-line codes are available for ICD-10 (http://www.who.int/classifications/apps/icd/icd10online/) and for ICD-9-CM (Clinical modifications). However, ICD-9-CM is still used for coding records for medical claims billing.

Injury

An injury is a physical manifestation of bodily harm resulting from contact with a surface, temperature extremes, objects, substances, or from bodily motion. In the US in 2005, the number one cause of death among persons aged 1–44 years was unintentional injury (National Center for Health Statistics, 2007). Injuries and poisoning were also the number one cause of hospitalization and days of hospital care and for visits to hospital emergency departments for individuals less than 18 years of age in 2006 (National Center for Health Statistics, 2009).

Coding of the external cause of injury is required whenever an injury is the principal diagnosis or directly related to the principal diagnosis. When coding multiple trauma cases, the codes should be listed in sequence of the condition that presents the most serious threat to life. While the level of coding detail will aid in providing more detail for developing prevention initiatives, the increased coding demands upon acute care and emergency room staff provides a challenge.

Disability

Impairment in functioning is termed disability. Disability can be physical or cognitive. Disability is measured in the Behavioral Risk Factor Surveillance System Survey through the following questions: "Are you limited in any way in any activities because of physical, mental, or emotional problems?" and "Do you now have any health problem that requires you to use special equipment, such as a cane, wheelchair, a special bed, or a special telephone?" Individuals responding "yes" to either question are classified as having a disability (U.S.D.H.H.S., 2000). *Physical disability* is also commonly measured in clinical settings address limitations in personal care (activities of daily living, ADL), routine needs (instrumental activities of daily living, IADL), or a chronic condition. Physical disability measures commonly used in clinical settings, including activities of daily living and instrumental activities of daily living, are limited in their consideration of the spectrum of disability. The International Classification of Functioning, Disability and Health (ICF) considers the impact of the environment on the person's functioning (WHO, 2001).

Cognitive disability is characterized both by a significantly below-average score on a test of mental ability or intelligence and by limitations in the ability to function in routine activities of daily life, such as communication, self-care, and getting along in social situations or school activities. Intellectual disability can be measured by intelligence quotient (IQ) or by the types and amount of support they need.

Health-Related Quality of Life

HRQoL is multidimensional construct which represents the domains thought to measure both health and healthy living. The impetus for the development of this measure was driven largely by the pharmaceutical industry whereby many similarly formulated drugs produced similar clinical outcomes (e.g., reduction in the rate of cancer occurrence) with similar costs, necessitating a more refined and comprehensive understanding of treatment impact of endpoints that would complement the interpretation of the main clinical effect. The most commonly used domains in HRQoL are: (1) signs and symptoms, (2) treatment effects, (3) functional health, (4) work life, (5) emotional health, (6) social and leisure activities, and (6) reproductive health. HRQoL is used to measure the outcome of care to supplement other information on the outcomes of care such as morbidity and mortality and the administrative measures of rates of readmission and adverse outcomes and length of stay. HRQoL is viewed as a patient-reported outcome. HRQoL is used as a measure because some outcomes of treatment may yield identical morbidity, mortality, and administrative measures, but are only distinguishable in terms of HRQoL. HRQoL is also important measure to understand the impact of persistent ill-health because numerous disorders are associated with short- and long-term disabilities and chronic recurrences where the classic WHO definition of health does not apply. Tracking HRQoL in different populations can identify subgroups with poor physical or mental health and can help guide policies or interventions to improve their health. In selecting a HRQoL for monitoring outcomes of care in a population, the health care manager should ascertain that the biological and physiological variables measured relate to the disease whose outcomes of care are being assessed. HRQoL measures can be validated through a construct validation approach such as comparison against a previously validated quality of life measure or against self-reported healthy days (Mielenz et al., 2006; Moriarty et al., 2003).

Classification Systems: Health Care Services

Features of the health care services, their organization, technology, and personnel (see chapter "An Epidemiologic Framework for the Delivery of Health Care Services") impact health either directly (availability of mammography) or indirectly (e.g., provide the electronic health record infrastructure for quality improvement initiatives). Classifying health care services aids in facilitating the evaluation of their effectiveness in improving the health of populations.

Classifying Organizational Features

Various classification schemes of the entities which provide services have been developed to better isolate their effects on population health. The entities could be entire systems, organizations, or smaller units, such as intensive care units, or physician or other health care organizations (e.g., home care types). Bazzoli et al. (2006) present a taxonomy which considers important hospital organizational characteristics include: membership in a health system, type of health system membership (e.g., centralized, decentralized, independent, etc.), and health network type (e.g., centralized, decentralized, independent, etc.). Features of the organization have been identified to promote safety in hospitalized patient populations as well as quality. Organizational classifications also apply to physician arrangements such as a group practice model, independent physician association, or solo physician practice. Schmittdiel et al. (2006) found that medical groups were able to organize and coordinate chronic care management better than IPAs because of their structures, processes, and cultural features. The North American Industry Classification System (NAICS) is the current standard used by federal statistical agencies to classify business establishments for the purpose of collecting, analyzing, and publishing statistical data related to the US business economy. The NAICS replaces the Standard Industrial Classification (SIC) system. NAICS provides a three-digit numeric coding scheme for all industry sectors including establishments that provide health care and social assistance for individuals delivered. These are grouped into the industry sector category Health Care and Social Assistance (HCSA). The codes consider only those establishment delivering care by trained professionals and may be further defined by the educational credentials of individuals providing care in that subsector. The scheme codes according to the continuum of care. Examples of health services and their codes are ambulatory health care services, NAICS 621; hospitals, NAICS 622; and nursing and residential care facilities, NAICS 623. Over 12% of the employed workforce and 8% of all establishments are in the HCSA classified in this category. With increased precision of classifying health service units, a more precise assessment of the impact of various organizational risk factors (e.g., structure, staffing) can be made.

Classifying Procedures

Procedures are a common, special form of health services. A procedure involves a particular technique used (e.g., a vaginal birth), the use of technology (administration of intravenous chemotherapy) or medical materials (e.g., laboratory test). The procedure is performed for diagnostic or therapeutic reasons. Procedures are typically coded in one of three ways. The International Classification of Disease (ICD-9-CM) system is used to classify procedures done in in-patient settings until 2013 when ICD-10-PCS (Procedural Coding System) will be adopted. The ICD procedure code is assigned by a registered health information management personnel. The Current Procedural Terminology (CPT®) coding system developed by the American Medical Association consists of five-digit numeric values used to represent the broad category and specific types of services provided by or performed by a nonphysician under the direct supervision of a physician. The broad categories of visits are: office visits, hospital visits, and consultations (CPT® code numbers 99201–99499). Specific procedures are also coded using the five-digit scheme (e.g., CPT Code 36415 Routine Venipuncture). The CPT procedure codes may be accompanied by a two-digit end-modifier to represent the circumstances affecting the performance of the procedure ("-----.47 anesthesia by a surgeon"). The CPT system, similar to the ICD classification system, continues to evolve.

It is used in private and federal health care systems. The health care manager is advised to be aware of what versions are currently in use. At the time of this writing, CPT-4 is the current version. CPT codes are specifically assigned by a physician. CPT codes are the required code sets for outpatient care. The Healthcare Common Procedure Coding System (HCPCS codes) is comprised of two levels. Level I uses CPT codes as a foundation to classify "nontechnical" or procedures not necessarily physician-specific such as wound care. According to the Center for Medicare and Medicaid Services, which developed the system and maintains it, Level II alpha numeric coding system (A to V) that classifies equipments, products, and supplies that are medical in nature are not accounted for in the HCPCS level I, CPT codes. For example, any catheter supplied is coded within the HCPCS range A4300–A4355 (depending upon the specific type). Procedure codes are able to be abstracted from patient care records, usually from a discharge abstract summary. These procedure codes can provide the basis of the numerator for constructing utilization rates. They are obtained from the hospital discharge record or outpatient billing record. For a more extensive discussion concerning health care coding and classification systems, the reader should consult Giannangelo (2006).

Control of Measurement Error

Error is defined as the difference between the true phenomenon and what is actually measured. Measurement error, therefore, is not perfectly capturing what is intended. Inherent in every measure, be it medical records, responses to surveys, or a laboratory test, is the possibility of error. In medical records, a frequent error is the omission of documentation of negative findings (e.g., not documenting that the person was *not* a smoker). One strategy for the control of error, assuming the validity of the measure is acceptable, should be aimed at reducing variation in measurement. Variability of response can emanate from transitory person factors (e.g., technician or participant illness), measurement format (e.g., letters to small), coder/technician/interviewer effects (e.g., coder using general not specific codes, differences in response to interview due to gender of interviewer; technician unable to calibrate correctly), and variations in the measurement environment (e.g., noise, temperature). Regardless of the measurement selected, a plan should be in place for the control of measurement error. The aspects to consider for controlling measurement error are displayed in Table 8. Reisch et al. (2003) evaluated the effectiveness of some of these steps, masking the abstractors as to the case or control status of the records. This was achieved by focusing the quality assurance evaluation conducted through double-review of charts for the first knowledge of symptoms and history of mammograms within a 3-year window prior to diagnosis.

Once the measurement is validated and the error control plan developed, an operations manual should be prepared that contains the following information: (1) how the measurement was developed (validated, piloted), (2) procedures for

Table 8 Strategies for the control of measurement error

- Avoid ambiguous or complex wording of questions
- Order questions according to major concepts of categories of items (e.g., group questions concerning health habits)
- Ensure that choices to questions are mutually exclusive
- Determine the reliability and validity of the measure in the population to be studied
- Have a written protocol for measurement
- Determine the credentials and training required for staff obtaining the measurements
- Develop a standard procedure for training data collection staff which includes:
  - Standardized training examples
  - Individual orientation
- Conduct a pilot study to determine the feasibility of administering the measure, its acceptability, and administration time
- Ensure that interviewers/abstractors are thoroughly trained and provided instructions when questions or respondents are not clear regarding the questions
- Institute procedures to ensure the completeness and accuracy of recording measurements, coding of information, and data entry
- Monitor staff's adherence to the data collection protocol which includes:
  - Ensuring that a random selection process is followed
  - Double review of first 5–10 charts abstracted or repeat surveys or samples
  - Onsite visits by study data managers/lead investigators
  - Monthly double review of random sample of data collected for key variables
  - Monthly conference calls
- Use and outside referent (person or lab standard) to compare abstractor, interviewer, or technician's data
- Ensure that data are collected (or are available) from all eligible records, specimens, or persons by performing simultaneous data collection and cleaning
- Ensure the security of data collected (locked file cabinets, secured specimen containers, password protected electronic files)
- Perform reliability checks among those performing measurements
- Review data collected in raw form and as summary statistics on a regular basis

the administration of the measurements, (3) training and credentials of those administering the measure, (4) methods for collecting data to assess the quality of the information obtained from the measure, and (5) the statistical procedures used to evaluate the reliability and validity of the measure over repeated measurements or over time. The operations manual should be easily accessible to all involved in the data collection, data management, and data analysis preferably in web-based or other searchable format.

Sources of Data for Epidemiological Studies

Directly obtaining information from surveys, data abstraction, laboratory measures, clinical assessments, or anthropomorphic information from a study participant are examples of primary data collection. A relatively inexpensive and rapid alternative to collecting measurements for planning, assessing, or evaluating the efficacy of health services is to utilize existing or secondary data sources. The National Vital Statistics System is the oldest system of data collected according to uniforms standards and procedures. The registration of vital events, births, deaths, marriages, divorces, and fetal deaths is authorized by the legal authority of the state, city, or territory in which the individual resides. The National Center for Health Statistics (NCHS) is another major source of US population-based data. The NCHS data are collected through personal interviews or examinations or by using systems containing data collected from vital and medical records. Some NCHS data systems and surveys are ongoing annual systems while others are conducted periodically. Table 9 summarizes publically available secondary source of data of interest to health care managers and planners. State and local governmental also have useful dataset which provide useful health information applicable to smaller areas:

- Statewide tumor registry (e.g., California Cancer Registry http://www.ccrcal. org/)
- Congenital malformations and birth defects registry (e.g., http://www.dshs.state. tx.us/birthdefects/default.shtm)
- Medicare and Medicaid National Claims History Files (http://www.cms.gov)
- World Trade Center Health Registry (http://www.wtcregistry.org)
- Millenium Cohort Study (Department of Defense, Smith et al., 2007; http:// www.millenniumcohort.org/)

Also private organizations and firms may collect and analyze health-related information:

- Center for Health System Change (National surveys with some regional estimates of consumers, physicians, and employers perceptions of the financing and delivery of health services http://www.hschange.com/)
- NutritionQuest (Dietary and physical activity forms, nutrient databases, http:// www.nutritionquest.com/)
- Quality Metric (Population health monitoring forms and databases http://www. qualitymetric.com/)
- MarketScan® data warehouse (patient-level data including inpatient, outpatient, drug, lab, etc. from employer-sponsored insurance claims data, http://pharma. thomsonhealthcare.com)

Regardless if the data source is public or private, the health care manager should be aware of any potential measurement error. The disadvantage of some national, state, and even city data sets containing health information is that generalization to smaller geographic areas may not be valid because of their sampling design. Shah et al. (2006) illustrate how even community areas within a city can be significantly differentially affected by disease, behavioral risk factors, and access to health care. Additionally, duplicate reports, differences in reporting/measurement periods, reporting delays, variations in understandability by population subgroups, and mis-classification all affect the validity of conclusions that may be drawn.

Table 9 Selected data sources for epidemiological studies

Name/website	Data source/methods	Applications of data	Planned sample	Planned periodicity
Ambulatory health care data http://www.cdc.gov/nchs/about/major/ahcd/ahcd1.htm	• Encounter forms complete by physicians practicing in private offices • Physician-level personal interviews	• Characteristics of patients' visits 1. Diagnoses and treatments • Prescribing patterns • Characteristics of practice	• 3,000 physicians in office-based practices • 25,000 patient visits	Annual
Area Resource File of DHHS, Health Resources and Services Administration http://www.arfsys.com	Collection of data from 50 sources including American Medical Association American Hospital Association US Census Bureau Centers for Medicare & Medicaid Services Bureau of Labor Statistics National Center for Health Statistics	• Hospital expenditures • Monitoring health care safety net • Manpower planning • Assessment of shortage areas • Planning for demand of healthcare services	U.S. at county level and Territories Guam, Puerto Rico, and the Virgin Islands	Updated according to data source, last complete update 2007
Behavioral Risk Factor Surveillance Survey (BRFSS) http://www.cdc.gov/brfss	• Telephone surveys	• Health care access • Health care insurance • Nutrition • Physical activity • Quality of life • Use of screening tests • Tobacco, alcohol use	• Random monthly samples to obtain representative sample of state and other US possessions	Annual reports
Census of the US population http://www.census.gov	• Personal interviews	• Demographic trends of gender, age, race, marital status by geographic location as small as a block in urban areas	• Count of everyone living in the USA	Every 10 years, mandated by the US Constitution The next census is in 2010

(continued)

Table 9 (continued)

Name/website	Data source/methods	Applications of data	Planned sample	Planned periodicity
Longitudinal study of aging http://www.cdc.gov/nchs/lsoa.htm	• Telephone interviews • Administrative match data: National Death Index cause-of-death and CMS Medicare files	• Changes in functional status, chronic conditions, comorbidity • Living arrangements, social support • Health care coverage and utilization • Death rates by social, economic, family, and health characteristics	• 9,447 persons age 70 and over at the time of Phase 2 of NHIS-D (1994–1996)	Ongoing
Medicare Provider Analysis and Review (MEDPAR) File http://www.cms.hhs.gov/ IdentifiableDataFiles/05_ MedicareProviderAnalysis andReviewFile.asp	• Claims for services provided to beneficiaries admitted to Medicare certified in-patient hospitals and skilled nursing facilities (SNF) compiled as stays comprised of 1 or more stays in a facility	• Demographic • Diagnosis • Surgical procedures • Use of hospital or SNF resources • Charge data by category • Days of care • Entitlement data		Annual calendar year and fiscal year since 1991
Minimal Data Set (MDS) http://www.medicare.gov/ NHCompare/home.asp	• Data abstracted by nursing facility personnel • Staff assessment of residents	• Health status of residents of nursing facility (NF) • NF resident physical function, cognitive function, social engagement	• Residents of federally certified NF (1.7 million NF residents)	90–100 days
National Health and Nutrition Examination Survey (NHANES) http://www.cdc.gov/nchs/nhanes.htm	• Personal interviews • Physical examinations • Laboratory tests • Nutritional assessments • DNA repository	• Disease or condition prevalence • Nutrition monitoring • Heart disease • Diabetes • Nutritional disorders • Environmental exposures monitoring • Children's growth and development • Infectious disease monitoring • Overweight and physical fitness	• ~5,000 persons per year all ages • Oversample adolescents • Oversample 60+ • Oversample Blacks and Mexican Americans • Pregnant women	Annual with capability for longitudinal follow-up

Survey	Method	Content	Sample	Frequency
National Health Interview Survey (NHIS) http://www.cdc.gov/nchs/nhis.htm	• Personal interview	• Health status and limitations • Utilization of health care • Injuries • Family resources • Health insurance • Access to care • Selected conditions • Health behaviors • Functioning • HIV/AIDS testing • Immunization	• ~40,000 households • Oversample Blacks & Hispanics	Annual
National Hospital Discharge Survey (NHDS) http://www.cdc.gov/nchs/about/major/hdasd/nhdsdes.htm	• Hospital records • Computerized data sources	• Hospitalized patient characteristics • Hospital characteristics • Length of stay • Primary and multiple diagnoses • Surgical and diagnostic procedures	• 500 hospitals • 300,000 discharges	Annual
National Hospital Ambulatory Survey (NHAMCS) http://www.cdc.gov/nchs/about/major/ahcd/nhamcsds.htm	• Encounter forms completed by physicians and other hospital staff • Facility and personal interviews	• Characteristics of patients' visits to hospital outpatient departments and emergency departments • Diagnoses and treatments • Prescribing patterns • Characteristics of facility	• 600 hospitals • 70,000 patient visits	Annual
National Nursing Home Survey (NNHS) http://www.cdc.gov/nchs/mhs.htm	• Long-term care providers • Interviews with facility administrators and staff familiar with facility/medical records	• Characteristics of nursing homes • Number and characteristics of residents and discharges • Medical diagnoses and functional status	• 1,500 nursing homes • 9,000 current residents • 9,000 discharges	Conducted 2004, 1999, 1997, and 1995

(continued)

Table 9 (continued)

Name/website	Data source/methods	Applications of data	Planned sample	Planned periodicity
National Home and Hospice Care Survey (NHHCS) http://www.cdc.gov/nchs/nhhcs.htm	• Home health agencies and hospices • Interviews with administrators and staff familiar with agency/medical records	• Characteristics of home health agencies and hospices • Number and characteristics of patients and discharges • Medical diagnoses and functional status	• 1,800 home health agencies and hospices • 10,800 current patients • 10,800 discharged patients	2007, 2000, 1998, 1996, 1994, 1992
Online Survey and Certification Automated Record (OSCAR) http://www.medicare.gov/NHCompare/home.asp	• State survey and certification process for nursing facilities (NF), observation of residents	• Characteristics of NF and staffing	• All licensed NF's	9–15 month cycles
The Third National Health and Nutrition Examination Survey (NHANES III) Linked Mortality File http://www.cdc.gov/nchs/about/major/nhanes/nh3data.htm	• NHANES III participants age 17 and older linked with death records from the National Death Index (NDI)	• Health and nutritional status	National estimate of civilian noninstitutionalized population 5,630 matched records	NHANES III 1988–1994 Death records through 12/31/00
Vital Statistics Cooperative Program (VSCP) http://www.cdc.gov/nchs/nvss.htm	• State vital registration systems • Linked birth/infant death program	• Life expectancy • Causes of death • Infant mortality • Prenatal care and birth weight • Nonmarital birth • Birth rates • Pregnancy outcomes • Occupational mortality • Teen pregnancy • Method of delivery • Preterm delivery • Multiple births • Prenatal mortality • Maternal smoking	• All births • All deaths • Reported fetal deaths 20+ weeks gestation • Counts of marriages and divorces	Annual

Summary

Because of the complexity associated with the emergence of health problems, precision in measuring exposure to both risk factors and types of health services used as well as health status is essential for precision in the decision-making process. The more accurately the health care manager can quantify exposure and outcome, the less likely she is to make a false claim about a causal relationship between the two. The soundness of the measurements used always should be a consideration when interpreting the magnitude of the health problems confronted, the factors that contribute to their emergence, and the strategies employed. The next chapters illustrate how epidemiologic measures can be applied.

Discussion Questions

Q.1. For a variety of reasons including lack of resources and public health infrastructure, the collection of accurate information about health in developing nations may be problematic. What approaches would you take to measuring health in a developing nation?

Q.2. The use of publically available questionnaires or items from them provides not only access to free and validated survey forms, but also normative data for comparisons for the responses. Select one of the data sources listed in Table 9. Search for and obtain one of the survey forms or section of a survey form used to obtain the data. Describe how you would use the data from the survey form to assess the health of the community in which your local hospital resides. What are the limitations of this survey form in assessing the health of the community?

Q.3. The ICD coding is the most universally accepted system for coding diseases, injuries, procedures, and signs and symptoms of disease. How can the ICD system be used in ascertaining the health of a Medicare population? What alternatives exist for assessing the health of a Medicare population?

Q.4. The Medicare population is comprised of individuals with many health care needs, primarily because of their age. Cite barriers to obtaining measurements of health in this population and propose methods for ensuring the quality of data collected.

References

Bazzoli, G.J., Shortell, S.M., and Dubbs, N.L., 2006, Rejoinder to taxonomy of health networks and systems: a reassessment, *HSR: Health Serv. Res.* **41**:629–639.

Centers for Disease Control and Prevention (CDC), 2008, Behavioral Risk Factor Surveillance System Survey Questionnaire. US Dept. of Health and Human Services, Centers for Disease Control and Prevention, Atlanta, GA.

Chen, H., Cohen, P., and Kasen, S., 2007, Cohort differences in self-rated health: evidence from a three-decade, community-based, longitudinal study of women, *Am. J. Epidemiol.* **166**:439–446.

Cook, L.S., White, J.L., Stuart, G.C.E., and Magliocco, A.M., 2003, The reliability of telephone interviews compared with in-person interviews using memory aids, *Ann. Epidemiol.* **13**:495–501.

DeSalvo, K.B., Fan, V.S., McDonell, M.B., and Fihn, S.D., 2005, Predicting mortality and health-care utilization with a single question, *HSR: Health Serv. Res.* **40**:1234–1246.

Edwards, S.L., Slattery, M.L., Murtaugh, M.A., Edwards, R.L., Bryner, J., Pearson, M., Rogers, A., Edwards, A.M., and Tom-Orme, L., 2007, Development and use of touch-screen computer-assisted self-interviewing in a study of American Indians, *Am. J. Epidemiol.* **165**:1336–1342.

Finch, B.K., Hummer, R.A., Reindl, M., and Vega, W.Λ., 2002, Validity of self-rated health among Latino(a)s, *Am. J. Epidemiol.* **155**:755–759.

Fleiss, J.L., Jr., Levin, B., and Paik, M.C., 2003, *Statistical Methods for Rates and Proportions*, 3rd ed., Wiley, New York.

Galea, S., and Tracy, M., 2007, Participation rates in epidemiologic studies, *Ann. Epidemiol.* **17**:643–653.

Giannangelo, K., 2006, *Healthcare Code Sets, Clinical Terminologies, and Classification Systems*, American Health Information Management Association, Chicago, IL.

Greenland, S., 2000, An introduction to instrumental variables for epidemiologists, *Int. J. Epidemiol.* **29**:722–729.

Hoffmeister, M., Chang-Claude, J., and Brenner, H., 2007, Validity of self-reported endoscopies of the large bowel and implications for estimates of colorectal cancer risk, *Am. J. Epidemiol.* **166**:130–136.

Idler, E.L., Russell, L.B., and Davis, D., 2000, Survival, functional limitations, and self-rated health in the NHANES I Epidemiologic Follow-up Study, 1992, *Am. J. Epidemiol.* **152**:874–883.

Kennedy, B.S., Kasl, S.V., and Vaccarino, V., 2001, Repeated hospitalizations and self-rated health among the elderly: a multivariate failure time analysis, *Am. J. Epidemiol.* **153**:232–241.

Lee, S.J., Moody-Ayers, S.Y., Landefeld, C.S., Walter, L.C., Lindquist, K., Segal, M.R., and Covinsky, K.E., 2007, The relationship between self-rated health and mortality in older black and white Americans, *J. Am. Geriatr. Soc.* **55**:1624–1629.

Link, M.W., Battaglia, M.P., Frankel, M.R., Osborn, L., and Mokdad, A.H., 2006, Address-based versus random-digit-dial surveys: comparison of key health and risk indicators, *Am. J. Epidemiol.* **164**:1019–1025.

Mielenz, T., Jackson, E., Currey, S., DeVellis, R., and Callahan, L.F., 2006, Psychometric proper-ties of the Centers for Disease Control and Prevention Health-Related Quality of Life (CDC HRQOL) items in adults with arthritis, *Health and Quality of Life Outcomes* 2006, **4**:66, http://www.hqlo.com/content/4/1/66.

Morgan, R.O., Teal, C.R., Reddy, S.G., Ford, M.E., and Ashton, C.M., 2005, Measurement in Veterans Affairs health services research: veterans as a special population, HSR: Health Serv. Res. **40**:1573–1583.

Moriarty, D.G., Zack, M.M., and Kobau, R., 2003, The Centers for Disease Control and Prevention's Healthy Days Measures – Population tracking of perceived physical and mental health over time, *Health and Quality of Life Outcomes* **1**:37, http://www.hqlo.com/content/1/1/37.

Natarajan, L., Flatt, S.W., Sun, X., Gamst, A.C., Major, J.M., Rock, C.L., Al-Delaimy, W., Thomson, C.A., Newman, V.A., and Pierce, J.P. for the Women's Healthy Eating and Living Study Group, 2006, Validity and systematic error in measuring carotenoid consumption with dietary self-report instruments, *Am. J. Epidemiol.* **163**:770–778.

National Center for Health Statistics, 2007, *Health, United States, 2007, with Chartbook on Trends in the Health of Americans*, Hyattsville, MD.

Oleske, D.M., Kwasny, M.M., Lavender, S.A., and Andersson, G.B.J., 2006, Risk factors for recurrent episodes of work-related low back disorders in an industrial population, *Spine* **31**:789–798.

Oleske, D.M., Kwasny, M.M., Lavender, S.A., and Andersson, G.B.J., 2007, Participation in occu-pational health longitudinal studies: predictors of missed visits and dropouts, *Ann. Epidemiol.* **17**:9–18.

Paul-Dauphin, A., Guillemin, F., Virion, J., and Briancon, S., 1999, Bias and precision in visual analogue scales: a randomized controlled trial, *Am. J. Epidemiol.* **150**:1117–1127.

Reisch, L.M., Fosse, J.S., Beverly, K., Yu, O., Barlow, W.E., Harris, E.L., Rolnick, S., Barton, M.B., Geiger, A.M., Herrinton, L.J., Greener, S.M., Fletcher, S.W., and Elmore, J.G., 2003, Training, quality assurance, and assessment of medical record abstraction in a multisite study, *Am. J. Epidemiol.* **157**:564–551.

Rosner, B., 2006, *Fundamentals of Biostatistics*, 6th ed., Duxbury Press, Belmont, CA.

Schmittdiel, J.A., Shortell, S.M., Rundall, T.G., Bodenheimer, T., Selby, J.V., 2006, Effect of primary health care orientation on chronic care management, *Ann. Fam. Med.* **4**:117–123.

Sechrest, L., 2005, Validity of measures is no simple matter, *HSR: Health Services Res.*, **40**: 1584–1604.

Shah, A.M., Whitman, S., and Silva, A., 2006, Variations in the health conditions of 6 Chicago community areas: a case for local-level data, *Am. J. Pub. Health* **96**:1485–1491.

Smith, B., Smith, T.C., Gray, G.C., and Ryan, M.A.K. for the Millennium Cohort Study Team, 2007, When epidemiology meets the internet: web-based surveys in the Millenium Cohort Study, *Am. J. Epidemiol.* **166**:1345–1354.

Smith, T.C., Smith, B., Jacobson, I.G., Corbeil, T.E., and Ryan, M.A.K., for the Millennium Cohort Study Team, 2007, Reliability of standard health assessment instruments in a large, population-based cohort study, *Ann. Epidemiol.* **17**:525–532.

Snow, A.L., Cook, K.F., Lin, P, Morgan, R.O., and Magaziner, J., 2005, Proxies and other external raters: methodological considerations, *HSR: Health Serv. Res.* **40**:1676–1693.

U.S. Department of Health and Human Services (U.S.D.H.H.S), 2000, *Healthy People 2010*, U.S.D.H.H.S, Washington, DC.

Van Griensven, F., Naorat, S., Kilmarx, P.H., Jeeyapant, S., Manopaiboon, C., Chaikummao, S., Jenkins, R.A., Uthaivoravit, W., Wasinrapee, P., Mock, P.A., and Tappero, J.W., 2006, Palmtop-assisted self-interviewing for the collection of sensitive behavioral data: randomized trial with drug use urine testing, *Am. J. Epidemiol.* **163**:271–278.

Wholey, D.R., Christianson, J.R., Finch, M., Knutson, D., Rockwood, T., and Warrick, L., 2003, Evaluating health plan quality 1: a conceptual model, *Am. J. Managed Care* **9**:SP53–SP64.

World Health Organization (WHO), 2001, *International Classification of Functioning, Disability and Health (ICF)*, http://www.who.int/classifications/icf/en/.

Chapter 3
Descriptive Epidemiological Methods

Learning Outcomes

After completing this chapter, you will be able to:

1. Construct rate measures to identify population subgroups at high risk for a health problem. Provide the information in tabular and graphic forms.
2. Select a health problem and using the appropriate descriptive epidemiologic measures to characterize it in terms of person, place, and time.
3. Construct and interpret odds ratios and relative risks to identify potentially modifiable risk factors.
4. Determine which risk factors, identified from a set of data, could be targeted for a prevention intervention.

Keyterms Adjusted rate • Crude rate • Incidence rate • Life expectancy • Mortality rate • Odds ratio • Population attributable risk • Prevalence rate • Relative risk • Specific rate

Introduction

The previous chapter discussed principles for ensuring the accuracy of the information obtained through the measurement process. These principles apply to both raw (primary) data and that which is calculated from the raw data (secondary data). Proper management of the documentation of the data collected, prevention of errors through well-designed data collection protocols, staff training in data collection procedures, and complete and detailed operations manuals support the reliability of the information obtained and ultimately help to ensure the validity of the information analyzed. These measurement fundamentals provide the basis for constructing the descriptive epidemiologic measures described in this chapter to aid in accurately assessing population health, potential for adverse exposures, and determining priorities for action.

D.M. Oleske (ed.), *Epidemiology and the Delivery of Health Care Services: Methods and Applications*,
DOI 10.1007/978-1-4419-0164-4_3, © Springer Science+Business Media, LLC 2009

Descriptive epidemiological methods characterize health events, health problems, and exposures in terms of person, place, time, and variability. These measures help answer the questions relative to the events, problems, and exposures: "Who is affected?" "Where?" "When?" and "How does this change over time?" There are numerous applications of descriptive epidemiological measures. Descriptive epidemiology measures are used to: identify populations and population subgroups or areas at particular risk, prioritize health problems, establish a baseline of the level of exposure of health problem for evaluating trends, and evaluating effectiveness of programs and policies in terms of progress toward achieving health goals.

This chapter will focus on those descriptive epidemiological measures commonly used in characterizing the health of a population. Application of the measures will be illustrated.

Types of Rate Measurements

To quantify the magnitude of disease, injury, disability, other health event, or exposure it must be measured. In epidemiology, the measurement of events is expressed in terms of occurrence relative to a referent population instead of only raw numbers. Descriptive epidemiologic measures of the frequency of health events in population are called rates. Table 1 displays some of the common rate measures used in assessing the health of populations. The basics of computing rate measures follow.

Incidence and Mortality Rate

An *incidence rate* is the occurrence of new or incident cases of a health event diagnosed within a defined period of time occurring in a population at risk for the event. A *mortality (or death) rate* is another descriptive measure representing the number of deaths occurring within a specified time in a population at risk for the death event. Both the incidence rate and the mortality rate are descriptive measures of risk. The generalized format for the computation of these rate measures is:

$$\text{Incidence rate} \left(\text{or mortality rate}\right) \text{per } 10^k = E_{(t)} / P_{(t)} \times 10^k$$

where E = number of events (or deaths) occurring in the population at risk during a specified period of time (usually a year) (t); P = average population at risk (or mid-year July 1 population) in the same geographic area at the same time t in which the events (or deaths) occurred; $10^k = k$ factor of 10 to represent the occurrence of the event as a whole number relative to the population from which it was derived.

The *numerator* may refer to the onset of an illness or represent all new cases of a health event (morbidity) or a death (mortality) occurring in a population. To identify a new or incident case of an illness or condition, knowledge of the time of onset of

Table 1 Common rate measures

Age-specific death rate per 100,0000	$= \dfrac{\text{No. of deaths in age group during a specific time period}}{\text{Midyearresident population * in age group during same time period} \times 100,000}$
Birth rate per 1,000 population	$= \dfrac{\text{No. of live births in a population}}{\text{Midyear resident population *} \times 1,000}$
Case fatality rate per 100 persons	$= \dfrac{\text{No. of deaths from a disease in a year}}{\text{No. diagnosed with disease in year} \times 100}$
Death rate per 100,000 population	$= \dfrac{\text{No. of deaths in a population in a year}}{\text{Midyear resident population*} \times 100,000}$
Fertility rate per 1,000 women aged 15–44 years	$= \dfrac{\text{No. of live births regardless of age of mother}}{\text{No. of women } 15-44 \text{ years} \times 1,000}$
Fetal death rate per 1,000 live births plus fetal deaths	$= \dfrac{\text{No. of fetal deaths with stated or presumed gestation of} > 20 \text{ weeks}}{\text{Sum of live births plus fetal deaths} \times 1,000}$
Hospital occupancy rate as a percent	$= \dfrac{\text{Total annual no. patients/365 days}}{\text{No. hospital beds, cribs, and pediatric bassinets on last day of reporting period} \times 100\%}$
Infant mortality rate per 1,000 live births	$= \dfrac{\text{No. of infant} (< 1 \text{year old}) \text{ deaths during a calendar year}}{\text{No. of live births during same year} \times 1,000}$
Maternal mortality rate per 100,000 live births	$= \dfrac{\text{No. of maternal deaths}}{\text{No. of live births} \times 100,000}$
Neonatal mortality rate per 1,000 live births	$= \dfrac{\text{Death of children under 28 days of age}}{\text{live births during some year} \times 1,000}$
Nursing home occupancy rate as a percent	$= \dfrac{\text{No. of residents at the facility reported on the day of the interview}}{\text{No. of reported beds} \times 100\%}$
Perinatal mortality rate per 1,000 live births plus late fetal deaths	$= \dfrac{\text{No. of late fetal deaths plus infant deaths within 7 days of birth}}{\text{Sum of live births plus late fetal deaths} \times 1,000}$
Postneonatal mortality rate per 1,000 live births	$= \dfrac{\text{No. deaths of children under 28 days of age}}{\text{No. live births during same year} \times 1,000}$
Relative survival rate expressed as a percent	$= \dfrac{\text{Observed survival rate for a patient group}}{\substack{\text{Expected survival rate forpersons in the general population of same age,} \\ \text{race, sex, and calendar year of observation} \times 100\%}}$

*July 1 in noncensus years, April 1 in census years

the event is essential. This can only be achieved if the population in a geographic area is already being monitored for changes in health status or will be involved in such monitoring. The ability to identify and define an incident event varies depending upon the condition. Death events and the cause(s) of death are identified from a death certificate (Fig. 1). For acute onset conditions, such as gastroenteritis, acute myocardial infarction, or nonfatal trauma, the identification of a new case from a medical record or registry can be pinpointed. Even with good clinical definition of a case, an incident case may be difficult to identify through administrative or medical records. An alternate source of morbidity incident cases is through a registry. Registries to maintain incidence information, be if for diseases (e.g., tumor registry), trauma cases, or for other conditions (e.g., birth defects) are difficult and costly to maintain. The emerging possibility of biomarkers used to identify accurately new cases, such as troponin testing for the presence of myocardial damage, offers the ability to tract and predict disease trends which may impact health utilization and decrease mortality from heart disease (Sanfilippo et al., 2008). When the onset is not readily apparent, as is the case with chronic conditions, mental disorders, and behavioral problems, surrogate measures are used. For example, an incident (or new) case of cancer is defined by the date of histological confirmation. The incidence rate of addiction to an illegal drug, such as heroin, may be approximated from the date of first presentation to a treatment center, adjusting for a time lag in first use (Hickman et al., 2001). In some circumstances, multiple new events may occur within the same population in the time period of observation. This is exemplified in the calculation of nonfatal injury rates. The numerator may consist of either the number of persons who experienced an injury or the number of injuries occurring, depending upon the intent of the reporting. Reasons for not identifying an incident case or properly classifying a death event include: varying in the severity of a condition, lack of access to health care, lack of availability of diagnostic services, miscoding of the death event, new syndrome not previously recognized, or increased reporting of cause unknown/unspecified in the case of deaths (e.g., Sudden Infant Death Syndrome [SIDS]) (Shapiro-Mendoza et al., 2006). Regardless of the definition or ascertainment method for the event, the numerator must be derived from the same population comprising the denominator.

The *denominator* should not include those who already have the condition or who are not susceptible to it by virtue of immunity, immunization, surgery, or other factors that excludes the potential for being exposed. For example, in computing the incidence rate of prostate cancer neither females nor individuals who had their prostate removed should be included in the denominator. The choice of a denominator for a rate measure depends on the manner in which the time of observation for the events is considered. The denominator for constructing rate measures of events occurring in community populations is derived from the decennial census or from interim population projections based on census data. In this circumstance, the identification of persons who are truly at risk for the health event is not practical. The average population at risk, the population at mid-year (July 1) for noncensus years or April 1 for census years, is used for denominator in computing the rate. For rates calculated for smaller populations, such as an outbreak, corrections are

U.S. STANDARD CERTIFICATE OF DEATH

LOCAL FILE NO.   STATE FILE NO.

1. DECEDENT'S LEGAL NAME (Include AKA's if any) (First, Middle, Last)   2. SEX   3. SOCIAL SECURITY NUMBER

4a. AGE-Last Birthday (Years) | 4b. UNDER 1 YEAR (Months / Days) | 4c. UNDER 1 DAY (Hours / Minutes) | 5. DATE OF BIRTH (Mo/Day/Yr) | 6. BIRTHPLACE (City and State or Foreign Country)

7a. RESIDENCE-STATE   7b. COUNTY   7c. CITY OR TOWN

7d. STREET AND NUMBER   7e. APT. NO.   7f. ZIP CODE   7g. INSIDE CITY LIMITS? □ Yes □ No

8. EVER IN US ARMED FORCES? □ Yes □ No   9. MARITAL STATUS AT TIME OF DEATH □ Married □ Married, but separated □ Widowed □ Divorced □ Never Married □ Unknown   10. SURVIVING SPOUSE'S NAME (If wife, give name prior to first marriage)

11. FATHER'S NAME (First, Middle, Last)   12. MOTHER'S NAME PRIOR TO FIRST MARRIAGE (First, Middle, Last)

13a. INFORMANT'S NAME   13b. RELATIONSHIP TO DECEDENT   13c. MAILING ADDRESS (Street and Number, City, State, Zip Code)

14. PLACE OF DEATH (Check only one: see instructions)

IF DEATH OCCURRED IN A HOSPITAL: □ Inpatient □ Emergency Room/Outpatient □ Dead on Arrival   IF DEATH OCCURRED SOMEWHERE OTHER THAN A HOSPITAL: □ Hospice facility □ Nursing home/Long term care facility □ Decedent's home □ Other (Specify):

15. FACILITY NAME (If not institution, give street & number)   16. CITY OR TOWN, STATE, AND ZIP CODE   17. COUNTY OF DEATH

18. METHOD OF DISPOSITION: □ Burial □ Cremation □ Donation □ Entombment □ Removal from State □ Other (Specify):   19. PLACE OF DISPOSITION (Name of cemetery, crematory, other place)

20. LOCATION-CITY, TOWN, AND STATE   21. NAME AND COMPLETE ADDRESS OF FUNERAL FACILITY

22. SIGNATURE OF FUNERAL SERVICE LICENSEE OR OTHER AGENT   23. LICENSE NUMBER (Of Licensee)

ITEMS 24-28 MUST BE COMPLETED BY PERSON WHO PRONOUNCES OR CERTIFIES DEATH   24. DATE PRONOUNCED DEAD (Mo/Day/Yr)   25. TIME PRONOUNCED DEAD

26. SIGNATURE OF PERSON PRONOUNCING DEATH (Only when applicable)   27. LICENSE NUMBER   28. DATE SIGNED (Mo/Day/Yr)

29. ACTUAL OR PRESUMED DATE OF DEATH (Mo/Day/Yr) (Spell Month)   30. ACTUAL OR PRESUMED TIME OF DEATH   31. WAS MEDICAL EXAMINER OR CORONER CONTACTED? □ Yes □ No

CAUSE OF DEATH (See instructions and examples)   Approximate interval: Onset to death

32. PART I. Enter the chain of events—diseases, injuries, or complications—that directly caused the death. DO NOT enter terminal events such as cardiac arrest, respiratory arrest, or ventricular fibrillation without showing the etiology. DO NOT ABBREVIATE. Enter only one cause on a line. Add additional lines if necessary.

IMMEDIATE CAUSE (Final disease or condition resulting in death) → a. _____ Due to (or as a consequence of): _____

Sequentially list conditions, if any, leading to the cause listed on line a. Enter the UNDERLYING CAUSE (disease or injury that initiated the events resulting in death) LAST   b. _____ Due to (or as a consequence of): _____

c. _____ Due to (or as a consequence of): _____

d. _____

PART II. Enter other significant conditions contributing to death but not resulting in the underlying cause given in PART I   33. WAS AN AUTOPSY PERFORMED? □ Yes □ No   34. WERE AUTOPSY FINDINGS AVAILABLE TO COMPLETE THE CAUSE OF DEATH? □ Yes □ No

35. DID TOBACCO USE CONTRIBUTE TO DEATH? □ Yes □ Probably □ No □ Unknown   36. IF FEMALE: □ Not pregnant within past year □ Pregnant at time of death □ Not pregnant, but pregnant within 42 days of death □ Not pregnant, but pregnant 43 days to 1 year before death □ Unknown if pregnant within the past year   37. MANNER OF DEATH □ Natural □ Homicide □ Accident □ Pending Investigation □ Suicide □ Could not be determined

38. DATE OF INJURY (Mo/Day/Yr) (Spell Month)   39. TIME OF INJURY   40. PLACE OF INJURY (e.g., Decedent's home; construction site; restaurant; wooded area)   41. INJURY AT WORK? □ Yes □ No

42. LOCATION OF INJURY: State: City or Town:

Street & Number: Apartment No.:   Zip Code:

43. DESCRIBE HOW INJURY OCCURRED: 44. IF TRANSPORTATION INJURY, SPECIFY: □ Driver/Operator □ Passenger □ Pedestrian □ Other (Specify)

45. CERTIFIER (Check only one): □ Certifying physician-To the best of my knowledge, death occurred due to the cause(s) and manner stated. □ Pronouncing & Certifying physician-To the best of my knowledge, death occurred at the time, date, and place, and due to the cause(s) and manner stated. □ Medical Examiner/Coroner-On the basis of examination, and/or investigation, in my opinion, death occurred at the time, date, and place, and due to the cause(s) and manner stated.

Signature of certifier: _____

46. NAME, ADDRESS, AND ZIP CODE OF PERSON COMPLETING CAUSE OF DEATH (Item 32)

47. TITLE OF CERTIFIER   48. LICENSE NUMBER   49. DATE CERTIFIED (Mo/Day/Yr)   50. FOR REGISTRAR ONLY- DATE FILED (Mo/Day/Yr)

51. DECEDENT'S EDUCATION-Check the box that best describes the highest degree or level of school completed at the time of death. □ 8th grade or less □ 9th - 12th grade; no diploma □ High school graduate or GED completed □ Some college credit, but no degree □ Associate degree (e.g. AA, AS) □ Bachelor's degree (e.g. BA, AB, BS) □ Master's degree (e.g. MA, MS, MEng, MEd, MSW, MBA) □ Doctorate (e.g. PhD, EdD) or Professional degree (e.g. MD, DDS, DVM, LLB, JD)   52. DECEDENT OF HISPANIC ORIGIN? Check the box that best describes whether the decedent is Spanish/Hispanic/Latino. Check the "No" box if decedent is not Spanish/Hispanic/Latino. □ No, not Spanish/Hispanic/Latino □ Yes, Mexican, Mexican American, Chicano □ Yes, Puerto Rican □ Yes, Cuban □ Yes, other Spanish/Hispanic/Latino (Specify) _____   53. DECEDENT'S RACE (Check one or more races to indicate what the decedent considered himself or herself to be) □ White □ Black or African American □ American Indian or Alaska Native (Name of the enrolled or principal tribe) _____ □ Asian Indian □ Chinese □ Filipino □ Japanese □ Korean □ Vietnamese □ Other Asian (Specify) _____ □ Native Hawaiian □ Guamanian or Chamorro □ Samoan □ Other Pacific Islander (Specify) _____ □ Other (Specify) _____

54. DECEDENT'S USUAL OCCUPATION (Indicate type of work done during most of working life. DO NOT USE RETIRED).

55. KIND OF BUSINESS/INDUSTRY

NAME OF DECEDENT / To Be Completed/ Verified By: FUNERAL DIRECTOR   To Be Completed By: MEDICAL CERTIFIER   To Be Completed By: FUNERAL DIRECTOR

Fig. 1 (a) Sample death certificate

Examples of properly completed medical certifications

CAUSE OF DEATH (See instructions and examples)		Approximate interval: Onset to death
32. PART I. Enter the chain of events--diseases, injuries, or complications--that directly caused the death. DO NOT enter terminal events such as cardiac arrest, respiratory arrest, or ventricular fibrillation without showing the etiology. DO NOT ABBREVIATE. Enter only one cause on a line. Add additional lines if necessary.		
IMMEDIATE CAUSE (Final disease or condition ——→ resulting in death)	a. Rupture of myocardium Due to (or as a consequence of):	Minutes
Sequentially list conditions, if any, leading to the cause listed on line a. Enter the	b. Acute myocardial infarction Due to (or as a consequence of):	6 days
UNDERLYING CAUSE (disease or injury that initiated the events resulting in death) LAST	c. Coronary artery thrombosis Due to (or as a consequence of):	5 years
	d. Atherosclerotic coronary artery disease	7 years

PART II. Enter other significant conditions contributing to death but not resulting in the underlying cause given in PART I		33. WAS AN AUTOPSY PERFORMED? ■ Yes □ No
Diabetes, Chronic obstructive pulmonary disease, smoking		34. WERE AUTOPSY FINDINGS AVAILABLE TO COMPLETE THE CAUSE OF DEATH? ■ Yes □ No

35. DID TOBACCO USE CONTRIBUTE TO DEATH?	36. IF FEMALE:	37. MANNER OF DEATH
■ Yes □ Probably □ No □ Unknown	■ Not pregnant within past year □ Pregnant at time of death □ Not pregnant, but pregnant within 42 days of death □ Not pregnant, but pregnant 43 days to 1 year before death □ Unknown if pregnant within the past year	■ Natural □ Homicide □ Accident □ Pending investigation □ Suicide □ Could not be determined

CAUSE OF DEATH (See instructions and examples)		Approximate interval: Onset to death
32. PART I. Enter the chain of events--diseases, injuries, or complications--that directly caused the death. DO NOT enter terminal events such as cardiac arrest, respiratory arrest, or ventricular fibrillation without showing the etiology. DO NOT ABBREVIATE. Enter only one cause on a line. Add additional lines if necessary.		
IMMEDIATE CAUSE (Final disease or condition ——→ resulting in death)	a. Aspiration pneumonia Due to (or as a consequence of):	2 Days
Sequentially list conditions, if any, leading to the cause listed on line a. Enter the	b. Complications of coma Due to (or as a consequence of):	7 weeks
UNDERLYING CAUSE (disease or injury that initiated the events resulting in death) LAST	c. Blunt force injuries Due to (or as a consequence of):	7 weeks
	d. Motor vehicle accident	7 weeks

PART II. Enter other significant conditions contributing to death but not resulting in the underlying cause given in PART I		33. WAS AN AUTOPSY PERFORMED? ■ Yes □ No
		34. WERE AUTOPSY FINDINGS AVAILABLE TO COMPLETE THE CAUSE OF DEATH? ■ Yes □ No

35. DID TOBACCO USE CONTRIBUTE TO DEATH?	36. IF FEMALE:	37. MANNER OF DEATH
□ Yes □ Probably ■ No □ Unknown	□ Not pregnant within past year □ Pregnant at time of death □ Not pregnant, but pregnant within 42 days of death □ Not pregnant, but pregnant 43 days to 1 year before death □ Unknown if pregnant within the past year	□ Natural □ Homicide ■ Accident □ Pending investigation □ Suicide □ Could not be determined

38. DATE OF INJURY (Mo/Day/Yr) (Spell Month) August 15, 2003	39. TIME OF INJURY Approx. 2320	40. PLACE OF INJURY (e.g., Decedent's home, construction site, restaurant, wooded area) road side near state highway	41. INJURY AT WORK? □ Yes ■ No

42. LOCATION OF INJURY: State: Missouri		City or Town: near Alexandria	
Street & Number: mile marker 17 on state route 46a	Apartment No.:		Zip Code:

43. DESCRIBE HOW INJURY OCCURRED: Decedent driver of van, ran off road into tree	44. IF TRANSPORTATION INJURY, SPECIFY: ■ Driver/Operator □ Passenger □ Pedestrian □ Other (Specify)

Fig. 1 (**b**) Sample properly completed cause of death section on death certificate (From Heron et al., 2008)

made to the denominator. The denominator may also be formed in consideration of how long the population at risk was observed. This denominator is expressed in terms of person time-units and an example is computed below:

Given a group of four persons observed for the following duration:

- Person A is observed for 5 days
- Person B is observed for 1 day
- Person C is observed for 1 week
- Person D is observed for 1 month (assumes the average month is 30.5 days)
- Denominator = 43.5 person-days

The *factor of* (10^k) used in the computation of a rate enables the relationship between the smaller number of events relative to a larger denominator to be more meaningful by converting the dividend to a whole number with one or two decimals to the right. The factor of 10 selected depends upon convention and the size of the population from which the events were derived. A factor of 100,000 is used for computing rates for community populations. Generally, a power of 10 is selected such that the lowest level of the variable for which the rate is calculated is one digit to the right of the decimal.

The events for the numerator must come from the same *time period* in which the denominator was observed. Incidence rates can be computed for short time periods – hours, days, or weeks, as for epidemics of infectious disease – or over longer periods. The time period is by convention 1 year for common community-based events. If the number of events in a given year is low (<10), events and the denominator are averaged over a period of time, usually 3–5 years.

Data from Barker et al. (2006) illustrate the calculation of incidence rates for two population subgroups using a person-years denominator:

Incidence rate of heart failure (HF) per 1,000 person years (PY) of observstion for 1990–1994 by age group 70–74 years =

$$\frac{56 \text{ HF cases}_{70-74y.o.}}{6,641 \text{ person-years}_{70-74y.o.}} \times 1,000 = 8.4 \text{ HF cases per } 1,000 \text{ PY}$$

Incidence rate of HF per 1,000 PY for age group 75–79 years =

$$\frac{48 \text{ HF cases}_{75-79 \text{ y.o.}}}{4,093 \text{ person-years}_{75-79y.o.}} \times 1,000 = 11.7 \text{ HF cases per } 1,000 \text{ PY}$$

The same factor of 10 must be used when calculating rates for all levels within a variable.

The use of the decimal in the representation of the rate value must also be consistent throughout the levels of the variables for which the rates are calculated.

Prevalence Rate

Prevalence rate is the total number of living persons (new or incident cases and preexisting cases) identified within a defined time period with the health condition divided by the average number of persons in the population or mid-year population in the same time period in which the total number of cases were selected. The prevalence rate, when referring to a disease in a specific period of time, is a measure of morbidity or disease burden in a population. The number of individuals with the health condition or factor examined who constitute the numerator also must be derived from the denominator and both should come from the same geographic area and in the same time period. Mathematically, this is represented as:

$$\text{Prevalence rate per } 10^k = \frac{\text{Total number of cases}_{(t)}}{\text{Total population at mid-year}_{(t)}} \times 10^k$$

The referent time (*t*) can be short, one-point in time (point prevalence), or over time (period prevalence). The prevalence rate is influenced by how many individuals develop the condition in a particular time frame (incidence rate), how long the condition lasts (duration), and/or how long individuals with the condition survive. Factors that influence the development of an incident case (e.g., changes in exposures that result in disease, changes in the way individuals access health care, or changes in diagnostic methods) also affect the prevalence. The validity of the prevalence rate is also a function of the size of the population studied, the precision in establishing the boundaries (neighborhood, community, geopolitical area) of the population at risk (e.g., by verifying address where a person usually sleep at night in the case of the prevalence of IV drug users, residency in a school district in the case of autistic children), the thoroughness of efforts to ascertain all living cases of the conditions (e.g., clinics, schools, self-reports, field case-finding, etc.), and the standardization of the procedures or accuracy of testing to classify the case. A prevalence rate of exposure can also be computed. In this context, the number of persons in a population exposed to a particular risk factor in a given time period is the numerator and the criteria for the selection of the denominator follow as above. The factor of 10 in computing this prevalence rate is commonly 100 or 100%. Figure 2 displays trended prevalence rates expressed as per 100 persons for selected health conditions and risk factors. Prevalence rates are useful in guiding planning, program evaluation, and for resource allocation because they represent the number of cases (or "burden of disease") relative to the number of persons with a particular condition in a geographic area. Figure 2 shows that the most dominant risk factor, and one that is rapidly increasing, among the vast majority of the US population is "overweight." The high prevalence of obesity in Black females and Native American boys in Fig. 3 illustrates the urgent need for intervention also in these younger population subgroups. A decreasing prevalence of a disease may reflect either a decrease in exposure to a factor is decreasing or that control measures are increasing in effectiveness. Data from the National Health and Nutrition Examination

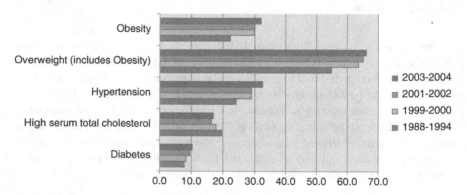

Fig. 2 Prevalence rate per 100 persons, selected conditions and risk factors, persons aged 20+ years, civilian noninstitutionalized population, United States, 1988–2004 (National Center for Health Statistics, 2007)

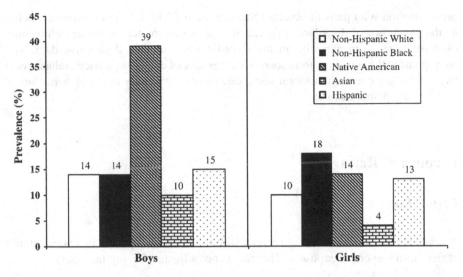

Fig. 3 Prevalence of obesity (body mass index ≥ 30 kg/m^2) among US adolescents, by ethnicity, National Longitudinal Survey of Adolescent Health, 1994–1996 data,Wang, Y., et al. The obesity epidemic in the United States—gender, age, socioeconomic, racial/ethnic, and geographic characteristics: a systematic review and meta-regression analysis, *Epidemiol. Rev.* 2007;29:6–28, by permission of Oxford University Press

Survey 1999–2004 revealed that despite an increase in the prevalence of diabetes, the prevalence of the population glycemic (HbA$_{1c}$ <7.0%) and blood pressure (<130/80 mm Hg) control in the diabetic population has also increased (Ong et al., 2008). This illustrates how the prevalence rate of disease or exposure establishes a baseline level to better understand if greater awareness of a condition, availability of or access to health care services (e.g., introduction of insurance coverage for mammography), or changes in the criteria for diagnosing the condition influence the emergence of trends observed.

Prevalence rates may be difficult to compute directly, particularly for health conditions that may not come to diagnostic attention because of lack of culturally appropriate initiatives for prevention services and opportunities for testing, lack of access to treatment, or because local surveillance programs have not fully implemented confidential reporting. Because prevalence is in part determined by the incidence rate of the disease, any limitation associated with the accuracy of defining a case also affects the accuracy of the prevalence rate. For example, estimates of human immunodeficiency virus (HIV) infection prevalence may be underestimated as cases may be initially asymptomatic and are more likely to occur among those who do not routinely seek medical care (Campsmith et al., 2008).

Prevalence rates may also be difficult to determine for emerging conditions for which specific diagnostic tests do not exist. Such is the case with autism which can include a spectrum of disorders including deficits in communication and socialization, developmental disabilities, and unusual behaviors such as rituals or preoccupation with parts of objects (Nicholas et al., 2008). In circumstances such as the psychosocial disorders, a prevalent case is determined by trained clinician diagnosticians, with expertise in the disorder under review descriptive data, as appropriate to the condition, from sources such as special education service evaluations, psychometric or neurobehavioral tests, description or observations of behaviors, and developmental histories.

Formats of Rates

Crude Rate

A *crude rate* is the total count of persons with the event or exposure in a population at risk for the event or exposure. This rate is not adjusted for any factors.

Specific Rate

A *specific rate* refers to a count of persons with an event in a segment of a population in relation to the total number of persons in that same segment of the population. The specific rate is commonly restricted to subgroups of the population by age, race, sex, or causes of death. Commonly health problems have unique patterns of specific rates, at the very least, by age. Figure 2 displays age-specific mortality. For HIV, the rates increase during middle age and then declines (Fig. 4a); for malignant neoplasms, the rates exhibit a steep increase with age (Fig. 4b); for diseases of the heart, the rates exhibit a J-shaped curved (Fig. 4c); for motor vehicle accidents, the rates demonstrate bimodality with peaks in the 18–24-year age groups and then increasing over age 75 years (Fig. 4d).

Summary Rate Measures

An *adjusted rate* is a summary descriptive epidemiologic measure which takes into account the variables that may emphasize or diminish the detection of the frequency of the health problem in a population examined. Adjusted rates are used to compare rates across time periods, geographic areas, or organizational units where differences in population characteristics are expected. The variables used in the adjustment are most commonly age, gender, and race. As illustrated in Fig. 2, age has a pronounced influence on the emergence and variation of health problems whether they are acute or chronic conditions or injuries. Age would, thus, be an important factor to account

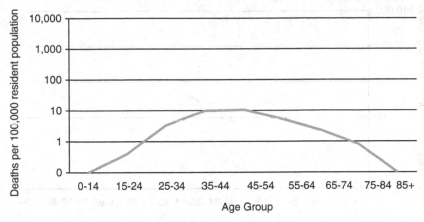

Death Rates for Human Immunodeficiency Virus (HIV), All Races, Both Genders, United States, 2005

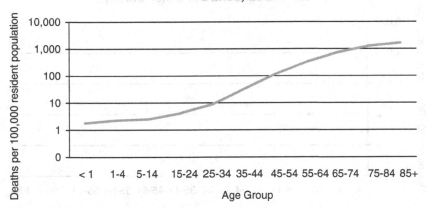

Death Rates for Malignant Neoplasms, All Races, Both Genders, United States, 2005

Fig. 4 (a) Age-specific mortality rates for human immunodeficiency virus (HIV) infection, all races, both genders, United States, 2005. (b) Age-specific mortality rates for malignant neoplasms, all races, both genders, United States, 2005

for when comparing annual injury rates between cities or states. Such comparisons can only be made when rates are adjusted for an important confounding factor. Adjustment to rates can be accomplished through arithmetic weighting procedures or statistical procedures.

The most common method for adjusting rates is the *direct standardization method*. The direct standardization method weights specific rates within strata (or groups) by the variable targeted to control for confounding, usually age. The weights are derived from the proportions of persons from a standard population or a standard

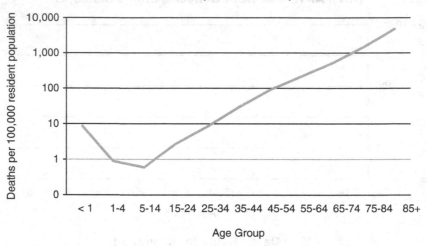

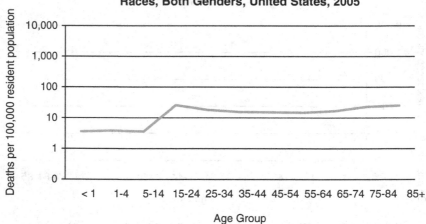

Fig. 4 (**c**) Age-specific mortality rates for diseases of the heart, all races, both genders, United States, 2006. (**d**) Age-specific mortality rates for motor vehicle accidents, all races, both genders, United States, 2006 (National Center for Health Statistics, 2008)

million population in the corresponding stratum (or group) (*i*). Any standard population can be used for the weighting, US population (1970, 1990, 2000), a 1991 Canadian population, a European population, or a world population depending upon the comparison intended. The US 2000 population is currently commonly in use for national comparisons over time or across geographic area. The formula for computing a one-factor adjusted rate using the direct method is as follows:

$$\text{Adjusted rate} = \sum_{i=x}^{y} \left[\left(\frac{event\ counts\ (i)}{population\,(i)} \right) \times 100{,}000 \times \left(\frac{standard\ population\ (i)}{\sum_{j=x}^{y} standard\ population\,(j)} \right) \right]$$

where i represents the level (or interval) of the variable targeted for adjustment. This formula is applied to the data Table 2. The stratum (age group)-specific rates of breast cancer mortality per 100,000 in the two race groups are given in this example. The breast cancer mortality rates in each age group (i) are then respectively weighted (i.e., multiplied) by the proportion of individuals in that age group by the US population in each age-group. The sums of these products (viz., columns "weighted rate...") are summed for each race group yielding the final summary or adjusted (age-adjusted in this example) rate.

The standardized adjusted rate computed in Table 2 is interpreted to mean that the mortality from breast cancer is higher among Black women than White women, even adjusting for differences in the distribution of age between the two groups. If adjustment for more than one factor is desired, the reader should consult the methods in Fleiss et al. (2003). An adjusted rate is a summary rate and plotted as an individual data point may not allow easy visualization of trends.

The leading causes of death in the U.S. are displayed in Table 3. The crude death rate is used to rank order the causes of death as a means of prioritizing target areas for research, intervention, or policy formulation (see chapter "Epidemiology and the Public Policy Process"). The age-adjusted rates are used to calculate the percentage change for a particular cause over time.

In addition to this arithmetic method of adjusting rates, there are *statistical methods for adjusting rates* for comparing them across geographic areas and times including ordinary least squares regression and Poisson regression models. Ordinary least squares and Poisson regression models are used in small area analysis; it is important to adjust for a wide variety of variables including age, sex, race, primary chronic condition, and multiple chronic conditions which could influence the utilization of health care (Wennberg et al., 2008). Joinpoint regression (National Cancer Institute, 2008) model is used to fit a series of joined straight lines on a log scale to estimate trends in adjusted rates to examine temporal trends. The resultant values from the regression are represented as annual percentage changes which equal to $100 \times (e^b - 1)$, where b is the slope of the regression line and the significance is evaluated using the appropriate statistical test, two-tailed.

Years of potential life lost (YPLL) is a summary measure of premature mortality. To compute the YPLL, the number of deaths for each age group, with eight groups (under 1 year, 1–14, 15–24, 25–34, 45–54, 55–64, 65–74 years) being the convention, is tallied. The midpoint for each group is determined (e.g., 0.5, 7.5, 19.5, 29.5, 39.5, 49.5, 59.5, 69.5) and subtracted from the age that they would have expected to live, which then represents the number of years of life lost (YLL). The average life expectancy in the USA is 75 years and the mid-point for each age group is subtracted from 75 years. For example, if a death from homicide occurred in the 15–24 years age group, 55.5 years of life would be considered lost (75 years − 19.5 (midpoint

Table 2 Calculation of age-adjusted mortality rate for breast cancer using the direct method

Age group (years)	White (W) female breast cancer mortality rate per 100,000[a] rW	Black (B) female breast cancer mortality rate per 100,000[a] rB	2000 US standard population by age group[b] n	Proportion of 2000 US standard population by age group p	Weighted rate white females p × rW	Weighted rate black females p × rB
Under 5 years	0	0	18,986,520	0.069134	0	0
5–9 years	0	0	19,919,840	0.072532	0	0
10–14 years	0	0	20,056,779	0.073031	0	0
15–19 years	0	0	19,819,518	0.072167	0	0
20–24 years	0.1	0.1	18,257,225	0.066478	0.006648	0.006648
25–29 years	0.6	1.8	17,722,067	0.06453	0.038718	0.116154
30–34 years	2.7	6.2	19,511,370	0.071045	0.191822	0.440479
35–39 years	6.9	15.1	22,179,956	0.080762	0.557258	1.219506
40–44 years	12.9	25.6	22,479,229	0.081852	1.055891	2.095411
45–49 years	20.9	39.5	19,805,793	0.072117	1.507245	2.848622
50–54 years	33.7	58.1	17,224,359	0.062718	2.113597	3.643916
55–59 years	48.9	72.4	13,307,234	0.048454	2.369401	3.508070
60–64 years	61.1	85.8	10,654,272	0.038794	2.370313	3.328525
65–69 years	75.9	88.1	9,409,940	0.034264	2.600638	3.018658
70–74 years	89.1	103.6	8,725,574	0.031772	2.830885	3.291579
75–79 years	110.8	121.4	7,414,559	0.026998	2.991378	3.277557
80–84 years	133.8	135.6	4,900,234	0.017843	2.387393	2.419511
85+ years	179.2	196.5	4,259,173	0.015509	2.779213	3.047519
Totals			274,633,642	1.000000	23.8004	32.26215

Age-adjusted breast cancer mortality rate per 100,000 population =

$$\sum(p \times r_i) \times 100,000 =$$

= 23.8 breast cancer deaths among White females per 100,000 population

= 32.3 breast cancer deaths among Black females per 100,000 population

[a]Source: Surveillance, Epidemiology, and End Results Program of the National Cancer Institute (2004)

[b]Source: U.S. Bureau of the Census, Census of Population (2000)

Table 3 Deaths and death rates for 2006 and age-adjusted death rates and percentage changes in age-adjusted rates from 2005 to 2006 for the 15 leading causes of death: United States, final 2005 and preliminary 2006 (Heron et al., 2008)

Rank[a]	Cause of death	ICD Code on the International Classification of Diseases, Tenth Revision, Second Edition, 2004	Number	Crude death rate	Age-adjusted death rate 2006	Age-adjusted death rate 2005	Percent change
…	All causes		2,425,901	810.3	776.4	798.8	−2.8
1	Diseases of heart…	(I00–I09,I11,I13,I20–I51)	629,191	210.2	199.4	211.1	−5.5
2	Malignant neoplasms…	(C00–C97)	560,102	187.1	180.8	183.8	−1.6
3	Cerebrovascular diseases…	(I60–I69)	137,265	45.8	43.6	46.6	−6.4
4	Chronic lower respiratory disease	(J40–J47)	124,614	41.6	40.4	43.2	−6.5
5	Accidents (unintentional injuries)	(V07–X59,Y85–Y86)2	117,748	39.3	38.5	39.1	−1.5
6	Alzheimer's disease…	(G30)	72,914	24.4	22.7	22.9	−0.9
7	Diabetes mellitus…	(E10–E14)	72,507	24.2	23.3	24.6	−5.3
8	Influenza and pneumonia…	(J10–J18)	56,247	18.8	17.7	20.3	−12.8
9	Nephritis, nephrotic syndrome and nephrosis…	(N00–N07,N17–N19,N25–N27)	44,791	15	14.3	14.3	0.0
10	Septicemia…	(A40–A41)	34,031	11.4	10.9	11.2	−2.7
11	Intentional self-harm (suicide)	(U03,X60–X84,Y87.0)	32,185	10.7	10.6	10.9	−2.8
12	Chronic liver disease and cirrhosis	(K70,K73–K74)	27,299	9.1	8.7	9	−3.3
13	Essential hypertension and hypertensive renal disease	(I10,I12,I15)[b]	23,985	8	7.6	8	−5
14	Parkinson's disease…	(G20–G21)	19,660	6.6	6.3	6.4	−1.6
15	Assault (homicide)…	(cU01–U02,X85–Y09,Y87.1)	18,029	6	6	6.1	−1.6
…	All other causes…	(Residual codes)	455,333	152.1	…	…	…

[a]Rank based on number of deaths

[b]Cause-of-death title has been changed in 2006 to reflect the addition of Secondary Hypertension (ICD-10 code I15)

[c]Beginning 2001 includes acts of terrorism

value) years = 55.5 YLL). The number of deaths in an age group is then multiplied by the number of YLL in that age group. The summary YPLL is then derived by summing the products of the YLL multiplied by the number of deaths in each age group over all the age groups. The YPLL can be calculated for all causes of death combined or for specific causes of death. The YPLL may be represented as a rate per 100,000 population under 75 years. The YPLL is a useful summary measure when examining or prioritizing health problems in communities that disproportionately affect younger persons or for assessing the impact of community-based interventions in geographic areas with a large minority or immigrant population which are typically younger than the population of the community as a whole. Table 4 displays the age-adjusted YPLL of major causes of death in the USA for 2000 and 2005. Note that mortality from unintentional injuries is ranked higher as a health concern using the YPLL method than its ranking computed using direct standardization. Additionally, the direction of the trends is different with the direct standardization method showing that unintentional injuries are declining whereas the YPLL method identifies an increasing trend in these categories of deaths. The YPLL rankings in Table 3 indicate that additional policies and/or public and community interventions are warranted aimed at violence prevention and injury control, particularly in the types of

Table 4 Percentage change in age-adjusted[a] years of potential life lost before age 75 (YPLL-75) for selected causes of death, all persons, US, 2000 and 2005 (Heron et al., 2008)

Cause of death	YPLL(75) per 100,000 population under 75 years of age		Percentage change 2000–2005
	2000	2005	
All causes	7,578.1	7,299.8	−3.67
Diseases of heart	1,253.0	1,110.4	−11.38
Ischemic heart disease	841.8	701.8	−16.63
Cerebrovascular diseases	223.3	193.3	−13.43
Malignant neoplasms	1,674.1	1,525.2	−8.89
Trachea, bronchus, and lung	443.1	392.9	−11.33
Colorectal	141.9	124.7	−12.12
Prostate	63.6	55.1	−13.36
Breast	332.6	296.2	−10.94
Chronic lower respiratory diseases	188.1	181.2	−3.67
Influenza and pneumonia	87.1	83.6	−4.02
Chronic liver disease and cirrhosis	164.1	152.6	−7.01
Diabetes mellitus	178.4	179.9	−0.84
Human immunodeficiency virus (HIV) disease	174.6	133.6	−23.48
Unintentional injuries	1,026.5	1,132.7	10.35
Motor vehicle-related injuries	574.3	564.4	−1.72
Suicide	334.5	347.3	3.83
Homicide	266.5	276.8	3.86

[a]Age-adjusted to the year 2000 standard population

communities previously described. The concept of premature mortality or YLL can be extended to include years lost due to a state less than full health (termed "disability") (YLD). The YLL and YLD when summed equal a Disability Adjusted Life Year (DALY). The DALY is a composite summary measure which is the sum of the years of life lost due to premature mortality (YLL) and the years lost due to disability for incident cases of a health condition. One DALY represents the loss of 1 year of full health. The DALY then is used to represent a "burden of disease" in a population which is a particularly good measure for health conditions which have multidimensional impairments (e.g., limitations of physical functioning, social functioning impairments, etc.) associated with them, such as mental illness (Ustun, 1999).

Life expectancy is the average number of years remaining to a person at a particular age who was born at a particular time. The remaining years of life are based upon the age-specific death rates in effect at the time the measure was constructed. The death rates are applied to survivors in each age or age group to obtain a probability of dying with the resultant tabulations presented as a life table from which the life expectancy measure is calculated. Thus, life expectancy is a measure of the mortality pattern across all age groups, infants, children, adults, and the elderly. The primary drivers of the summary life expectancy values are the magnitude of rates occurring early in life. Populations with high infant mortality and/or high mortality during adolescent or young adult years will have markedly lower life expectancies. Life expectancy is a proxy summary measure of overall mortality level in a population or a population subgroup as well as is a proxy measure of the quality of life of a nation. Table 4 displays the life expectancies for various member countries of the World Health Organization according to country income level.

Ratio Measures

The *risk ratio* compares two rate measures of risk (e.g., incidence or mortality rates). Generally, the group with the higher risk (rate) for the health problem evaluated or the group in which exposure to the risk factor is greatest is placed in the numerator. The rate of the lower-risk group or the group with less or no exposure is in the denominator. The rate in the numerator and the rate in the denominator typically will be an adjusted rate so that the effect of the major confounding variable is eliminated and the two populations can be appropriately compared. The male–female risk ratio for mortality due to HIV infection is computed using the age-adjusted death rates from Table 5:

$$\text{Risk ratio} = \frac{\text{rate in the higher risk group or exposed group}}{\text{rate in the lower risk or non-exposed group}}$$

$$= \frac{19.4 \text{ age-adjusted HIV death rate per } 100,000 \text{ among blacks}}{2.2 \text{ age-adjusted HIV death rate per } 100,000 \text{ among whites}}$$

$$= 8.82$$

Table 5 Life expectancy and selected morbidity measures and risk factors for World Health Organization (WHO) member nations by region and income group (WHO, 2008)

WHO group	Life expectancy[a] at birth (years) both sexes	Prevalence of tuberculosis[a] (per 100,000 population)	Prevalence of HIV among adults aged ≥15 years (per 100,000 population)[b]	Infant mortality rate per 1000 live births, both sexes[c]	Low birth weight newborns (%)[d]	Access to improved sanitation (%)[e]
Region						
African region	51	547	4,459	84	14	33
Region of the Americas	75	44	442	18	9	87
South-East Asia Region	64	289	289	52	26	37
European Region	74	54	342	14	8	92
Eastern Mediterranean Region	64	152	192	62	17	60
Western Pacific Region	74	199	89	20	8	63
Income group						
Low income	59	362	1,039	73	22	78
Lower middle income	71	188	239	27	9	88
Upper middle income	69	121	1,484	22	10	95
High income	80	17	249	6	7	100
Global	67	219	662	49	16	60

[a] 2006
[b] 2005
[c] 2007
[d] 2000–2002
[e] 2006
See World Health Organization (2008) for list of countries within region and income groupings

The computed risk ratio means that blacks are 8.82 times more likely to die from HIV infection than whites. Since this ratio compares two age-adjusted rates, the risk ratio is not due to differences in the age distribution between blacks and white. A risk ratio of twofold or greater for a health problem between the two groups compared indicates disparity of particular concern. Rank-ordered, a twofold greater risk of death is noted as follows: in blacks relative to whites for HIV (8.82), homicide (5.70), and diabetes (2.08); and for males relative to females for suicide (4.09), homicide (3.84), HIV (2.70), motor vehicle accidents (2.44), and chronic liver disease (2.14) (Table 6).

The *relative risk (RR)* is computed from a cross-tabulated format. In Table 8 the members of the sample studied are cross classified into exposure-outcome cells whereby the rows represent exposure levels, usually a nominal level of measurement, exposed vs. not exposed, and columns represent the outcome, usually also a nominal level of measurement, outcome present vs. absent.

The true measures of risk are typically only derived from studies with a longitudinal component or where the population at risk is known. The RR can be estimated from an *odds ratio (OR)*. When estimating the RR, the OR is calculated as the ratio of the odds of an event occurring given exposure to the odds of an event when exposure is absent. The RR and the OR computed from the same sample are approximately equal when the prevalence of the event is low. Note that in Table 9 the computed RR and the OR are in the same positive direction and are approximately equal.

The RR and the OR are both descriptive ratio measures used to appraise the strength of an association between exposure and an event. As ratio measures, the valid values of the RR and the OR range from 0 to $+\infty$. An RR or an OR of 1 means that the chances of the event (or exposure) are the same between the two groups compared, the exposed and the nonexposed.

Table 6 Age-adjusted death rates per 100,000 population for selected causes of death, by gender and race, United States, 2005 (Heron et al., 2008)

Cause of death	Age-adjusted death rate per 100,000 population			
	Males	Females	Blacks	Whites
All causes	951.1	677.6	1,016.5	785.3
Diseases of heart	260.9	172.3	271.3	207.8
Malignant neoplasms	225.1	155.6	222.7	182.6
Cerebrovascular disease	46.9	45.6	65.2	44.7
Chronic lower respiratory disease	51.2	38.1	30.6	23.4
Influenza and pneumonia	23.9	17.9	21.7	20.2
Chronic liver disease and cirrhosis	12.4	5.8	7.7	9.2
Diabetes mellitus	28.4	21.6	46.9	22.5
Human immunodeficiency virus (HIV) disease	6.2	2.3	19.4	2.2
Motor vehicle-related injuries	21.7	8.9	14.5	15.6
Suicide	18.0	4.4	5.2	12.0
Homicide	9.6	2.5	21.1	3.7

Table 7 Risk ratios of age-adjusted rates per 100,000 population for selected causes of death by gender and race, United States, 2005

	Risk ratio of	
Cause of death	Male to female	Black to white
All causes	1.40	1.29
Diseases of heart	1.51	1.31
Malignant neoplasms	1.45	1.22
Cerebrovascular disease	1.03	1.46
Chronic lower respiratory disease	1.34	0.67
Influenza and pneumonia	1.34	1.07
Chronic liver disease and cirrhosis	2.14	0.84
Diabetes mellitus	1.31	2.08
Human immunodeficiency virus (HIV) disease	2.70	8.82
Motor vehicle-related injuries	2.44	0.93
Suicide	4.09	0.43
Homicide	3.84	5.70

Table 8 Formulae for computation of relative risk and odds ratio

	Event		
	Yes	No	Total
Exposure			
Yes	a	b	a + b
No	c	d	c + d

Relative risk of event = Incidence rate in high risk group/Incidence rate in low risk group
$$= [a/(a+b)]/[c/(c+d)]$$
Odds ratio of exposure yielding an event $= (a/b)/(c/d)$

Table 9 Relative risks and odds ratios of medical error from shifts (Rogers et al., 2004)

Average hours worked on scheduled day	No. of shifts	No. of errors (%)	Odds ratio	Relative risk
<8.5	771	12 (1.6)	1.00 (referent)	1.00 (referent)
8.5–12.5	2,484	77 (3.1)	2.02	1.99
12.5 or more	2,057	103 (5.0)	3.33	3.22
Total	5,312	192 (3.5)	–	–

Using formula from Table 8 to compute odds ratio and relative risk of medical error:

	Error		
Average hours worked	Yes	No	Total
8.5–12.5 h	77(a)	2,407 (b)	2,484 (a + b)
<8.5	12 (c)	759 (d)	771 (c + d)

Odds ratio $= (a/b)/(c/d) = (77/2,407)/(12/759) = 2.02$
Those odds of those 8.5–12.5 h reporting a medical error are 2.02 times those working less than an 8.5 h day
Relative risk $= (77/2,484)/(12/759) = 1.99$
The risk of medical error is 1.99 times greater in those working a 8.5–12.5 h than those working less than 8.5 h

Because the RR and the OR are estimates of a true value calculated from samples, a confidence interval, usually 95% is computed to assess the reliability of the sample estimates. A *confidence interval* is an interval that is generated from a random sample of an underlying population such that if the sampling was repeated numerous times and the parameter was calculated from each sample according to the same method the samples would contain some interval probability of values in which the true parameter (in this example the RR or the OR) would lie.

The *population attributable risk* (PAR) utilizes ratios to estimate the proportion of the risk of exposure due to a particular factor. This measure has importance as it assesses the theoretically achievable reduction in risk if the risk factor were entirely removed from a population. It is for this reason that the PAR is a useful measure of the efficacy of population-based preventive interventions when multiple risk factors are involved in the emergence of a disease as is the case of chronic conditions. The calculation of the PAR is illustrated in Table 10. The PAR can also be estimated from the OR. Thus, when resources are limited, the PAR can aid in determining which interventions may have the greatest impact upon a population. The PAR of 56% means that 56% of the risk of diabetes is due to weight gain. This indicates that the greatest opportunity for preventing diabetes mellitus is to control weight gain to no more than 7 kg (15.4 lbs) after age 21 years. However, 44% of the risk of diabetes is due to other factor(s). Caution in the interpretation of the PAR is advised as different risk factors may be subject to different levels of bias in the classification of the different exposures evaluated as well as there may be a number of individuals exposed who may not respond to the intervention proposed. Also, the calculated PARs presented in Table 10 are "unadjusted." Methodologies exist for examining combinations of risk factors and the impact of interpreting a PAR when selectively removing exposure to a risk factor while leaving all other exposures unchanged (Walter, 1998).

Table 10 Computation of population attributable risk (Data from: Koh-Banerjee et al., 2004)

Subgroup	% of men	RR_{DM}	PAR (%)
Weight gain of ≥7 kg since age 21 years	55	3.3	56
Waist gain of ≥2.5 cm over 9 years	56	1.4	20

RR_{DM} = relative risk of diabetes mellitus

$$\text{Population Attributable Risk (PAR\%)} = \frac{Pe(RR-1)}{1+Pe(RR-1)} \times 100\%$$

where Pe = proportion controls exposed; RR = relative risk for exposed compared with unexposed where the risk among unexposed is 1
Thus,

$$PAR_{\text{weight gain}\geq 7kg} = \frac{0.55(3.3-1)}{1+0.55(3.3-1)} \times 100\% = 56\%$$

Summary

This chapter presented common descriptive epidemiologic measures useful in planning health care services, and for evaluating policies and programs. Rate measures prioritize health problems within a population or across time or geographic areas. They also can be used to evaluate trends within population subgroups. Summary descriptive measures provide a quick assessment of the health of populations.

Boxed Example 1 Consequences of Long-Term Survival from Cancer

---

Problem: There is an increasing prevalence of cancer survivors because of increases in the early detection of cancer and advances in effective treatment. Cancer therapy is often intensive (invasive surgery, high-dose chemotherapy and radiation therapy, multimodality therapy) and potentially results in long-term psychological and physical late effects and even damage to normal tissue affecting physical performance which results in participation restrictions in activities of daily living (see Conceptual Model).

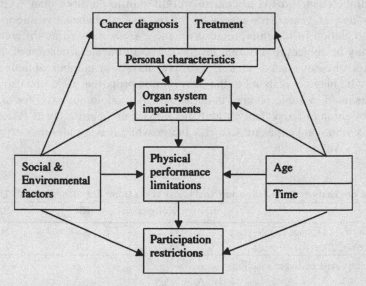

Reprinted from *Ann. Epidemiol.* Vol. 16. Ness, K.K. et al. 197–205. Copyright 2006 with permission from Elsevier.

Method and Data: Data from the National Health and Nutrition Examination Survey (NHANES 1999–2002) were used to analyze the information for those who were noninstitutionalized persons age 20+ years at the time of the home interview. Complex multistage samples design was used. Physical performance limitation was ascertained if the responded states "some difficulty," "much difficulty," or "unable to do" one or more of 11 physical performance activities (e.g., getting out of bed, stooping, etc.), without special equipment or one or more of seven routine activities (e.g., dressing, preparing meals, etc.) or a positive response to having "difficulty walking without using any special equipment."

Results: The overall prevalence of cancer history was 8.7%. The prevalence of any restriction in routine activities was: 13.0% for those without cancer, 30.5% for those <5 years post cancer diagnosis, 31.3% for those 5+ years cancer survivor. The prevalence of any performance limitation was: 21.2% for those without cancer, 52.7% for those <5 years post cancer diagnosis, 54.4% for those 5+ years cancer survivor.

Source: Ness et al. (2006).

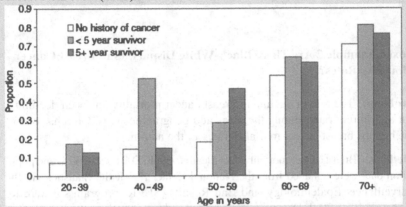

Proportion of adult participants in NHANES 1999–2002 with physical performance limitations.

Reprinted from Ann. Epidemiol., Vol.16, Ness, K.K., et al., 197–205, Copyright 2006, with permission from Elsevier.

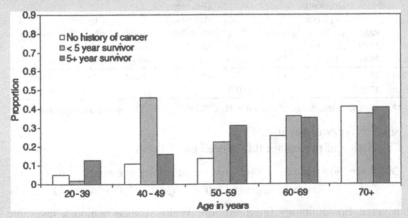

Proportion of those with participation restrictions reported among adult participants in NHANES 1999–2002. Reprinted from Ann. Epidemiol., Vol.16, Ness, K.K., et al., 197–205, Copyright 2006, with permission from Elsevier.

Boxed Example 1 (continued)

Managerial Epidemiology Interpretation: Prevalence measures are estimates of the burden of disease and are the most useful in planning for health services utilization. Both new and long-term cancer survivors experience physical performance limitations and participation restrictions at a greater rate than the general population. Rehabilitation intervention offered soon after active cancer therapy is completed may benefit those particularly for those under 60 years of age as a means of preventing and mitigating long-term disability. The manager may also need to re-formulate the conceptual model and consider other variables which could affect long-term disability. Additional descriptive epidemiologic data may be necessary for the under 60 year age group.

Boxed Example 2 Are There Black-White Disparities in Breast Cancer Mortality Rates?

Problem: The rate of decline in breast cancer mortality has been declining, but at different rates among the races and geographic areas. Ohio has one of the highest breast cancer mortality rates in the nation.

Methods: Breast cancer mortality data (deaths with ICD-9 code of 174) and population data were obtained from the National Center for Health Statistics via the Surveillance, Epidemiology, and End Results (SEER) program software for the period 1970–2001. Data were age-adjusted to the 2000 US standard population. The Breslow-Day statistic was used to evaluate the significance between the rates.

Data and Results: Breast Cancer Mortality in Ohio 1970–1974 and 1996–2001 by Race, Women, 30–74 Years

Race	Rate[a] 1970– 1974	Difference (%) Black vs. Whites in 1970– 1974	p-value for difference	Rate[a] 1997– 2001	Difference (%) Blacks vs. Whites in 1997– 2001	p-value for difference	Change (%) 1970– 1974 vs. 1997–2001	p-value for difference
Whites	47.7	−0.8	0.18	35.4	41.8	<0.001	−25.8	<0.001
Blacks	47.3			50.2			6.1	0.17

[a]Age-adjusted standardized rates per 100,000 using US 2000 standard population

Source: Tyczynski et al. (2006).

Calculation of percentage difference is as follows:

Difference (%) = (Rate comparison group − rate in referent group)

/Rate referent group × 100% = (50.2 − 35.4)/35.4 × 100% = 41.8%

Managerial Epidemiology Interpretation: White women exhibit a favorable rate of decline in breast cancer mortality whereas among Black women the rate increased but was not significantly different from 30 years ago. Reasons for

Boxed Example 2 (continued)

the high rates in Black females include an increased incidence of breast cancer, a potentially increasing higher tumor grade of the cancer, and a lack of access to health care for screening, initial treatment and follow-up care due to lack of insurance and/or availability of screening services and health care providers. Health care managers should give priority attention to ensuring that follow-up of any abnormal screening mammography test is done particularly quickly, especially for population subgroups at high risk for breast cancer mortality.

Ratios aid in evaluating the degree of the relationship between exposure and outcome. Descriptive measures, in general, are useful in identifying the components of the health care system that could be modified to by identifying populations at risk because of their demographic composition, exposure, or geographic location. The type of epidemiologic measure used depends upon the objective of the assessment, the nature of the health problem being evaluated, and the type of data available for the assessment.

Discussion Questions

Q.1. Compare the rankings of the causes of mortality in Tables 4 and 6. What accounts for the differences in ranking of causes of mortality? Which table of data would you use in determining what should be priority areas for health care services in a community comprised of immigrants and racial or ethnic minorities?

Q.2. How can mortality data be used in prioritizing which level health care services would be appropriate for a community (see also Tables 3, 5–6, 10, and Fig. 4)? What are the limitations of mortality data in prioritizing health problems for which to develop health care services in a community?

Q.3. Data from the National Health and Nutrition Examination Survey 1999–2004 found the prevalence of diagnosed diabetes to significantly increase from 5.1% in the period 1988–1994 to 6.5% in the period 1999–2002. During these same time periods undiagnosed diabetes and impaired fasting glucose remained unchanged (Ong et al., 2008). What factors could have accounted for the overall increase in prevalence in diagnosed diabetes?

References

Barker, W.H., Mullooly, J.P., and Getchell, W., 2006, Changing incidence and survival for heart failure in a well-defined older population, 1970–1974 and 1990–1994, *Circulation* **113**:799–805.

Campsmith, M.L., Rhodes, P., Hall, H.I., and Green, T., 2008, HIV prevalence estimates—United States, 2006, *M.M.W.R.* **57**:1073–1076.

Fleiss, J.L., Levin, B., and Park, M.C., 2003, *Statistical Methods for Rates and Proportions*, 3rd ed., Wiley, Hoboken, NJ.

Heron, M., Hoyert, D.L., Xu, J., Scott, C., and Tejada, B., 2008, Deaths: Preliminary Data for 2006, *National Vital Statistics Reports* **vol. 56**, no. 16. National Center for Health Statistics, Hyattsville, MD.

Hickman, M., Seaman, S., and de Angelis, D., 2001, Estimating the relative incidence of heroin use: application of a method for adjusting observed reports of first visits to specialized drug treatment agencies, *Am. J. Epidemiol.* **153**:632–41.

Koh-Banerjee, P., Wang, Y., Hu, F.B., Spiegleman, D., Willett, W.C., and Rimm, E.B., 2004, Changes in body weight and body fat distribution as risk factors for clinical diabetes in US men, *Am. J. Epidemiol.* **159**:1150–1159.

National Cancer Institute, 2008, *Joinpoint Regression Program, Version 3.3* (August 16, 2008), http://srab.cancer.gov/joinpoint.

National Center for Health Statistics, 2007, Health, United States, 2007, With Chartbook on Trends in the Health of Americans, Hyattsville, MD.

Ness, K.K., Wall, M.M., Oakes, J.M., Robison, L.L., and Gurney, J.G., 2006, Physical performance limitations and participation restrictions among cancer survivors: a population-based study, *Ann. Epidemiol.* **16**:197–205.

Nicholas, J.A., Charles, J.M., Carpenter, L.A., King, L.B., Jenner, W., and Spratt, E.G., 2008, Prevalence and characteristics of children with autism-spectrum disorders, *Ann. Epidemiol.* **18**:130–136.

Ong, K.L., Cheung, B.M.Y., Wong, L.Y.F., Wat, N.M.S., Tan, K.C.B., and Lam, K.S.L. 2008, Prevalence, treatment, and control of diagnosed diabetes in the U.S. National Health and Nutrition Examination Survey 1999–2004, *Ann. Epidemiol.* **18**:222–229.

Rogers, A.E., Hwang, W., Scott, L.D., Aiken, L.H., and Dinges, D.F., 2004, The working hours of hospital staff nurses and patient safety, *Health Affairs* **23**:202–212.

Sanfilippo, F.M., Hobbs, M.S.T., Knuiman, M.W., and Hung, J., 2008, Impact of new biomarkers of myocardial damage on trends in myocardial infarction hospital admission rates from population-based administrative data, *Am. J. Epidemiol.* **168**:225–233.

Shapiro-Mendoza, C.K., Tomashek, K.M., Anderson, R.N., and Wingo, J., 2006, Recent national trends in sudden, unexpected infant deaths: more evidence supporting a change in classification or reporting, *Am. J. Epidemiol.* **163**:762–769.

Tyczynski, J.E., Hill, T.D., and Berkel, H.J., 2006, Why do postmenopausal African-American women not benefit from overall breast cancer mortality decline? *Ann. Epidemiol.* **16**:180–190.

U.S. Department of Health and Human Services (USDHHS), Centers for Disease Control and Prevention, 2007, *Health, United States, 2007: with Chartbook on Trends in the Health of Americans* (August 16, 2008), http://www.cdc.gov/nchs/data/hus/hus07.pdf.

Ustun, T.B., 1999, The global burden of mental disorders, *Am. J. Pub Health* **89**:1315–1318.

Walter, S.D., 1998, Attributable risk in practice, *Am. J. Epidemiol.* **148**:411–413.

Wang, Y., and Beydoun, M.A., 2007, The obesity epidemic in the United States—gender, age, socioeconomic, racial/ethnic, and geographic characteristics: a systematic review and meta-regression analysis, *Epidemiol. Rev.* **29**:6–28.

Wennberg, J.E., Fisher, E.S., Goodman, D.C., and Skinner, J.S., 2008, *Tracking the Care of Patients with Severe Chronic Illness: The Dartmouth Atlas of Health Care 2008*, The Dartmouth Institute for Health Policy and Clinical Practice, Dartmouth, NH.

World Health Organization (WHO), 2008, *World Health Statistics*, WHO Press, Geneva, Switzerland.

Chapter 4
Epidemiological Study Designs for Evaluating Health Services, Programs, and Systems

Learning Outcomes

After completing this chapter, you will be able to:

1. Compare and contrast the advantages and disadvantages of observational study designs in the identification of new risk factors for health problems.
2. Differentiate among the common epidemiological study designs regarding the level of evidence they provide.
3. Describe how a randomized clinical trial can aid in evaluating the effectiveness of an intervention to promote health in a community.
4. Determine a program's effectiveness using epidemiological methods.

Keyterms Case-control study • Cohort • Cross-sectional study • Descriptive study • Evaluation • Longitudinal study • Meta-analysis • Quasi-experimental design • Randomized clinical trial

Introduction

Program evaluation is vitally important to improve the performance of health care organizations, health systems, and public health services. According to Clement and Wan (2001): "evaluation is a means by which a program, service, or a process is examined and an informed judgment is made concerning the extent of success in reaching predetermined goals." These authors describe that evaluation is integral in the delivery of health care by: "(1) assuring the delivery of a high quality of health care; (2) serving as a toll for monitoring care and controlling costs; and (3) promoting accountability for public and private program expenditures." Evaluation is an aid to managerial decision-making in regarding the current and future allocation of resources to the various phases of a program – planning, design, implementation, and monitoring. Clement and Wan also propose evaluations that can be done for a variety of purposes including: "to improve the delivery of care, to test an innovation, to determine the effectiveness of regulatory policy, to assess the appropriateness of continuing or altering an intervention, or to compare

D.M. Oleske (ed.), *Epidemiology and the Delivery of Health Care Services: Methods and Applications,*
DOI 10.1007/978-1-4419-0164-4_4, © Springer Science+Business Media, LLC 2009

health system effectiveness across nations." Driving the need for more evaluation at every level of health care services, private or public, is the ever increasing costs of health care such that continued increased spending may not necessarily produce the desired outcomes. The alternative of not spending or limiting resources may yield ethical dilemmas. Program evaluation provides a more systematic review of the use of resources (people, facilities, financial) as interventions for achieving health care goals and hence improves the efficiency and effectiveness of health care services. The ability to interpret and apply findings from program evaluations and study designs is also a critical competency for an evidence-based practitioner according to Brownson et al. (1999), whether that individual is an epidemiologist or a health care manager.

An epidemiological model of the delivery of health care services (see chapter "An Epidemiologic Framework for the Delivery of Health Care Services") guides in identifying the information that is required for program evaluation. Specifically, epidemiology "provides a framework for planning, monitoring the health of a population, identifying changes in risk factors over time, and prioritizing health problems requiring correction (Clement and Wan, 2001)." Epidemiologic measures and study designs are the basis of the analytic approaches for evaluating if programs are effective in preventing and controlling disease, disability, injury, and other health problems in populations receiving health care services. This chapter presents an overview of the conceptual dimensions of program evaluation and the issues involved in selecting the appropriate study design for determining the most effective health care delivery strategies.

Dimensions of Evaluation

The conduct of an evaluation for an intervention, program or policy requires that several conceptual issues in the design and conduct of analysis be addressed (Clement and Wan, 2001). The conceptual issues are as follows:

- Determine the population targeted (for the intervention; to who the program applies).
- Identify the aspects of health care to be evaluated.
- Identify and develop the evaluation criteria, standards, and measures.
- Specify the design and analytic approaches appropriate to the evaluation.
- Identify who will conduct the evaluation and how it is to be financed.
- Assess the impact of the evaluation.
- Identify the major findings and implications.

Following the epidemiological framework for the delivery of health care (see chapter "An Epidemiologic Framework for the Delivery of Health Care Services"), the first design consideration is the determination of the population targeted for the intervention that could be people, organizations, or communities. Epidemiologic measures (mortality, adverse event rates, etc.) are utilized to identify those entities most in need (e.g., communities near toxic waste disposal sites, patients at risk for medical error, safety net hospitals, etc.) and therefore who can most benefit from the intervention. Ensuring the adequacy of the sample size and its representativeness of the population who are the intended beneficiaries of the intervention are fundamental to the validity of the evaluation.

The success of interventions, programs, or policies to improve or benefit the health of population is highly influenced by the context of the health care delivery system in which they are delivered or implemented. It is for this reason that aspects of the health system should be considered in each evaluation. These aspects include the:

- Quality of care
- Safety of the care processes and their delivery (see chapter "Delivering Health Care with Quality: Epidemiological Considerations")
- Accessibility, acceptability, and availability of resources for the inception and continuation of the intervention (see chapter "An Epidemiologic Framework for the Delivery of Health Care Services" for definitions)
- Continuity of care (maintaining monitoring and treatment as appropriate between successive episodes of contact with the health care system)
- Continuity of communication (during the intervention and through the dissemination of evaluation findings)
- Effectiveness of the health care services (the degree to which stated or accepted goals are achieved in the ordinary setting in which the intervention is conducted)
- Efficiency of health services delivery (the ability to achieve the desired goal with minimal resources)

It may not be feasible to consider all of the above for many reasons. For example, an evaluation of a needle exchange program was limited by whether or not the participants had access to care to evaluate if/when seroconversion for HIV occurred as well as the reports of participation in a NEP prone to socially desirable responses (Safaeian et al., 2001). When aspects of the conceptual dimensions cannot be addressed, the findings of an evaluation report should address how the evaluation outcomes or benefits could have been altered by one or more of the contextual aspects.

The Evaluation Process

Evaluation is a dynamic, iterative, and continuous process linked to optimizing benefit of an intervention relative to a specific health problem identified in a population in need. According to Clement and Wan (2001), there are four interrelated components of the evaluation process: planning, implementation, intervention, and monitoring/feedback (Fig. 1). The planning process is covered in "Strategic Planning and Its Epidemiological Basis," but planning for any intervention begins when a problem is identified through epidemiologic data. Criteria are then established

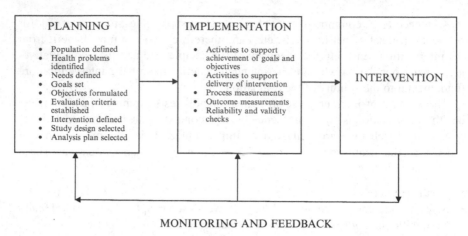

MONITORING AND FEEDBACK

Fig. 1 The evaluation process: a reiterative model (Adapted from Clement and Wan, 2001)

based upon those data and other data as necessary to characterize the need which has given rise to the problem. The data which characterize the need may also be used in the evaluation process. For example, if epidemiologic data identify a high prevalence of obesity in a population and this health problem is addressed through a health promotion program, the change in the prevalence of obesity may be used as an evaluation criterion. Implementation focuses on the establishment of mechanisms to ensure adequate scope of coverage, integrity, and safety of the intervention in the target population. Intervention is the delivery of the change activities be it at the individual, community, or policy levels. Interventions examined through the evaluation process are specific in that they are tailored to the population in need of the intervention (effectiveness) which in contrast to interventions testing efficacy which restrict the population to certain eligibility criteria to determine if it will actually produce the desired outcomes. Monitoring and feedback need to be ongoing throughout the evaluation process. If progress toward goals is not being met, then corrective mechanisms need to be instituted to address deficiencies in the implementation of the program processes ("implementation" component) and then addressed in the evaluation process and subsequently monitored in the reiterative process.

Conceptual Framework for Specifying Evaluation Criteria

The conceptual framework for specifying evaluation criteria according to Clement and Wan (2001) is based upon the original model put forth by Donabedian (1966) to evaluate medical care. This model categorizes evaluation criteria in three categories: structural, process, and outcome measures that can be used to determine the achievement of program, health service, or health system objectives. Structural measures represent the features of the organization, its personnel performing an intervention (such as ratio of primary care physicians to population served), the location where a service is given, and the resources required to plan, design, deliver, and monitor the intervention. Capital, material, technical, and human resources expended on a program are all structural criteria. Process measures are the tasks associated with the implementation and receiving of the intervention. Process measures consider either provider delivered interventions or patient/client's activities in obtaining care or compliance with care guidelines. Outcome measures are specified by the criteria attributable to the hypothesized success of the intervention and would necessarily include some measure of health but also other measures such as satisfaction with care. Outcomes according to Donabedian (1966) remain the ultimate effectiveness measures of care. Ideally, program evaluation should consider criteria from each of these domains to be measured during the implementation of an intervention.

Analytical Approaches to Evaluation: An Epidemiological Perspective

The conduct of evaluation studies is an essential component of the evaluation process. An epidemiological perspective is crucial in this process because the success of a program in achieving its goals is influenced by the characteristics of the population served, their health care needs, and their ability to utilize health care services. Since programs are instituted in defined populations, epidemiological methods can be used to quantify the health needs, the criteria for evaluating the intervention aimed at addressing the problem causing the needs, and measure and analyze program outcomes. Epidemiologic study designs provide a framework for the evaluation process and the analytic methods are used to measure the success of the intervention relative to epidemiologic measures. A description of the epidemiologic study designs and statistical methods commonly used in program evaluation follow.

Study Designs

Once it is determined what aspect of the health care delivery system will be evaluated, the study design can be selected for the evaluation plan. A study design is the template by which a sample is drawn to test a hypothesis or explore a research question. Figure 2 displays the common study designs used in epidemiology according to the level of evidence provided. Characterizing a phenomenon in terms of its magnitude and variability is considered the most basic level of evidence. The highest level of evidence is provided by the randomized clinical trial (RCT). The epidemiologic study designs commonly used in program evaluation are often those used in

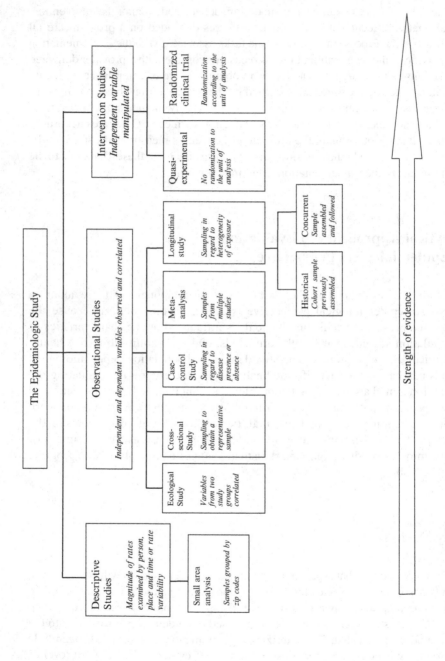

Fig. 2 Common epidemiologic study designs according to level of evidence provided

epidemiologic research to identify risk factors and how they can be controlled or modified. The initial and most crucial decision in the choice of a study design is a consideration of the timing of the evaluation relative to the stage of the program operations. If the program has been in operation for some time, an observational study may be implemented. If the program is introduced simultaneous with the evaluation process, an experimental design is more appropriate. Another consideration influencing the study design is how the sample can be selected relative to the exposure or program introduction and when was the outcome determined.

The strategy in selecting among these choices is to use the design to build upon existing evidence regarding the relationship among study variables. For example, if the relationship is well known between exposure and a health outcome and can be repeated using different observational designs, and intervention study would be warranted. The intervention study would aid in confirming the relationship adding to the body of evidence to confirm the "dose" of the intervention, the timing of its introduction (before the event) before the outcome. The common epidemiological study designs used in program evaluation as well as epidemiologic research are presented.

Descriptive Study Designs

A *descriptive study* seeks to obtain information about the magnitude or variation of a health problem or exposure through rate measures graphed, plotted, or otherwise visualized by selected characteristics representing person, place, or time. Descriptive studies are commonly used to generate hypothesis for testing using other study designs. In the context of program evaluation, descriptive studies are used in the needs assessment or planning phase of program evaluation. There are three major types of descriptive study designs, simple descriptive and variability studies.

A *simple descriptive study* design represents the magnitude, frequency, and variability of health problems or exposures as rate measures in terms of line (arithmetic or semi-log) graphs, bar charts, or maps according to personal characteristics (age, gender, race, etc.), time, and/or place. Figure 3 is an example of a descriptive study example which consists of line graphs plotting the prevalence of obesity in both males and females in major population subgroups between 1971 and 1974 and 2003 and 2004. The doubling of the prevalence of obesity among Black non-Hispanic women signals a health problem requiring immediate population-based intervention. A descriptive study in which gonorrhea rates are mapped by 20th percentiles by census block group identifies areas of highest risk (Fig. 4). Descriptive studies are utilized to help isolate priority areas of concern and/or important trends over time.

Small-area analysis (SAA) is a type of descriptive study intended to examine the significance of variability of rate measures where the geographic unit is restricted to a community area defined by the aggregation of population according to zip code. SAA assigns the population at risk (or denominator) and determines the

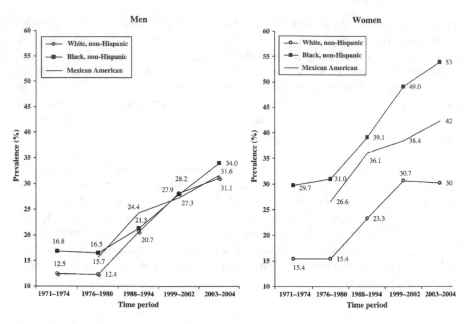

Fig. 3 Trends in the prevalence of obesity (body mass index ≥30 kg/m²) in US adults, by gender and ethnicity, National Health and Nutrition Examination Survey, 1971–2004 (Wang and Beydoun, The obesity epidemic in the United States—gender, age, socioeconomic racial/ethnic, and geographic characteristics: a systematic review and meta-regression analysis, *Am. J. Epidemiol.* 2007;29:6–28 by permission of Oxford University Press)

numerator from the population based upon zip codes used to define the area(s) using data sources appropriate to the study hypothesis. For example, in examining hospital utilization rates, populations can be assigned based upon the hospital they most frequently used in some period of time or the place of residence at the time of death (Wennberg et al., 2008). Administrative records of hospital discharges (e.g., the Medicare MedPAR beneficiaries file of fee-for-service claims data) are used when making population assignments to the denominator based upon hospitals used. Administrative records can also be used to assign populations to a denominator according to place of residence (e.g., Medicare Denominator file which provides demographic data). Numerator data (e.g., utilization, deaths) may be derived from administrative databases as well (e.g., Medicare Physician/Supplier Part B claims file) or through vita records (zip code residence of decedent or mother delivering a newborn). Through this descriptive analysis marked variations in health care delivery for selected treatment and diagnostic procedures independent (adjusted for) of population demographic characteristics (Fisher et al., 2003; Stukel et al., 2005). Figure 5 illustrates the variability in the utilization of end of life care. The conclusions drawn graphically as well as statistically are that marked variation in the utilization of care exists, even among hospitals which have high national prestige rankings. SAA overcomes some of the limitations of descriptive studies by characterizing variability in smaller geographic areas thereby attempting to account

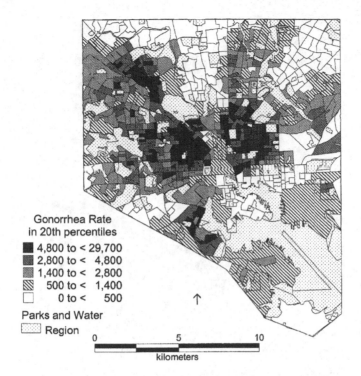

Gonorrhea Rate
in 20th percentiles

■ 4,800 to < 29,700
■ 2,800 to < 4,800
▨ 1,400 to < 2,800
▨   500 to < 1,400
□   0 to <   500

Parks and Water
▨ Region

0   5   10

kilometers

Fig. 4 Reported gonorrhea case rates per 100,000 per census block group reported in 20th percentiles, Baltimore City, Maryland, 1994–1999 (Jennings et al., Geographic identification of high gonorrhea transmission areas in Baltimore, Maryland, *Am. J. Epidemiol.* 2005;161(1):73–80 by permission of Oxford University Press)

for individual-level associations through various adjustment procedures to better represent variation due to these personal characteristics.

Cluster analysis is another approach to identify significant variation of rate measures using statistical techniques in groups, usually supplemented with some mapping technique, to identify grouped events or exposures in consideration of time unit. These include the spatial scan statistic (Kulldorff, 1997), hierarchical geostatistical logistic model, and a multilevel models (HLM, Scientific Software International, Inc., Lincolnwood, IL). Geographic clustering technique allows targeting health services intervention at areas more precisely than at the state, county, or census tract level. For example, geographic cluster analysis had identified an area where women aged 50 years or older were twice as likely to be diagnosed with late-stage breast cancer compared with the rest of the state and, therefore, should be a priority area for breast health and screening services (Schootman et al., 2007). Jennings et al. (2005) use cluster detection controlling for race and ethnicity for reported gonorrhea cases by census block group to devise strategies for more (Fig. 6). Cluster analysis uses the descriptive rates from Fig. 4 to more precisely identify areas to target for deploying more precisely targeted health care service intervention of any level.

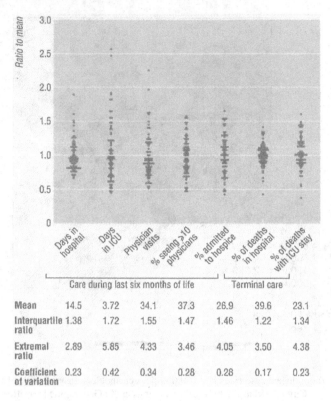

Mean	14.5	3.72	34.1	37.3	26.9	39.6	23.1
Interquartile ratio	1.38	1.72	1.55	1.47	1.46	1.22	1.34
Extremal ratio	2.89	5.85	4.33	3.46	4.05	3.50	4.38
Coefficient of variation	0.23	0.42	0.34	0.28	0.28	0.17	0.23

Fig. 5 Distribution of rates and statistical measures of variation for end of life care among 77 cohorts assigned to hospitals with national reputations for high quality. ICU = intensive care unit (Reproduced from "Use of hospitals, physician visits, and hospice care during last six months of life among cohorts loyal to highly respected hospitals in the United States," J.E. Wennberg, et al. *BMJ*. 328: 607 copyright notice 2004 with permission from BMJ Publishing Group Ltd.)

Descriptive epidemiologic studies are typically derived from vital data and census information which is readily available. For this reason, descriptive studies can be quick and easy to do. Descriptive studies are limited in that secondary data sources are often used, namely they examine data that have been previously collected for some other purpose and for this reason may be dated.

Observational Study Designs

Observational study designs explore associations between (and among) exposures and health outcomes to evaluate the: (1) significance of the association, (2) strength of the association, (3) direction (positive or negative) of the statistical parameter (odds ratio, relative risk, beta coefficient, correlation coefficient) representing the association, (4) temporality of the exposure occurring prior to the outcome in a latency period considered reasonable to cause the outcome, (5) evidence for the variation in likelihood of outcome relative to exposure, and

Fig. 6 Geographic clusters of gonorrhea cases per census block group, Baltimore City, Maryland, 1994–1999 (Jennings et al., Geographic identification of high gonorrhea transmission areas in Baltimore, Maryland, *Am. J. Epidemiol.* 2005;161(1):73–80 by permission of Oxford University Press)

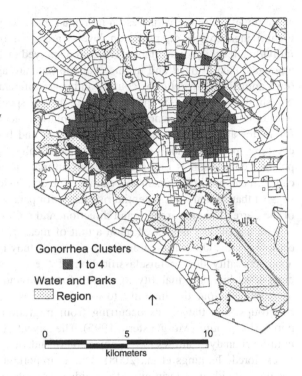

(6) persistence after consideration of confounding factors. The common thread of this category of studies is that the exposure is not manipulated, only documented through information collected through survey forms, biological samples, administrative records, and other sources and associations with selected outcomes are analyzed. For this reason, observational studies are sometimes referred to as correlational studies in the social science literature. A useful summary of the points addressed in this section regarding observational study designs is found in the STROBE statement (Von Elm et al., 2007). The acronym STROBE represents the aim of the collaborators which is: STrengthening the Reporting of OBservational studies in Epidemiology. The STROBE collaboration developed a recommended checklist of items that should be addressed in reports of observational studies. This aids not only in critiquing the published study, but also serves as a guide for planning observational studies.

The common observational epidemiologic study designs are ecologic, cross-sectional, case-control, longitudinal, and meta-analysis. These are described below.

Ecologic Study Design

An *ecologic study* uses variables from two study groups (one of which is the group rate measure of the health problem under study) and examines their correlation, the strength of the correlation, and the direction of the correlation to make inferences about the effect of the variables on individual risk. Aggregate variables or environmental measures (e.g., pollution levels) are used because information at the individual level is not available. The data displayed in Table 1 represent the type of aggregate data utilized and in this example data are aggregated for each variable (e.g., animal fat, cigarette) by country and from different sources within the country. Not shown, but utilized in the analyses are the sex-specific age-standardized (to the world population) incidence rates of pancreatic cancer averaged over 1993–1997 for males and females, separately. Figure 7a and b displays the results of the ecologic correlation analysis whereby a statistically significant moderately strong positive correlation is observed between animal fat consumption and pancreatic cancer incidence in both men and women. The conclusions of this ecologic analyses suggest that animal fat is potential risk factor for pancreatic cancer; the significance of the correlation, its strength and direction, and uniformity in both sexes.

The use of data not based upon a unit of measurement is one limitation of an ecologic study. Other limitations of an ecologic study include deriving conclusions about causality due to misclassification of the exposure variables under study, cross-level bias, the inability to control for confounding, inability to distinguish temporal relation, the inability to examine exposure effects among population subgroups, and the biases occurring from migration to exposure levels across population groups (Morgenstern, 1995). The advent of new statistical software for multilevel analysis allows the combination of individual and community factors to be explored (Jennings et al., 2008). This is important in program evaluation and design as it aids in determining if individual or ecologic factors should be targeted for intervention and program evaluation.

Cross-Sectional Study Design

A *cross-sectional study* derives information from a random sample to estimate population parameters of interest for exposures (e.g., percentage of smokers or individuals who have had screening mammography in past year, etc.) or health problems (e.g., proportion of obese individuals, mean blood pressure, proportion of individuals with coronary artery disease, etc.). This study design is also used to assess the strength of the relationship between exposure to a risk factor and its hypothesized health problem through cross-classifying the members of the sample into exposure-disease categories or cells. The source of data used in cross-sectional studies most often is from some form of survey, namely telephone or person interviews, self-administered questionnaires, or medical record review. Some cross-sectional studies also may obtain information derived from biological measurements or clinical examinations and link these to various demographic characteristics. Examples of cross-sectional studies of particular importance for planning and evaluating health services utilization are the Behavioral Risk Factor Surveillance Survey (BRFSS) (see chapter "Measurement Issues in the Use of Epidemiologic Data") and the Center for Studying Health System Change Community Tracking Surveys (CTS) (http://www.hschange.com). Recently, data from the BRFSS revealed a decline in

Table 1 Data for an ecologic study: animal fat, alcohol consumption, mean of nine periods (1964–1994), food balance sheet, FAO[a], cigarette consumption, Mean of 1970, 1980, and 1990, WHO[a,b] and sex-specific age-standardized (world) incidence rates of pancreatic cancer, 1993–1997

Countries	Fat (% E^a) Animal	Total	Male Rate	Female Rate	Alcohol (% E)	Vegetable (g/day)
Denmark	34.3	43.9	7.2	5.8	6.24	174
New Zealand	29.9	36.4	6.4	5.0	5.11	232
Finland	29.5	37.1	8.8	6.3	4.79	106
UK	27.3	38.8	6.7	4.9	5.86	223
Hungary	27.2	34.2	–	–	6.49	237
France	26.3	38.3	5.9	3.2	7.64	326
Switzerland	26.2	40.4	7.4	5.0	6.09	233
Norway	25.9	38.4	7.5	5.8	2.76	147
Belgium	25.0	38.6	4.4	3.8	6.97	253
Austria	24.6	38.7	8.0	5.3	7.43	204
Germany	24.0	36.7	6.3	5.1	8.43	192
Czech Republic	23.0	32.2	11.3	7.0	7.63	218
Australia	23.0	33.0	6.5	4.7	5.61	187
Poland	22.5	29.1	8.7	5.6	3.36	304
Canada	22.3	36.9	7.3	5.6	4.36	267
Netherlands	22.0	38.5	6.2	4.7	4.97	207
Sweden	22.0	36.8	5.9	3.9	4.59	138
Argentina	19.7	31.5	6.8	5.0	0.30	192
USA	18.1	36.2	7.9	6.0	4.96	270
Malta	17.2	29.9	8.3	4.0	2.42	300
Hong Kong	17.1	33.1	4.0	2.7	1.88	202
Yugoslavia	16.3	26.8	6.9	5.2	4.03	221
Italy	15.4	33.5	8.8	5.6	5.66	435
Cuba	14.1	23.0	3.6	2.9	1.36	104
Spain	13.5	34.0	6.0	3.7	6.25	395
Portugal	12.1	28.0	4.4	4.3	9.12	368
Israel	11.9	32.1	6.8	4.5	1.30	366
Japan	10.1	21.9	9.4	5.4	4.87	305
Colombia	9.6	19.2	4.6	4.4	2.29	106
Ecuador	9.6	26.1	3.9	3.6	1.46	86
Costa Rica	8.4	21.5	4.3	3.7	2.45	56
China	6.8	13.7	5.3	4.2	1.48	179
Thailand	5.9	14.6	1.6	1.2	2.75	99
Korea	5.7	13.2	7.4	4.5	7.78	424
India	3.7	14.5	2.0	1.4	0.25	132
Mean	18.6	30.9	6.4	4.5	4.54	225
SD	8.0	8.4	2.1	1.3	2.44	98

[a] FAO, Food and Agriculture Organization; WHO, World Health Organization; %E, percent of total energy; NAY, no./adult/year.
[b] Data shown are ranked by the descending order of animal fat consumption (Data from: Zhang et al., 2005)

the proportion of women aged 40 years and older who reported having had a mammogram in the 2 years preceding the survey (Ryerson et al., 2007). Although this annual survey relies on self-reported information, the same survey format is utilized in all time periods. Concerns regarding decreasing access to breast-imaging

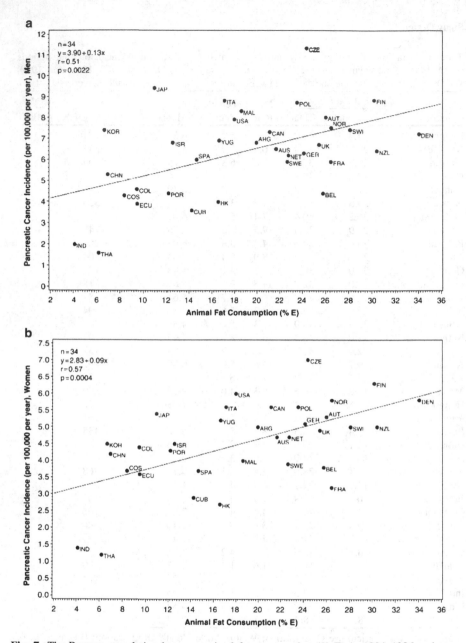

Fig. 7 The Pearson correlation between animal fat consumption (% E) in 1984–1986 and age-standardized pancreatic cancer incidence in 1993–1997 (**a**) for men (**b**) for women. % E, percent of total energy; ARG, Argentina; AUS, Australia; AUT, Austria; BEL, Belgium; CAN, Canada; CHN, China; COL, Colombia; COS, Costa Rica; CUB, Cuba; CZE, Czech Republic; DEN, Denmark; ECU, Ecuador; FIN, Finland; FRA, France; GER, Germany; HK, Hong Kong; IND, India; ISR, Israel; ITA, Italy; JAP, Japan; KOR, Korea; MAL, Malta; NET, Netherlands; NOR, Norway; NZL, New Zealand; POL, Poland; POR, Portugal; SPA, Spain; SWE, Sweden; SWI, Switzerland; THA, Thailand; UK, United Kingdom; USA, United States; YUG, Yugoslavia (Reprinted from *Annals of Epidemiology* 15(7), Zhang, J., et al., "Animal fat consumption and pancreatic cancer incidence: evidence of interaction with cigarette smoking," 500–508, Copyright 1999 with permission from Elsevier)

facilities, increasing financial constraints regarding payment for mammograms or malpractice concerns may have contributed to the decline. The CTS database contains periodic national surveys of households and physicians in 60 communities across the USA. Household surveys query changes in health care access, utilization, insurance, perceptions of the quality of care, and payment of medical bills. Physician surveys include responses to questions regarding source of practice revenue, quality of care, care practices, and practice arrangements. Among the significant findings from this database is that over 20% of the US population in 2007 reporting delaying or obtaining needed medical care within the past 12 months as compared with 14% of the population in 2003.

The sample evaluated from a cross-sectional study design is from one point in time and yields prevalence data. Thus, the cross-sectional study has limited use for determining causality not being able to discern if the exposure truly occurred before the health problem. A cross-sectional study obtains information from a sample and cross-classifies individuals according to exposure-health condition status. Cross-classification is used to estimate a population parameter for a risk factor or health condition (e.g., proportion who are obese; proportion with diabetes) and to determine the extent to which an exposure or risk factor is associated with a particular health condition. Information (both exposure and health conditions) for cross-sectional studies is typically collected by some form of a survey, namely telephone or personal interviews, self-administered questionnaires, or medical record reviews. Cross-sectional studies may also obtain information derived from biological measurements and clinical examinations. Some cross-sectional studies employ selective over-sampling or weighting of population subgroups because of their difficulty in recruiting for study. If applicable, the statistical analyses should then report how the sampling and weighting of the sample to ensure its representativeness relative to the population from which it is drawn is taken into account.

Disadvantages of cross-sectional studies include the exposure events that are subject to the recall bias of the study participant and the inability to precisely establish exposure before the health event under study occurred. Another bias of the cross-sectional study is that it may represent only survivors, and hence may underestimate the effect of exposures by missing incident cases of the condition under study.

Case-Control Study Design

A *case-control study* design compares the prevalence of exposure in those who have the outcome under investigation to those who do not. Controls are individuals who represent the population that the cases were derived from except that they are without the health problem under investigation. Controls may be selected by some random process and/or matched by certain characteristics such as age (within 5 years), sex, and geographic location (to control for environment and/or socioeconomics). For studies involving matching, the criteria should be specified along with the number of controls selected per case.

Controls are selected from the same population as the cases, except for they do not have the health event under investigation. Community controls are ideal.

Random digit dialing (RDD) has been the major technique in selecting population controls (and samples for cross-sectional studies) (Hartge et al., 1984). Changes in telephone technology (e.g., caller identification, answering machines, etc.) have affected response rates. An alternate strategy for control selection proposed by Stone et al. (2007) is as follows: (1) define a geographic area, (2) obtain addresses from a commercial Internet database (e.g., http://www.melissadata.com), (3) randomly select the required number of addresses, (4) obtain information about occupants of addresses from a commercial Internet database (e.g., http://www.accurint.com), (5) contact occupants of interest by mail followed by a telephone call. Enhancement of participation of controls may be achieved with a modest financial incentive (Coogan and Rosenberg, 2004). In planning control selection, an increased number of unlisted or nonpublished phone number, phone calls, in-person visits, and letters sent to nonresponders to request a phone number with time/date of contact is expected over time. Control participants particularly difficult to reach are Hispanic, unmarried, aged 50–64 years and have less than a college education. Individuals easier to interview are those who have first-degree relative with cancer (Rogers et al., 2004).

Selection bias and response bias are common in case-control studies. Selection bias occurs when cases or controls differentially participate in a study because of their association with a disease outcome as for example, parents of children with leukemia being more likely to participate in a study examining the significance of maternal exposure to ionizing radiation. Selection bias is a particular concern when exposure and disease are highly correlated. Response bias emerges depending upon the perceived social impact of or concern over the exposure and/or the condition. Socially undesirable conditions or exposures (e.g., chemically dependent individuals, use of illegal drugs) lower the likelihood of a truthful response. Highly emotionally charged conditions (e.g., childhood cancers) may yield high participation rates, but trigger over-reporting of exposures especially among cases. Higher nonparticipation rates of control subjects may occur relative to cases who may have a vested interest in the study results.

Longitudinal Study Design

A *longitudinal study* (or *prospective study*) compares the rate of an event in exposed and nonexposed groups to risk factor(s) under investigation, neither of which had the event at the time the observation began (Time$_0$). Eligibility criteria should be clearly defined regarding in particular to who is free of the outcome under study and the specification of the validity of exposure measurement over time. Thus, in reality, two time measurements are required to establish the sample for a longitudinal study. At the first time measurement, all members who have the potential for being exposed, regardless if they have been exposed or not, are assembled. Individuals with the event of interest are identified and removed from the study. In the second time measurement, the remaining sample is followed over time and the events during this time are systematically ascertained. The first time measurement yields a prevalence estimate. The second measurement yields an incidence measurement. Because the initial sample may be acquired over several time periods, the possibility that diagnostic methods may influence how a case is identified for inclusion or excluded. However, this potential bias is more of a concern in samples constructed which focus on a specific disease or problem type where treatment regimens may influence the rate and types of outcomes observed (Ellison, 2006).

To determine the rate of occurrence of the event under study, the sample must be observed over a sufficient amount of time so as to accurately capture most or all of the intended outcome events. The frequency of efforts to ascertainment of the outcome measurement should be grounded upon knowledge of the natural history of the disease or health problem being studied. Oleske et al. (2007a) measured recovery outcomes in a longitudinal study of low back pain at 1, 2, 6, and 12 months after enrollment. The follow-up intervals were based upon known epidemiological data of the natural history of recovery from low back pain, with the acute phase within the first 60 days and symptoms continuing to either resolve or decrease after 6 months. The methods and frequency of follow-up are particularly important to precisely capture exposure information that varies over time (time varying covariates) (e.g., hours per day exposed to ergonomic risk factors during work tasks) and known to effect the outcome(s) under study and to minimize losses to follow-up for a more accurate determination of study outcome(s). Depending upon the objectives of the study, follow-up data collection may consist of telephone interviews, self-administered surveys (mail, web-based), and/or clinical measurements. At the conclusion of the study, the follow-up time should be reported in terms of total person-years observed and median time of follow-up regardless of the number of phases or intervals in which follow-up data were collected for example "46,026 women accrued 665,407 person-years of follow-up, with a mean follow-up of 14.5 years" (Lacey et al., 2006) (see chapter "Descriptive Epidemiological Methods").

A special type of longitudinal study is a *cohort study*. This type of study design examines morbidity or mortality rates of groups of individuals called a cohort because they are initially all defined by a common event, exposure, a time period or a combination thereof (e.g., multiple-events, event-exposure) as they pass through all or part of their lifespan. The purpose of this type of study design is to determine if there are age, period, or generation effects affecting the slopes of the rates evaluated (see Boxed Example 1). Cohort studies are also useful in what is termed "outcomes research." When used in this context, the sample may be retrospectively assembled and is more heterogeneous than those in a RCT (see "Randomized Clinical Trial" below). Cohort studies formed for this purpose may either be used to verify the efficacy of the protocol for a particular type of treatment used in a clinical trial or to help refine the understanding of the treatment protocol ("exposure factors") that may be the best alternative to test vs. standard care in a specific group of patients. An example of a time-based cohort used for outcomes research would be the follow-up of asthma patients who were first hospitalized during a specific time period to determine how the use of inhaled corticosteroids affected the use of subsequent hospitalization (Donahue et al., 1997). Longitudinal studies examining the specific etiologic or prognostic risk factors (factors that influence the course of a disease over its natural history) may be easily constructed from disease registries designed to maintain data for those diseases or special conditions. Cancer registries are utilized for ascertaining the survival of various cohorts of cancer patients in terms of survival rates relative to various treatment regimes (see National Cancer Institute Surveillance and End Results at http://seer.cancer.gov). A tuberculosis registry can provide information on predictors (e.g., compliance with treatment guidelines) of recurrent disease (Selassie et al., 2005). Twin registries can aid in differentiating the genetic and in utero, shared and external environmental influences upon behavioral and biological risk factors (Austin et al., 1987). Longitudinal studies are important not only for identifying risk factors for health problems, but also for aiding in the predicting of health services utilization or nonutilization. The identification of pre-hypertension (130-139/84-89 mm Hg) as a risk factor for coronary can aid in targeting treatment services in high risk socio-demographic groups with possible greater impact on excess mortality from cardio-vascular disease (Allaire et al., 1999; Gu et al., 2008).

The designation of a time interval for follow-up of the study participants, particularly with respect to the construction of a cohort is a critical design element of

Boxed Example 1 Trajectory of Depression in an Urban Population

Problem: The incidence and prevalence of affective disorders are difficult to determine. Many who have the condition do not seek appropriate treatment and become at risk for recurrent episodes.

Methods: Adult residents were recruited by a telephone survey from the NYC metropolitan area between March and July 2002. The Brief Symptom Survey was used to assess retrospective recall of depression symptoms. Trained staff used computer-assisted telephone devices to conduct the interviews in English, Spanish, Mandarin, and Cantonese using translated and back-translated questionnaires. In households, adults were randomly selected based upon those whose birth date was closest to the interview date, with up to ten attempts made to complete an interview. The overall response rate was 34%; persons 65+ years included at least two waves was 11.6% of the sample whereas this age group comprised 16.5% of the population.

Data and Results: Baseline $(T_0)^*$ 6 months (T_1) 18 months (T_2)

Boxed Example 1 (continued)

Data and Results:

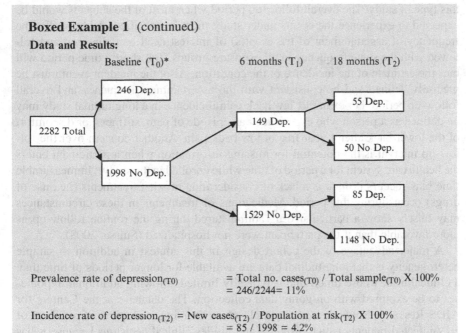

Prevalence rate of depression$_{(T0)}$ = Total no. cases$_{(T0)}$ / Total sample$_{(T0)}$ X 100%
                                                         = 246/2244= 11%

Incidence rate of depression$_{(T2)}$ = New cases$_{(T2)}$ / Population at risk$_{(T2)}$ X 100%
                                                         = 85 / 1998 = 4.2%

Managerial Epidemiology Interpretation: The incidence rate is calculated from the total sample minus the cases present at baseline. The lower percentage of persons 65+ years in the sample compared with the general population may underestimate the absolute prevalence and incidence of depression. Treated depression can have a good prognosis and reduce the incidence of recurrent depression in a population. Social support networks, known to promote mental health, may be effective community-based intervention for this condition which may be recurring or persistent. Health care managers may consider sponsoring community support groups for patients discharged from hospitals for an acute episode of depression.

_____

* Numbers do not add up to numbers at previous wave because not all participants completed all waves.
Source: Beard et al. (2008).

this type of study. The overall follow-up period when most of the subjects would be expected to experience the events under study must be specified. Additionally, the frequency of ascertainment of the event(s) of interest need be delineated and followed with the same frequency in all exposure groups. Too short a time period will bias the estimate of the incidence of the condition. Also, the incident event must be precisely defined and be consistent with the ascertainment frequency and overall follow-up period. For example, low back pain incidence in a longitudinal study may be defined as a person who experienced an episode of pain, stiffness, or discomfort of the lower back after 1 year free of low back pain. Another concern over the follow-up interval is the potential for missing information when a participant enters the health care system for a period of time while enrolled in the study. "Immeasurable time bias" occurs if there is a lack of consideration of what treatments (i.e., use of drugs) occur during this period. Medications or treatments in these circumstances may falsely show a particular drug administered during the routine follow-up as more favorable than if the participant were not hospitalized (Suissa, 2008).

A major advantage of the cohort design in this context in addition to sample heterogeneity is that longitudinal data are available for longer periods of time than a clinical trial, whose timeframe is typically limited, allowing additional hypotheses to be explored with on-going data collection. The database at the Centers for AIDS Research Network is an example of an ongoing evaluation of a cohort of HIV-infected patients which provides and guides clinical decisions because it has sufficient power for evaluating the effects of surrogate or intermediate outcomes and effects of treatment discontinuation (Kitahata et al., 2008). Other advantages of a longitudinal design include the ability to: (1) investigate the natural history of the disease under study, (2) determine disease prevalence, (3) determine disease incidence and/or mortality, (4) more precisely quantify exposure and exposure variation over time, (5) investigate multiple exposures and multiple outcomes, (6) examine exposure-disease interactions, (7) determine that exposures of interest prior to outcome(s) examined, and (8) investigate if outcomes vary with different levels of exposure and exposure interactions.

Challenges in the conduct of longitudinal studies include: (1) the construction and assembly of large sample required to provide valid measures of risk of the condition examined relative to exposure(s), (2) the long-time period required for follow-up to determine the impact of exposure, particularly for chronic conditions, (3) the cost of this type of study given the size and time requirements, and (4) the possibility of attrition due to migration, withdrawal, loss to follow-up, or aging of the study sample which would in itself potentially affect the risk of the outcome occurring. There are also significant challenges in recruiting a cohort willing to be only observed for a longer period of time as well as minimizing attrition of the cohort as they are followed over time. Recruitment strategies vary according to the population targeted for study. For example, face-to-face interactions are highly effective as a strategy for recruiting elderly persons in a longitudinal study than other methods (Samelson et al., 2008). The recording of contact information about individuals at the beginning of the study that are familiar with the whereabouts of the student participant in the event of inability of study staff to contact him/her is essential in addition to complete contact information for the study participant. Regular follow-up with the study participant through phone-calls, newsletters about the study, postcard or email reminders about follow-up appointment dates and locations help to reduce the likelihood of losses. Locating participants whose contact information may not have been updated can be assisted through a variety of proprietary firms with large national databases of addresses which include published, nonpublished, and governmental records as sources of information (e.g., http://www.accurint. com). Davis et al. (2008) provide a scheme for retrospectively constructing a cohort (see Fig. 8). The features of this approach, if exposure data and other characteristics

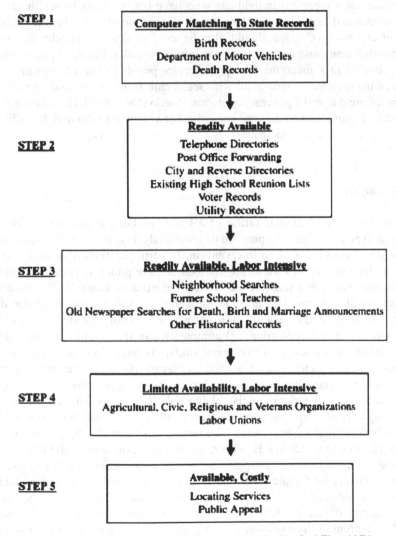

STEP 1

Computer Matching To State Records

Birth Records
Department of Motor Vehicles
Death Records

STEP 2

Readily Available

Telephone Directories
Post Office Forwarding
City and Reverse Directories
Existing High School Reunion Lists
Voter Records
Utility Records

STEP 3

Readily Available, Labor Intensive

Neighborhood Searches
Former School Teachers
Old Newspaper Searches for Death, Birth and Marriage Announcements
Other Historical Records

STEP 4

Limited Availability, Labor Intensive

Agricultural, Civic, Religious and Veterans Organizations
Labor Unions

STEP 5

Available, Costly

Locating Services
Public Appeal

Fig. 8 Example of steps involved in constructing a cohort: the Hanford Thyroid Disease Study (Reprinted from Davis et al., 2008 with permission from Elsevier)

of the study sample are sufficiently valid, are that it gains design efficiency in reducing some of the follow-up time required in ascertaining the outcome. Although in the context of a cohort retrospectively assembled, these authors' strategy provides a useful guidance for other studies with a longitudinal component.

Lastly, a major potential source of bias in a longitudinal study is the source of the sample. Ideally, the sample should be recruited from the community and be representative of it. Examples of longitudinal studies which recruited a community-based sample are the Framingham Heart Study and the Rancho Bernardo Study (Allaire et al., 1999; Langenberg et al., 2005). Cohort samples based upon industrial populations despite the availability of health claims and employee information may represent individuals who have better access to health care or are healthier and hence may underestimate the magnitude of a health problem (Tsia et al., 2008). Caution should also be used in drawing conclusions from cohorts other than those derived from community samples. For example, if selecting a cohort from a government hospital service population or a health plan, the health of the enrollee or individual who seeks care from a particular service site may be different than the general population (Mello et al., 2003). However, as with all studies, longitudinal studies are comprised of volunteers who may be different from those who do not participate.

Meta-Analysis

Meta-analysis is the summarization of a large number studies, usually of one particular type of design. The purpose of meta-analysis is to aid in the determination of the effectiveness of an intervention, in particular those that may impact changing the delivery of care to populations or have policy implications. Meta-analysis involves both a qualitative as well as quantitative analysis. The quantitative aspects of meta-analysis are: (1) the statistical summarization of the data from the multiple studies examined in terms of calculating the size of the effect of the risk factor or intervention, (2) computation of the confidence interval for each point estimate associated from each study, (3) determination of the statistical significance of heterogeneity among studies in relation to the study hypothesis, and (4) a graphical display of size of the samples. The meta-analysis displayed in Fig. 9 illustrates that the relative risk (RR) shows that increased physical activity over all forms of intensity statistically reduces the likelihood of hip fracture for both males and females. The largest sample in the study was contributed by Hoidrup et al. (2001). However, all the point estimates of the RR's are in the same direction (test of heterogeneity was nonsignificant, $p = 0.43$, and $p = 0.37$, respectively for females and males) although the result of all studies did not each show a statistically significant reduction (i.e., the upper limit of the confidence interval contained 1.0). Meta-analysis is also useful when all studies regarding a program intervention do not yield the same finding, even when the same study design is used.

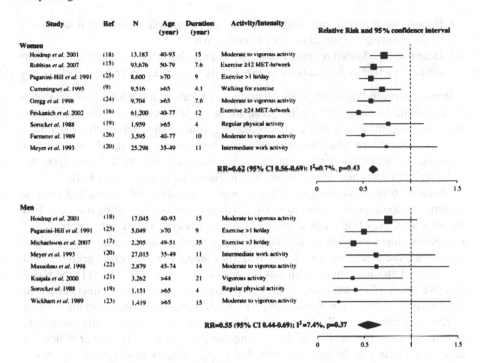

Fig. 9 Meta-analysis of 13 prospective studies for the association between physical activity and hip fracture. MET = metabolic equivalent (Reprinted from Moayyeri, 2008 with permission from Elsevier)

The qualitative aspect of the meta-analysis is the decision criteria involved in which comprises the systematic review of the literature. The general steps and criteria for the selection of a study are to be included in a meta-analysis. These are as follows:

1. State databases to be searched (e.g., PubMed, SciSearch, and EMBASE)
2. List all words and terms searched for primary and secondary endpoints of the study and various combinations of terms (e.g., activity: "motor activity," "physical activity," "exercise"; hip fractures: "fractures, bone," "fractures, hip," "osteoporosis," "bone density," "densitometry, X-ray," "accidental falls," "calcaneus ultrasonography")
3. Restrict the analysis of publications with same study design and variables examined. Search references of these publications for other relevant articles.
4. Ask experts in the field for additional references.
5. Include studies that have the same operational definitions of the main study independent variables (exposure or intervention).
6. If a longitudinal study, ensure all included studies had a minimum follow-up period.
7. Determine a time interval for selecting study (e.g., excluding studies before a certain time when diagnostic criteria substantially changed).
8. Determine if any study populations should be excluded (e.g., different populations and population subgroups have a different relation between body mass index and risk of diabetes).

9. Include most recent, one study with the largest sample, longest follow-up if a study results are reported in more than one article.
10. Determine if adjusted or crude rate measures only should be included (e.g., exclude studies in which only results for adjusted body mass index were presented).

Criteria regarding the "quality" of an article to include in a meta-analysis may also be used. In determining the "quality" of an article a scoring system is developed by the study investigator to determine a priori the inclusion of an article such as adequacy of details regarding how the diagnosis was made were presented, adequacy of response or participation rate. Guidelines for including an article based upon the statistical quality of the article are offered in Bailar and Mosteller (1988).

Because this study design analyzes pooled existing data compiled from a systematic, comprehensive review of the existing published literature, it is classified herein within the observational studies group and is considered retrospective even though the meta-analysis itself could be comprised of intervention studies. The results of a meta-analysis are viewed with the same caution as cross-sectional and case-control studies. Thus, the disadvantages of a meta-analysis are: (1) the retrospective nature of the analysis, (2) the computation of an "average" effect combined over many population types and time periods, (3) biases emerging from the pooling of results using potentially different study protocols (e.g., dosing, data collection, follow-up time), (4) stability of the findings or the impact of time over which the individual studies included were compiled (e.g., changes in diagnostic methods, changes in health of the populations studies), (5) the potential bias regarding the selection of studies included for the analyses, and (6) lack of uniform criteria for sufficiency or how many individual studies are required for valid conclusions to be drawn (avoiding a Type I or Type II error). With the volumes of health care research published daily, it may be difficult to draw conclusions from any one article and a series of articles investigating a particular relationship may even provide contradictory results. Therefore, a meta-analysis, by pooling study results to increase the available sample size for analysis, offers a number of advantages that include: (1) the generalizability of findings because of the large number of studies evaluated, (2) the reduction of the likelihood of a Type II error, namely a false negative finding, because of the larger size of the overall sample, (3) the exploration of a risk factor(s) or treatment effect(s) in population subgroups that would otherwise not be able to be evaluated in a single study, and (4) the generation of new hypotheses, particularly about duration and timing of exposure or intervention, because of the large size of the sample examined.

Intervention Study Designs

An intervention study is one in which manipulation of the independent variable occurs. The units of analysis of the effects of the intervention may or may not be randomized and differentiate whether or not the study is a quasi-experimental design or true experimental design. Intervention studies may or may not have a longitudinal component depending upon when the outcome of interest is to be measured. When applied to epidemiology and managerial epidemiology practice, intervention studies are used to test strategies for reducing risk factors or prognostic factors or for evaluating the efficacy of new programs.

A *quasi-experimental design* involves manipulation of the independent variable, but the unit of analyses is not randomly assigned to a study group either because a comparable study group is not available, some cross-contamination of the intervention within an organization can occur from the ways individuals interact or are organized may occur, or that randomization to the units of measurement are not feasible because a sampling frame of individuals within a sampling element is not available.

The randomization or other form of assignment (e.g., ranking of percentage of eligible students or patients of a particular category) of the elements, such as schools, clinics, communities, hospital wards, home care agencies which contain the units targeted for measurement of the intervention effects, is one type of quasi-experimental design. This type of design is often used for testing programmatic interventions intended for large populations for whom randomized is not feasible, but immediate favorable outcomes are desired such as health promotion projects, clinical practice guidelines, use of coaches or other facilitators to improve staff performance, or even an intervention intended to change the entire organizational culture such as some quality improvement or leadership initiative. The students, staff, or patients within the elements randomized or otherwise assigned are measured. The classic studies of the effects of fluoridated water upon the reduction of dental caries exemplify this form of quasi-experimental study design (Bailey et al., 2008). Even when a whole community is intentionally assigned to health promotion intervention, the intervention may not reach all participants as they may be economically or socially disadvantaged or otherwise not able to be affected by the intervention.

A *time-series design* is another type of quasi-experimental design. This design examines the outcome across multiple time periods and at least one period before and after the intervention. This design is schematically represented as:

$$O_1, O_2, O_3, \dots O_i \text{ X } O_{i+1}, O_{i+2}, O_{i+3} \dots O_{i+n}$$

where X = the intervention, i = the period being measured for each n interval. For example, if the intervention is expected to have an effect within 1 year, monthly measurements of the outcome would be taken for at least 12 months before and 12 months after. The multiple measurements before and after are intended to determine the presence of any background trends occurring either prior to or subsequent to the introduction of an intervention, for example, if a downward trend in the outcome was occurring well before the intervention was introduced. This design is commonly seen in evaluating a new policy, law, or program (the "intervention"). Statistical analyses are utilized to determine if the rate of change over time is significant relative to the timing of the introduction of the intervention. The strength of the interpretation of results from this design is only as valid as the estimation of the interval after which the outcome is expected to occur. The determination of the optimal follow-up interval is even a larger challenge for program or policy evaluation as compared with longitudinal studies of disease outcomes because the natural history of the disease can at least be estimated from the pathobiology of the condition. This design provides more accurate interpretation of change than a pre-post (or before-after) study design as more time points are considered in the evaluation.

The most common *experimental study design* utilized in the health care is the *RCT*. The purpose of the RCT is to determine the efficacy of an intervention. Efficacy is the degree to which the desired beneficial outcome from the application of the intervention occurs under optimal conditions. In addition to manipulation of the independent variable, the unit of measurement of the outcome of interest is the same unit that is randomized. In human trials, eligible consenting subjects are assigned on a random basis to one of *n*-number of study groups. Consent means both to participation ("informed consent") and the sharing of health information for recruitment and or study participation (HIPAA approval, see also chapter "Epidemiology and the Public Policy Process"). The random assignment of study subjects is an attempt to ensure assignment to study groups in a nonbiased manner. The random assignment is also a means of equalizing the distribution of unknown or unmeasured factors which could affect the study outcome. The RCT may have a longitudinal observational component whereby the study outcome may not be determined immediately after the intervention. An RCT is also referred to as a Phase III clinical research design. The National Institutes of Health (NIH) Center for Scientific Review (http://cms.csr.nih.gov) defines the Phase III designs as follows:

> ...prospective clinical investigations for the purpose of investigating the efficacy of the biomedical or behavioral intervention in large groups of human subjects (from several hundred to several thousand) by comparing the intervention to other standard or experimental interventions as well as to monitor adverse effects, and to collect information that will allow the intervention to be used safely.

RCTs have the potential for a number of biases including selection bias (including only certain study populations, or participation is influenced by the health or diagnosis of participants), compliance (to treatment) bias, attrition, and withdrawals. Attrition and withdrawal can reduce the sample size leading to a Type II error. Another limitation of most RCTs is the lack of representativeness in terms of race and ethnicity. Lack of trust due to historical abuse of research participants (e.g., Tuskegee study), lack of access to health care settings where clinical trials are conducted, cultural eligibility barriers (e.g., literacy, language), and economic barriers are barriers to enrollment in RCTs. These same factors which affect recruitment also influence retention of minorities in studies. Underwood and Alexander (2000) summarize the factors affecting recruitment and retention of minorities in clinical research. They underscore the importance of building trust between the research team and minority community as the key to higher participation rates.

Because of the rigor required in RCTs and their purpose, this study design is seldom used in program evaluation. The RCT design is more appropriate for determining what intervention may be most effective in a program or used as a basis for policy formulation (see Boxed Example 2).

Boxed Example 2 Evaluating the Efficacy of an Intervention Study

Problem: High rates of breast cancer mortality exist among black and women of low socioeconomic groups largely most present with late stage of the disease. Higher rates of breast cancer incidence exist among women who are first degree relatives. Increasing knowledge about the importance of breast cancer screening may lower the disparities.

Methods: A randomized clinical trial comparing intensive education on breast cancer screening standard clinic education was conducted to determine the impact upon breast cancer screening behaviors of first degree female relatives of breast cancer survivors. A low-income tri-ethnic group of female breast cancer survivors, postactive treatment, aged 21–64 years were randomized to one of the two study groups after informed consent. The breast cancer screening behaviors of first degree relatives were ascertained between 3 and 6 months after the breast cancer survivor completed her participation in the study group.

Data and results (Source: Oleske et al., 2007)

	Clinical breast exam scheduled		
Study group	Yes	No	Total
Intensive education	10	35	45
Standard clinic education	4	47	51

Null Hypothesis: The likelihood of receiving a clinical breast exam is the same between the two study groups.

EpiInfo™ was used to generate the following results:

Relative Risk (RR) = $10/45 \div 4/51 = 2.83$

Odds Ratio (OR) = $10/35 \div 4/47 = 3.36$

$P = 0.046$

Managerial Epidemiology Interpretation: The RR and the OR are used to determine the strength of the relationship between exposure and an outcome except for that the RR uses risk measures. In this case, both the OR and RR are positive and of similar magnitude and represent a statistically significant association ($p = 0.046$). This is expected as the OR is an estimate of the RR. Those relatives in the intensive education group were 2.83 times more likely to have scheduled a clinical breast exam than those in the standard clinic education group. This association is statistically significant and the null hypothesis is rejected. The health care manager from these data concludes that intensive education of the breast cancer survivor to spread the message in the community of the importance of breast cancer screening is highly effective in producing a favorable breast cancer screening behavior among her first degree relatives. This may aid in avoiding some of the late stage presentations of breast cancer by high-risk low income women.

Sample Considerations in Study Designs

The sample size and sample disposition are critical to any epidemiologic study design. The final sample assembled for analysis drives the nature of the conclusions drawn for both program evaluation and epidemiologic research.

The elements considered in determining the *sample size* is how large an error will be tolerated in estimating the magnitude of a problem or the effects of the intervention. There are different methodologies for calculating samples sizes for different study designs, matched and unmatched samples, statistical methods used, and number of variables independent and dependent considered. Common to all determinations of sample size required for a study regardless of design, the following elements must be specified in advance for the computation:

- Determination of the level of measurement of the unit of analysis (categorical or continuous)
- The test statistic used for determining the final evaluation or study outcomes
- Amount of change important to detect as a result of the intervention
- The power required to test the study hypothesis
- The analysis plan (matched sample, independent samples, multiple study groups of different sizes)
- The significance level (or Type I error)

For the specifics of calculations, the reader should refer to texts which give the details of the determination of the adequacy of a sample to be acquired to form conclusions from the results of a program evaluation or research study. For details concerning formulae for the computation of sample size for descriptive studies, the reader should consult Levy and Lemeshow (2008) and for observational and intervention studies Fleiss et al. (2003).

Regardless of the study design utilized in evaluation or a research study, the *disposition of the study sample* should be examined and reported. The disposition of the study sample should be reported according to the following categories:

- Eligible to be screened
- Unable to contact for screening
- Refused screening
- Ineligibles (those excluded, did not meet inclusion criteria)
- Eligible to participate after screening
- Refused participation before entry into study
- Investigator removal of sample due to insufficient exposure information
- Lost to follow-up (for studies with a longitudinal component)
- Moved out of study area
- Withdrawals (refusal to continue to participate [may represent adverse experience of study participation])
- Investigator removal of sample due to missing key outcome information
- Final analytic sample (completed the number of required follow-up visits and have completed exposure/intervention and outcome information [in studies with a longitudinal component, typically have at least the baseline and final follow-up visit])

The various reasons for nonparticipation in a study indicate that the definition of a refusal rate depends upon the denominator. It may be preferable to report a participation rate (the number who participate/those who were screened who met the study eligibility criteria × 100%). Displayed in Figs. 10 and 11 are templates for the disposition of a study sample, a cross-sectional study and randomized intervention study, respectively. In Fig. 10, the final sample utilized for analysis is 1,189 who have met all the study eligibility criteria and had information to evaluate the relationship between "exposure" and outcomes of interest. In Fig. 11, the resultant study sample available for analysis was also determined by the number of eligible study units who remained or were available for observation for the entire study period (187 and 192 households, respectively). A graphical representation of the disposition of the study sample aids in determining what may be potential sources of sample bias that may affect the conclusions drawn from the program evaluation or research study.

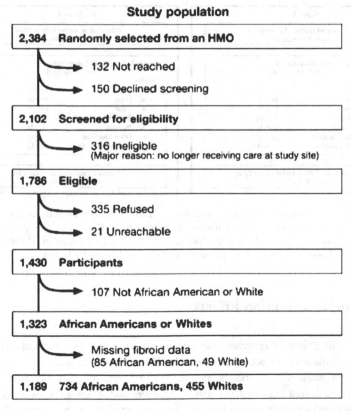

Fig. 10 Disposition of a study sample for a cross-sectional study (Reprinted from Baird et al., "Association of physical activity with the development of uterine leiomyoma," *Am. J. Epidemiol.* 2009;165(2):157–163 by permission of Oxford University Press)

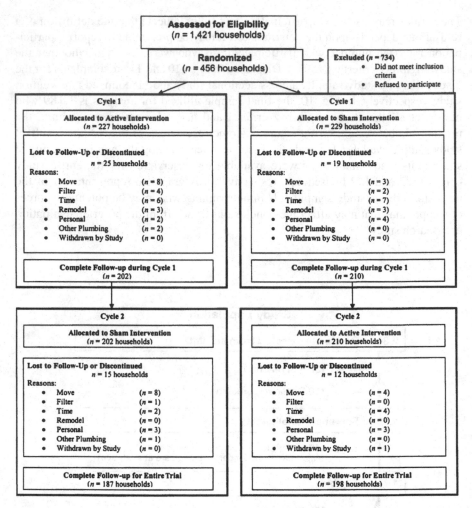

Fig. 11 Disposition of a study sample for a randomized controlled trial of in-home drinking water intervention to reduce gastrointestinal illness (Reprinted from Colford et al., "A randomized, controlled trial of in-home drinking water intervention to reduce gastrointestinal illness," 2005; 161(5):472–482, *Am. J. Epidemiol.* by permission of Oxford University Press)

Analyzing Intervention Effects

Analysis of the effects of program intervention commonly uses statistical methodologies and/or some form of economic analysis. The selection of a statistical method to analyze intervention effects depends upon the study design selected, the sampling strategy used in the design (e.g., matched sampling, independent sample), the level of measurement applied for evaluating outcomes, the number of outcomes measured, and the number of potential confounding or effect modifying variables considered (see chapter

"Measurement Issues in the Use of Epidemiologic Data"). The program itself is usually represented as a nominal level measurement (intervention present or absent; assigned to intervention or comparison group). Similarly, program outcomes or the dependent variables commonly also focus on the presence or absence of a condition at the conclusion of the program. For these reasons, the discussion of statistical measures in study designs used for program evaluation will focus on logistic regression, survival analysis, Cox proportional hazards regression, and survival analysis. When program outcomes are continuous, multiple linear regression may be the preferred analytic method and the reader should consult text for biostatistical methods such as those described in Rosner (2006). When an economic analysis is used to supplement program or health system evaluation, the reader should consult Glandon (2001) for the two most common analytic approaches used, **cost-benefit analysis** and **cost-effectiveness analysis**. Cost-benefit analysis (CBA) is a plot of the dollars expended for a program (or other intervention) versus the quantified benefits of a program represented as society's monetary value of the outcome (e.g., the cost of lives saved). Cost-effectiveness analysis plots the costs in dollars of a program (or intervention) versus the actual outcomes of a program expressed which are also expressed in quantifiable health outcome terms such as infant mortality rate, quality-adjusted life years rather than the monetary measures of outcomes used in CBA. For both analytic methods, the total costs must be compiled, both direct (e.g., salaries, equipment) as well as indirect (e.g, the time spent caregiving, travel time to assist in caregiving). In economic analyses, epidemiologic data provide data used for both the benefits and effectiveness components of these equations as well as aiding in modeling the sensitivity parameters (upper and lower bounds of estimated morbidity, mortality or utilization) for the estimates.

Logistic regression is a statistical method used to evaluate an intervention when the outcome variable is categorical (binary or ordinal), the independent variable (intervention) is dichotomous, and covariates can be categorical or continuous. This model requires that all the outcomes have been observed for the same amount of time in both study groups. This model estimates the odds ratio (OR) from the antilog of the logistic equation:

$$OR = e^{\beta x}$$

When performed using only one exposure variable at one level and a dichotomous outcome, the antilog of a univariate logistic regression model will yield the same value as the OR computed from a 2 × 2 table (see chapter "Descriptive Epidemiological Methods"). The test significance of the OR evaluates the null hypothesis of an exposure or risk factor represented as $\beta X_i = 0$. Because the OR is a point estimate of the true OR, the statistical significance of the OR can also be determined from computing the 95% confidence interval (CI). The general format for the computation of the 95% CI is:

$$UCL \text{ for } OR = e^{\beta + 1.96[SE(\beta)]}$$

$$LCL \text{ for } OR = e^{\beta - 1.96[SE(\beta)]}$$

Logistic regression can be performed using the statistical software packages Minitab 15 and SAS (PROC LOGIST) can be used for both binary and ordinal analyses. If the upper and lower 95% CI contain 1.0, the OR is not significantly different from an OR = 1. The wider the CI, the less precise is the estimate of the OR, even if statistically significant. A small sample size and few events in the exposure category contribute to the imprecision.

Survival analysis is used in program evaluation when the outcome of interest does not occur immediately after the intervention and the individuals who come in to the intervention enter and complete the program at different points in time. Survival analysis compares graphically and statistically the probability of an event (e.g., smoking cessation) between one or more groups in consideration of the amount of time each member of the group was observed. The most common method for constructing survival estimates is the product-limit method (Kaplan and Meier, 1958) whereby the survival function (s) at a given time (t) represents the probability of surviving $t \geq 0$ multiplied by the proportion of individuals surviving just before $t+1$.

The steps to obtain $s(t)$ using the product-limit method are: (1) define the number of persons at risk for the event at the beginning of the interval; (2) compute the number of persons experiencing the event in the first time interval; (3) divide the number experiencing the events by the total number starting (who were alive not experiencing the event) the interval (the conditional probability); (4) compute the probability of surviving beyond this point by repeating steps 1–3 and multiplying the conditional probability from each successive time interval. The survival function $s(t_i)$ is computed as the cumulative probability of overall survival as follows:

$$s(t_i) = (1 - E_1 / p_0)_{t0} \times (1 - E_2 / p_1)_{t1} \times (1 - E_3 / p_2)_{t2} \ldots (1 - E_i / p_i)_{t+1}$$

A graph of the cumulative probability of survival constructed by multiplying the probability of survival (s) through time (t) in interval $(i - 1)$ in which an event (E_i) occurred in the population at risk (p) in the time interval before the occurrence of the next event is called a product-limit or Kaplan-Meier survival curve. The estimated s within each time interval is calculated by dividing the number of events by the population at risk during the time interval. The time interval in which the event occurs becomes the next "plateau" in the curve extending over time until the next event occurs or the observation period ends. The data in Table 2 were used to construct Figure 4. The estimated survival curve in the figure self-rated health group (SRHG) excellent, very good or good using the above formula is computed as follows:

$$s(5.5\text{mos.}) = (1 - 1/8) = 0.8750$$
$$s(12.2 \text{ mos.}) = s(5.5\text{mos.}) \times (1 - 1/3) = 0.583$$
$$s(12.6 \text{ mos.}) = s(12.2 \text{ mos.}) \times (1 - 1/2) = 0.292$$

If the survival is computed and compared for two or more groups, the members of each group must be monitored according to the same intervals over time to accurately ascertain the time of the occurrence of the event under study. If the outcome was observed, that observation is termed "uncensored"; if the outcome was not observed by the time the study ended, the observation is "censored" at the time

Table 2 Data for survival analysis computation for low back pain recurrence according to self-rated health

(a) Subjects followed to determine low back pain recurrence, follow-up time, and self-rated health

Subject number	Self-rated health group[a]	Follow-up time to low back pain recurrence or drop out (months)	Low back pain recurrence[b]
1	1	6.2	No
2	1	12.2	Yes
3	1	12.0	No
4	1	13.0	No
5	1	12.6	Yes
6	1	12.0	No
7	1	11.9	No
8	1	5.5	Yes
9	2	8.8	Yes
10	2	6.2	Yes
11	2	5.9	Yes
12	2	5.2	Yes
13	2	9.6	Yes
14	2	12.4	Yes
15	2	11.8	No

[a] 1 = Excellent, very good, good, 2 = fair, poor
[b] Yes = 1 (uncensored event), No = 0 (censored event)

(b) Data organized from (a) to compute Kaplan–Meier estimates

Self-rated health group	Time (months)	Number at risk	Number failed	Survival probability
1	5.5	8	1	0.875
1	12.2	3	1	0.583
1	12.6	2	1	0.292
2	5.2	7	1	0.857
2	5.9	6	1	0.714
2	6.2	5	1	0.571
2	8.8	4	1	0.429
2	9.6	3	1	0.286
2	12.8	1	1	0.000

observation was concluded. A logrank statistical test compares the equality of the curves. Figure 12 displays Kaplan–Meier survival curves for low back pain recurrence by self-rated health group. The group with the higher self-rated health had a better survival than those with a lower self-rated health. The graphical and statistical analysis comparing two or more survival curves can be performed in Minitab 15 selecting the statics tab for *Reliability/Survival > Distribution Analysis (Right Censoring) > Parametric Distribution Analysis*. The validity of the survival estimate is enhanced by following a cohort long enough to enable documentation of all the events of interest ("uncensored" observations). Too many censored observations at the end of the study time may invalidate the results of the study. Survival analyses can be performed by most statistical software including freeware (http://seer.cancer.gov/seerstat/tutorials/survival3/). Caution should be used in interpreting any

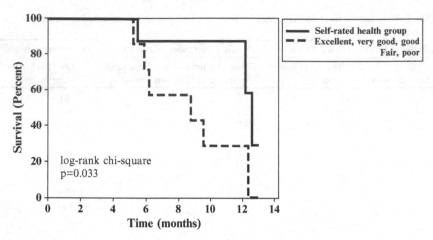

Fig. 12 Kaplan–Meier survival curves for recurrence of low back pain by self-rated health group

survival curves because the conditions that exist at the time in which the cohort was originally constructed (e.g., use of certain treatment and support modalities, better nutrition, etc.) may not apply to cohorts more recently constructed. Hence, survival analyses may underestimate the probability of some outcomes such as mortality. There are a number of statistical methods for testing the equality of survival curves (i.e., the null hypothesis is that survival is equal among the study groups) depending upon when the events occur over the time period observed.

Cox proportional hazards regression is a statistical test which compares two intervention groups with respect to the risk of an outcome (continuous or dichotomous) using some time metric to estimate hazard ratios and confidence intervals while adjusting for covariates. The assumption of proportional hazards is required to draw valid conclusions associated with this test. This assumption is evaluated by examining the graphs of survival curves constructed using the Kaplan–Meier methodology described above, namely proportional hazards are required for the validity of the Cox regression results. The model constructs the probability of outcome m at time t_j represented as $m(t)$, given that the population at risk $p(t)$ for the outcome at the beginning of an intervention has been observed for n intervals to time t_{j+n} as a hazard function $h(t)$:

$$h(t) = m(t)/p(t)$$

The Cox model then is represented as a regression equation:

$$h_i(t)/h_0(t) = e^{\beta i\, Xi}$$

where h = the hazard or probability of an outcome m at time t with (i) or without exposure (0) with coefficients (β_i) for an exponential set of variables (X_i). The ratio of the hazards in the above equation is the relative risk. Using the above formula and using data from Table 9.2, the relative risk (RR) of recurrence of low back pain in the self-rated health group poor, fair using SPSS Cox Regression is computed

Where:

$h_0(t)$ = the baseline hazard for a person with no recurrence assigned a value of 0 and assuming no time dependent covariates

$$\text{Recurrence} = \{ \begin{array}{l} 1 \text{ yes} \\ 0 \text{ no} \end{array}$$

$$\text{Self-rated health group} = \{ \begin{array}{l} 1 \text{ Poor, fair} \\ 0 \text{ Excellent, very good, good} \end{array}$$

β = coefficient of the self-rated health group = 1.597

RR (comparing recurrence to non-recurrence) = $e^{(1.597)}$ = 4.938

Those in the poor, fair self-rated health group are 4.938 times more likely to experience a low back pain recurrence within 13 months of follow-up. Since only 40% of the events are censored, the estimate of the RR has acceptable validity. This analysis can be also performed using the statistical software package SAS (PROC PHREG). This method should only be used if a small proportion of the observations are censored. Cox regression is the preferred method of comparing interventions when the members of the groups are not observed for the same period or when time varying covariates such as length of time enrolled in a program (Cox, 1972). An example of the application of the Cox model would be to determine the extent to which a global measure of self-rated health predicts hospitalization for cardiovascular disease in a cohort of elderly subjects followed over a 14-year period (Kennedy et al., 2001).

Summary

Evaluation and the concepts of study design and selection of analytic methods underlying it are not only essential to primary epidemiologic research, but also to program evaluation. Given the amount of resources involved in the launch of any new program or policy, evaluation needs to be incorporated and initiated as planning begins. The evaluation process itself may require the investment of resources, the amount of which varies depending upon what aspects of the health system are being evaluated, and the degree of involvement of multiple partnerships in conducting the program. Depending on who or what is requiring the evaluation or study should be the source of the funding for the evaluation. For example, if a health program is government-mandated then support for the evaluation should be supported by the appropriate government agency. Programs with wide-spread impact such as the WIC (Women, Infant and Children's) Program (http://www.fns.usda.

gov/wic/) require that all the major aspects of evaluation be considered, quality, access, availability, continuity, acceptability, efficiency, be considered in the design of an evaluation in addition to effectiveness by a multidisciplinary group of medical and nonmedical professionals and public members to accomplish the assessment. The understanding of the level of evidence, advantages and disadvantages of a study design and accompanying analytic methods, provides the building blocks for epidemiologic practice in program evaluation. Information from evaluations can be used for a wide range of purposes from determining the impacts of various health care alliances to aiding in deciding what services should continue or how treatments could be modified to be more effective.

Discussion Questions

Q.1. Use a statistical software package of your choice to analyze the data from Table 1 and replicate the correlation coefficients from the ecologic study results in Fig. 5a and b. Would you come to the same conclusions that alcohol is a potential risk factor for pancreatic cancer in males and females? Would you come to the conclusion that vegetable consumption is protective against pancreatic cancer? What are the limitations of this study design in drawing conclusions about potential risk factors or protective factors for any health problem? Cite some examples when use of this study design would be appropriate.

Q.2. Assuming a large managed care plan serves a population the represents a microcosm of America, select one leading chronic condition in the USA. Outline the evaluation plan for a program implemented by a managed care plan to lower the prevalence of this condition among its members.

Q.3. The "Know Your Body" program for reducing coronary heart disease risk factors in black youth was implemented in nine schools in the District of Colombia (Bush et al., 1989). Schools were randomly assigned to a control or an intervention group and focused on enrolling black students who were in grades 4–6 at baseline. Students enrolled in the study were followed for 3 years. Why were black youth targeted for this program? Why were schools randomized to the study group instead of students? What activities could be undertaken to maximize initial participation of students in the study program? Continued participation?

Q.4. The Third National Health and Nutrition Examination Survey (NHANES III) Linked Mortality File is a rich source of information regarding a wide variety of health and risk factors associated with mortality (see also chapter "Measurement Issues in the Use of Epidemiologic Data"). What type of study design(s) is (are) used in the compilation of this data file? What are sources bias using this database in computing odds ratios of potential risk factors (see also chapter "Descriptive Epidemiological Methods") relative to the study design?

References

Allaire, S.H., LaValley, M.P., Evans, S.R., O'Connor, G.T., Kelly-Hayes, M., Meenan, R.F., et al., 1999, Evidence for decline in disability and improved health among persons aged 55 to 70 years: The Framingham Heart Study, *Am. J. Pub. Health.* **89**:1678–1683.

Austin, M.A., King, M., Bawol, R.D., Hulley, S.B., and Friedman, G.D., 1987, Risk factors for coronary heart disease in adult female twins: genetic heritability and shared environmental influences, *Am. J. Epidemiol.* **125**:308–318.

Bailar, J.C., III, and Mosteller, F., 1988, Guidelines for statistical reporting in articles for medical journals, *Ann. Intern. Med.* **108**:266–273.

Bailey, W., Barker, L., Duchon, K., and Maas, W., 2008, Populations receiving optimally fluoridated public drinking water–United States, 1992–2006, *M.M.W.R.* **57**:737–41.

Baird, D.D., Dunson, D.B., Hill, M.C., Cousins, D., and Schectman, J.M., 2007, Association of physical activity with development of uterine leiomyoma, *Am. J. Epidemiol.* **165**:157–163.

Beard, J.R., Tracy, M., Vlahov, D., and Galea, S., 2008, Trajectory and socioeconomic predictors of depression in a prospective study of residents of New York City, *Ann. Epidemiol.* **18**:235–243.

Brownson, R.C., Gurney, J.G., and Land, G., 1999, Evidence-based decision making in public health, *J. Pub. Health Manag. Pract.* **5**:86–97.

Bush, P.J., Zuckerman, A.E., Theiss, P.K., Taggart, V.S., Horowitz, C., Sheridan, M.J., and Walter, H.J., 1989, Cardiovascular risk factor prevention in black schoolchildren: two-year results of the "Know Your Body" program, *Am. J. Epidemiol.* **129**:466–482.

Clement, D.G., and Wan, T.T.H., 2001, Evaluating health services, programs, and systems: an epidemiological perspective, In *Epidemiology and the Delivery of Health Care Services: Methods and Applications*, 2nd ed., D.M. Oleske (ed.), Plenum, New York.

Colford, J.M., Wade, T.J., Sandhu, S.K., Wright, C.C, Lee, S., Shaw, S., Fox, K., Burn,S., Benker, A., Brookhart, M.A., van der Laan, M., and Levy, D.A., 2005, A randomized, controlled trial of in-home drinking water intervention to reduce gastrointestinal illness, *Am. J. Epidemiol.* **161**:472–482.

Coogan, P.F., and Rosenberg, L., 2004, Impact of financial incentive on case and control participation in a telephone interview, *Am. J. Epidemiol.* **160**:295–298.

Cox, D.R., 1972, Regression models and life-tables, *J.R. Statist. Soc.* **B34**:187–220.

Davis, S., Onstad, L., Kopecky, K.J., Wiggins, C., and Hamilton, T.E., 2008, Locating members of a cohort identified retrospectively from limited data in 50-year-old records: successful approaches employed by the Hanford Thyroid Disease Study, *Ann. Epidemiol.* **18**:187–196.

Donabedian, A., 1966, Evaluating the quality of medical care, *The Milbank Mem. Fund Quart.* **44**:166–203.

Donahue, J.G., Weiss, S.T., Livingston, J.M., et al., 1997, Inhaled steroids and the risk of hospitalization for asthma, *J.A.M.A.* **277**:887–891.

Ellison, L.F., 2006, An empirical evaluation of period survival analysis using data from the Canadian Cancer Registry, *Ann. Epidemiol.* **16**:191–196.

Fabio, A., Loeber, R., Balasubramani, G.K., Roth, J., Fu, W., and Farrington, P., 2006, Why some generations are more violent than others: assessment of age, period, and cohort effects, *Am. J. Epidemiol.* **164**:151–160.

Fisher, E.S., Wennberg, D.E., Stukel, T.A., Gottlieb, D.J, Lucas, F.L., and Pinder, E.L., 2003, The implications of regional variations in Medicare spending. Part 2: Health outcomes and satisfaction with care, *Ann. Intern. Med.* **138**:288–298.

Fleiss, J.L., Levin, B., and Paik, M.C., 2003, *Statistical Methods for Rates and Proportions*, 3rd ed., Wiley, Hoboken, NJ.

Glandon, G.L., 2001, The contribution of epidemiological information in economic decision making. In *Epidemiology and the Delivery of Health Care Services: Methods and Applications*, 2nd ed. (D.M. Oleske, ed.), pp. 309–328, Plenum, New York.

Gu, Q., Burt, V.L., Paulose-Ram, R., Yoon, S., and Gillum, R.F., 2008, High blood pressure and cardiovascular disease mortality risk among U.S. adults: the Third National Health and Nutrition Examination Survey Mortality Follow-up Study, *Ann. Epidemiol.* **18**:302–309.

Hartge, P., Brinton, L.A., Rosenthal, J.F., et al., 1984, Random digit dialing in selecting a population based control group, *Am. J. Epidemiol.* **120**:825–833.

Hoidrup, S., Sorensen, T.I.A., Stroger, U., Lauritzen, J.B., Schroll, M., and Gronbaek, M., 2001, Leisure-time physical activity levels and changes in relation to risk of hip fracture in men and women, *Am. J. Epidemiol.* **154**:60–68.

Jennings, J.M., Louis, T.A., Ellen, J.M., Srikrishnan, A.K., Sivaram, S., Mayer, K., Solomon, S., Kelly, R., and Celentano, D.D., 2005a, Geographic prevalence and multilevel determination of community-level factors associated with herpes simples virus type 2 in Chennai, India, *Am. J. Epidemiol.* **167**:1495–1503.

Jennings, J.M., Curriero, F.C., Celentano, D., and Ellen, J.M., 2005b, Geographic identification of high gonorrhea transmission areas in Baltimore, Maryland, *Am. J. Epidemiol.* **161**:73–80.

Kaplan, E.L., and Meier, P., 1958, Nonparametric estimation from incomplete observations, *J. Am. Statist. Assoc.* **53**:457–481.

Kennedy, B.S., Kasl, S.V., and Vaccarino, V., 2001, Repeated hospitalizations and self-rated health among the elderly: a multivariate failure time analysis, *Am. J. Epidemiol.* **153**:232–241.

Kitahata, M.M., Rodriguez, B., Haubrich, R., Boswell, S., Mathews, W.C., Lederman, M.M., Lober, W.B., Van Rompaey, S.E., Crane, H.M., Moore, R.D., Bertram, M., Kahn, J.O., Saag, M.S., 2008, Cohort profile: the Centers for AIDS Research Network of Integrated Clinical Systems, *Int. J. Epidemiol.* **37**:948–955.

Kulldorff, M., 1997, A spatial scan statistic, *Commun. Stat. Theory Meth.* **26**:1481–1496.

Lacey, J.V., Leitzmann, M., Brinton, L.A., Lubin, J.H., Sherman, M.E., Schatzkin, A., and Schairer, C., 2006, Weight, height, and body mass index and risk for ovarian cancer in a cohort study, *Ann. Epidemiol.* **16**:869–876.

Langenberg, C., Bergstrom, J., Laughlin, G.A., and Barrett-Connor, E., 2005, Ghrelin, adiponectin, and leptin do not predict long-term changes in weight and body mass index in older adults: longitudinal analysis of the Rancho Bernardo Cohort, *Am. J. Epidemiol.* **162**:1189–1197.

Levy, P.S, and Lemeshow, S., 2008, *Sampling of Populations: Methods and Applications*, 4th ed., Wiley, Hoboken, NJ.

Luft, H.S., Rappaport, K.M., Yelin, E.H., and Aubry, W.M., 2006, Evaluating medical effectiveness for the California Health Benefits Review Program, *HSR: Health Serv.Res.* **41**:1007–1026.

Mello, M.M., Stearns, S.C., Norton, E.C., and Ricketts, T.C., 2003, Understanding biased selection in Medicare HMOs, *Health Serv. Res.* **38**:961–992.

Moayyeri, A., 2008, The association between physical activity and osteoporotic fractures: a review of the evidence and implications for future research, *Ann. Epidemiol.* **18**:827–835.

Morgenstern, H., 1995, Ecologic studies in epidemiology: concepts, principles, and methods, *Ann. Rev. Public Health.* **16**:61–81.

Oleske, D.M., Kwasny, M.M., Lavender, S.A., and Andersson, G.B.J., 2007a, Participation in occupational health longitudinal studies: predictors of missed visits and dropouts, *Ann. Epidemiol.* **17**:9–18.

Oleske, D.M., Galvez, A., Cobleigh, M.A., Ganshow, P., and Ayala, L.D., 2007b, Are tri-ethnic low-income women with breast cancer effective teachers of the importance of breast cancer screening to their first-degree relatives? *Breast J.* **13**:19–27.

Rogers, A., Murtaugh, M.A., Edwards, S., and Slattery, M.L., 2004, Contacting controls: are we working harder for similar response rates, and does it make a difference? *Am. J. Epidemiol.***160**:85–90.

Rosner, B., 2006, *Fundamentals of Biostatistics*, 6th ed., Duxbury/Thomson/Brooks/Cole, Belmont, CA.

Ryerson, A.B., Miller, J., Eheman, C.R., and White, M.C., 2007, Use of mammograms among women aged >40 years – United States, 2000–2005, M.M.W.R. **56**:49–51.

Safaeian, M., Brookmeyer, R., Vlahov, D., Latkin, C., Marx, M., and Strathdee, S.A., 2001, Validity of self-reported needle exchange attendance among injection drug users: implications for program evaluation, *Am. J. Epidemiol.* **151**:169–175.

Samelson, E.J., Kelsey, J.L., Kiel, D.P., Roman, A.M., Cupples, L.A., Freeman, M.B., Jones, R.N., Hannan, M.T., Leveille, S.G., Gagnon, M.M., and Lipsitz, L.A., 2008, Issues in conducting epidemiologic research among elders: lessons from The MOBILIZE Boston Study, *Am. J. Epidemiol.* **168**:1444–1451.

Schootman, M. J., Jeff, D.B., Gillanders, W.E., Yan, Y., Jenkins, B., and Aft, R., 2007, Geographic clustering of adequate diagnostic follow-up after abnormal screening results for breast cancer among low-income women in Missouri, *Ann. Epidemiol.* **17**:704–712.

Selassie, A.W., Pozsik, C., Wilson, D., and Ferguson, P.L., 2005, Why pulmonary tuberculosis recurs: a population-based epidemiological study, *Ann. Epidemiol.* **15**:519–525.

Suissa, S., 2008, Immortal time bias in pharmacoepidemiology, *Am. J. Epidemiol.* **167**:492–499.

Stone, M.B., Lyon, J.L., Simonsen, S.E., White, G.L., and Alder, S.C., 2007, An internet-based method of selecting control populations for epidemiologic studies, *Ann. Epidemiol.* **165**.109–112.

Stukel, T.A., Lucas, F.L., and Wennberg, D.E., 2005, Long-term outcomes of regional variations in intensity of invasive vs medical management of Medicare patients with acute myocardial infarction, *J.A.M.A.* **293**:1329–1337.

Tsai, S.P., Ahmed, F.S., Wendt, J.K., Bhojani, F., and Donnelly, R.P., 2008, The impact of obesity on illness absence and productivity in an industrial population of petrochemical workers, *Ann. Epidemiol.* **18**:8–14.

Underwood, S.M., and Alexander, G.A., 2000, Participation of minorities and women in clinical cancer research, *Ann. Epidemiol.* **10**:S1–S2.

Von Elm, E., Altman, D.G., Egger, M., Pocock, S.J., Gotzsche, P.C., and Vandenbroucke, J.P. for the STROBE Initiative, 2007, The strengthening the reporting of observational studies in epidemiology (STROBE) statement: guidelines for reporting observational studies, *Bull. World Health Org.* **85**:867–827.

Wang, Y., and Beydoun, M.A., 2007, The obesity epidemic in the United States—gender, age, socioeconomic, racial/ethnic, and geographic characteristics: a systematic review and meta-regression analysis, *Epidemiol. Rev.* **29**:6–28.

Wennberg, J.E., Fisher, E.S., Stukel, T.A., Skinner, J.S., Sharp, S.M., and Bronner, K.K., 2004, Use of hospitals, physician visits, and hospice care during last six months of life among cohorts loyal to highly respected hospitals in the United States, *B.M.J.* **328**:607–611.

Wennberg, J.E., Fisher, E.S., Goodman, D.C., and Skinner, J.S., 2008, *Tracking the Care of Patient with Severe Chronic Illness: the Dartmouth Atlas of Health Care 2008*, The Trustees of Dartmouth College, Lebanon, NH.

Zhang, J., Zhao, J., and Berkel, H.J., 2005, Animal fat consumption and pancreatic cancer incidence: evidence of interaction with cigarette smoking, *Ann. Epidemiol.* **15**:500–508.

Chapter 5
Screening and Surveillance for Promoting Population Health

Learning Outcomes

After completing this chapter, you will be able to:

1. Distinguish between screening and surveillance activities.
2. Interpret the accuracy of a screening test.
3. Identify limitations associated with screening for a health problem.
4. Plan a surveillance system based upon known risk factors for a health problem.
5. Identify limitations of a surveillance system.

Keyterms Positive predictive value • Screening • Surveillance • Surveillance system • Syndrome surveillance

Introduction

In managing the health of populations, prevention measures may not be feasible or highly effective. Moreover, prevention strategies for many health conditions may not be well known. For this reason, screening and surveillance are important strategies in managing population health in communities and in populations receiving health care services. Fundamental to the success of both screening and surveillance in terms of improving population health is knowledge of the natural history of the health problem and the ability to accurately detect the problem early.

Screening

The primary purpose of screening is to identify early signs and symptoms of a disease or health problem to implement early treatment or program intervention to reduce the likelihood of the emergence of disease or health problem and/or mortality from the disease in an individual. Screening in populations is only undertaken when

D.M. Oleske (ed.), *Epidemiology and the Delivery of Health Care Services:*
Methods and Applications,
DOI 10.1007/978-1-4419-0164-4_5, © Springer Science+Business Media, LLC 2009

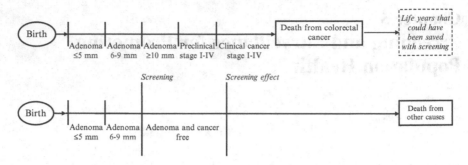

Fig. 1 Impact of screening upon the clinical course of colorectal cancer (Adapted from: Zauber et al., 2008)

Table 1 Examples of common screening tests and condition targeted for screening

Test	Targeted condition
Clinical breast exam	Breast cancer
Denver II (formerly Denver Developmental Screening Test, DDST)	Identification of children from birth to 6 years of age who may require additional evaluation to promote healthy development
Digital rectal exam	Prostate cancer
Fecal occult blood test	Colon cancer
Mammography	Breast cancer
Papanicolaou test	Invasive cervical cancer
Phenylketonuria Screening (PKU)	A rare genetic condition caused by a defect in the enzyme phenylalanine hydroxylase (PAH) which cases a build-up of phenylalanine resulting in mental retardation and behavioral abnormalities
Prostate specific antigen	Prostate cancer
Rapid HIV	Human Immunodeficiency Virus

there is proven benefit to the screening and the natural history of the disease is well established as for example with colorectal cancer (see Fig. 1). Screening may employ a technology (e.g., mammography), laboratory testing (e.g., prostatic specific antigen [PSA] blood test), a survey form (e.g., *Center for Epidemiologic Studies Short Depression Scale* [CES-D 10], Radloff, 1977), skill-based testing (e.g., *The Denver II*, Frankenburg et al., 1992), clinical assessment (e.g., digital rectal exam for prostate cancer), or a combination thereof. Table 1 lists examples of common screening tests and the condition targeted for the screening.

The value of a screening test is determined by its ability to distinguish a diseased from nondiseased state. Ideally, the screening test should have 100% specificity, 100% sensitivity, and 100% positive predictive value (PPV). Manufacturers provide information on the accuracy of screening tests produced. The computation of the values to assess a screening test was presented in chapter "Descriptive Epidemiological Methods." Criteria that should be considered when choosing a screening test follow principles presented in chapter "Epidemiological Study

Designs for Evaluating Health Services, Programs, and Systems" for Program Evaluation and are also useful in this selection process:

- Relatively inexpensive
- Easy availability
- High accuracy
- Can alter the course (severity, mortality) of a disease or health problem
- Acceptable to target population
- Convenient for staff
- Results are quickly available

Another approach to evaluating the accuracy of a screening test is to prepare a receiver operating characteristic (ROC) curve. This graphical technique is used when test measures are ordinal and the outcome (disease) measure is nominal, a likelihood ratio (LR) for each level of the test is computed and the area under a ROC curve is used to assess criterion validity. An ROC curve is a plot of the true positive rate (sensitivity) vs. the false positive rate (1-specificity) for each level of the test. The test level where an LR of 1.0 is exceeded is defined as the threshold for positivity or the cut point at which the value for the test will significantly predict the outcome. Statistical software is available to easily construct LRs and ROC curves using statistical software such as SPSS Inc.'s *Predictive Analytic Software* portfolio (http://ww.spss.com). The greater the area under the curve (AUC), the greater is the accuracy of the test measure in predicting the outcome represented by AUC = 1, perfect prediction and where AUC = 0.5 is random prediction. Figure 2 evaluates the value of the Body Mass Index (BMI) in screening for overweight in adolescents using ROC curves. Both ROC curves in Fig. 2 illustrate that use of BMI is a good method for screening for overweight in adolescents, with BMI providing a more accurate prediction of excess fatness in adolescent males than in females.

Not all screening is conducted to prevent disease. There are certain genetic conditions that are required by States for screening. It is established public health practice to screen newborns from a blood spot for selected endocrine (e.g., hypothyroidism), metabolic (e.g., phenylketonuria [PKU]), hematologic (e.g., sickle cell), and functional (e.g., hearing) disorders (Therrell et al., 2008). Although the conditions for which newborn screen is done are not currently preventable, many newborns can avoid severely disabling or fatal consequences to intervention if screening is conducted soon after delivery. Nutritional interventions, namely avoiding high protein foods in infancy, can prevent mental retardation in children with PKU. Treatment with a thyroid hormone, levo-thyroxine, can prevent mental retardation in children with congenital hypothyroidism.

Screening and screening tests can be conducted in a variety of settings, both traditional (in provider offices, clinics, health departments or hospitals) and nontraditional (schools, pharmacies, shopping malls, airports) (Boxed Example 1). Increasingly, screening tests are available for over-the-counter purchase for self-administration and at nontraditional health service settings (pharmacies offering cholesterol testing, liver function testing, diabetes screening, and hemoglobin A1C testing). Although these trends are important in engaging communities in healthy behaviors,

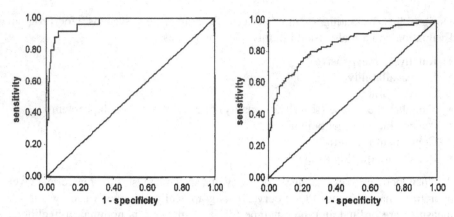

Fig. 2 (a) Receiver operating characteristics curve for male adolescents. BMI was significantly better than chance as a diagnostic test for excess fatness [X (0.97 ± 0.02; $n = 200$)]. The $45°$ represents chance as a diagnostic test (area under the curve = 0.5). Excess fatness cutoff = 25%. (b) Receiver operating characteristics curve for female adolescents. BMI was significantly better than chance as a diagnostic test for excess fatness [X (0.85 ± 0.02; $n = 274$)]. The $45°$ represents chance as a diagnostic test (area under the curve = 0.5). Excess fatness cutoff = 30% (From Neovius et al., 2004, with permission American Journal of Clinical Nutrition by Neovius, M.G., et al. Copyright 2004 by American Society for Nutrition. Reproduced with permission of American Society for Nutrition in the format textbook via Copyright Clearance Center.)

screening is not a substitute for regular contacts with a health care provider with whom the results should be shared, validated with a physical exam, and compared over time. A comprehensive review of the state of the evidence regarding screening practices for cancer in adults, cardiovascular, and respiratory diseases, infectious diseases, injury and violence, mental health and substance abuse, metabolic conditions, musculoskeletal conditions, obstetric and gynecologic conditions, vision disorders, and conditions in children is available in *The Guide to Clinical Preventive Services* (U.S. Preventive Services Task Force, 2008).

Boxed Example 1   Mammography or MRI in Detecting Breast Cancer in Younger Women?

Problem: The value of detecting tumors by mammographic screening in younger women is controversial because they have denser breasts than postmenopausal women. Yet, it is important to conduct screening in women who have a family history of breast cancer or are carriers of the BRCA1 or BRCA2 or other mutations as these conditions are after associated with a diagnosis at a younger age.

Methods and Data: Women ages 25–70 years with a genetic risk of breast cancer (cumulative lifetime risk of 15% or more) were recruited from six cancer clinics in the Netherlands. Surveillance was conducted by means of clinical breast exam by an experienced physician every 6 months and imaging studies performed annually.

Results (Data from: Kriege et al., 2004):

	Sensitivity (%)	
Screening method	Invasive breast cancer	Specificity (%)
Clinical breast examination (CBE)	17.9	98.1
Mammography	33.3	95.0
MRI	79.5	89.8

Magnetic resonance imaging (MRI) has a higher sensitivity rate than either CBE or mammography in detecting invasive breast cancer. The high sensitivity means that more True Positive cases are identified or that cases that test positive really have the disease. The False Negative rate is the lowest for MRI (100% − % Sensitivity = % False Negative; 100% − 79.5% = 20.5%). This means that fewer true positive cases are missed. The specificity is of similarly high magnitude among the three screening methods. This means there is a high percentage of cases that test negative that are truly negative.

Managerial Epidemiology Interpretation: The health care manager should understand that CBE is least likely to identify true positive cases of breast cancer, but is most likely to correctly classify true negatives. Mammography is not as effective in detecting breast cancer in young high risk women as MRI. MRI may be the screening method of choice for breast cancer in high risk young women.

The formulation of screening goals for a community, health plan membership, physician practice, or other population group should be undertaken by a health services manager practicing with epidemiologic principles. These should be crafted in consideration of national screening goals. Displayed in Table 2 are the *Healthy People 2010* screening goals for the USA.

Challenges to the Benefit of Screening

Large scale community-based screening, such as sexually transmitted disease (STD) walk-in clinics, offers various free services, including confidential and/or anonymous testing for human immunodeficiency virus (HIV). In community-based screening, tests with high specificity and high sensitivity may yield large numbers of persons with false positive or false negative results. Test results are influenced by test-kit handling, storage conditions, clinic/laboratory quality assurance protocols, test inventory lot quality, test operator training and proficiency, external controls, and patient characteristics. Also, different testing methods for the same condition using different bodily fluids may yield different results. For example, OraQuick® oral fluid testing (OraSure Technologies, Bethlehem, Pennsylvania) was found to

Table 2 Selected health goals from *healthy people 2010* and supporting details for screening populations, United States (Source: U.S.D.H.H.S. (2000))

Goal 3-11b	Women aged 18 years and older who received a Pap test within the preceding 3 years
National data source:	National Health Interview Survey (NHIS), CDC, National Center for Health Statistics (NCHS)
State data source:	Behavioral Risk Factor Surveillance System (BRFSS), CDC, National Center for Chronic Disease Prevention and Health Promotion (NCCDPHP)
Measure:	Percent (age adjusted)
Baseline:	79 (1998)
Numerator:	Number of women aged 18 years and older who report receiving a Pap test within the past 3 years
Denominator:	Number of women aged 18 years and older
Population targeted:	US civilian, noninstitutionalized population
Questions used to obtain the national data:	From the 1998 National Health Interview Survey: Have you ever had a pap smear test? *[If yes:]* When did you have your most recent pap smear test? Was it a year ago or less, more than 1 year but not more than 2 years, more than 2 years but not more than 3 years, more than 3 years but not more than 5 years, or over 5 years ago?
Goal 3–12	*Increase the proportion of adults who receive a colorectal cancer screening examination*
Goal 3-12a	*Adults aged 50 years and older who have received a fecal occult blood test (FOBT) or stool blood test within the preceding 2 years*
National data source:	National Health Interview Survey (NHIS), CDC, NCHS
State data source:	Behavioral Risk Factor Surveillance System (BRFSS), CDC, NCCDPHP
Measure:	Percent (age adjusted)
Baseline:	35 (1998)
Numerator:	Number of adults aged 50 years and older who report receiving fecal occult blood testing within the preceding 2 years
Denominator:	Number of adults aged 50 years and older
Population targeted:	US civilian, noninstitutionalized population
Questions used to obtain the national data:	From the 1998 National Health Interview Survey: A blood stool test is when the stool is examined to determine whether it contains blood. Have you ever had a blood stool test? *[If yes:]* When did you have your most recent blood stool test? Was it a year ago or less, more than 1 but not more than 2 years, more than 2 years but not more than 3 years, more than 3 years but not more than 5 years, or more than 5 years ago?
Goal 3-12b	*Adults aged 50 years and older who have ever received a sigmoidoscopy*
National data source:	National Health Interview Survey (NHIS), CDC, NCHS
State data source:	Behavioral Risk Factor Surveillance System (BRFSS), CDC, NCCDPHP
Measure:	Percent (age adjusted)
Baseline:	37 (1998)

(continued)

Table 2 (continued)

Goal 3-11b	Women aged 18 years and older who received a Pap test within the preceding 3 years
Numerator:	Number of adults aged 50 years and older who report ever receiving a sigmoidoscopy
Denominator:	Number of adults aged 50 years and older
Population targeted:	US civilian, noninstitutionalized population
Questions used to obtain the national Data:	From the 1998 National Health Interview Survey: A proctoscopic examination is when a tube is inserted in the rectum to check for problems. Have you ever had a proctoscopic examination?
Goal 3–13	*Increase the proportion of women aged 40 years and older who have received a mammogram within the preceding 2 years*
National data source:	National Health Interview Survey (NHIS), CDC, NCHS
State data source:	Behavioral Risk Factor Surveillance System (BRFSS), CDC, NCCDPHP
Measure:	Percent (age adjusted)
Baseline:	67 (1998)
Numerator:	Number of women aged 40 years and older who report receiving a mammogram within the past 2 years
Denominator:	Number of women aged 40 years and older
Population targeted:	US civilian, noninstitutionalized population
Questions used to obtain the national data:	From the 1998 National Health Interview Survey: A mammogram is an X-ray taken only of the breasts by a machine that presses the breast against a plate. Have you ever had a mammogram? *[If yes:]* When did you have your most recent mammogram? Was it a year ago or less, more than 1 year but not more than 2 years, more than 2 years but not more than 3 years, more than 3 years but not more than 5 years, or over 5 years ago?

have high false positive rates (or lower specificity) than finger-stick rapid testing whole-blood specimens for HIV. Out of 1,720 screened with oral fluid rapid testing, 343 false positive results occurred (Cummiskey et al., 2008). The efficacy of screening may also be mitigated by the strength of other risk factors acting upon intermediate steps in the causal pathway for a disease. Heavy cigarette smoking (≥ 40 pack-years) is highly associated with carcinoma in situ (Terry et al., 2000). The persistence of intermediate risk factors (e.g., heavy cigarette smoking) for an intermediate step of a disease may diminish the time-window for detecting an early phase of the disease, such as the early detection of adenomas in heavy cigarette smokers.

Some screening may not be able to be conducted anonymously or without bias. Such is the challenge with screening for obesity, particularly childhood obesity. Parental consent, overrepresentation of younger children, a lower response among adolescents, concerns over social stigma may all affect participation in screening for obesity (Crosbie et al., 2008).

Because screening may yield variability in specificity and sensitivity, either due to explained or unexplained variance, health care managers should have plans in place if results are unacceptable. These include monthly evaluation of screening specificity and sensitivity relative to manufacturer's reported results, repeat screening testing, utilizing confirmatory testing, and selecting a different manufacturer.

Surveillance

Surveillance is the systematic process of identifying, collecting, orderly summarization, analysis, and evaluation of data about specific diseases or health problems with the prompt dissemination of finding to those who need to know and those who need to take action. Response by the health system includes communication of risk identified from surveillance to the public, introduction of countermeasures such as recall of products, treatment of individuals who could transmit the disease, or the administration of immunizations. Surveillance can focus on the identification of: awareness of specific medical conditions (e.g. stroke events), behavioral risk factors (factors leading to the increased risk of a health problem because of an action or task) (e.g., needlestick injury surveillance, adverse drug events), birth defects, chronic diseases, clinical syndromes clustering (because of their potential for bioterrorism), dental caries, health-related quality of life (HRQoL), infectious diseases, indicators of the potential for infectious diseases in humans (e.g., surveillance of dead birds in identifying emergence of West Nile Virus), injuries, preventive service utilization, procedure utilization (e.g., assisted reproductive technology), and health problems whose prevalence is expected to markedly increase over time (e.g., epilepsy) (Centers for Disease Control, 2008; Chowdhury et al., 2007; Pelletier et al., 2005; Piriyawat et al., 2002; Wright et al., 2008; Zahran et al., 2005), and other health problems (e.g., nonfatal maltreatment of infants).

The process of surveillance begins with the definition of the "case." A case is initially defined by what is unusual about the disease, usually clinically by a set of signs and symptoms and their onset focused on unusual findings (e.g., mid-lobe lung consolidation pneumonia-like presentation on chest X-rays in SARS cases) and related to some common exposure (e.g., travel to a location where other known cases were identified). The case definition can then be further refined clinically (i.e., fewer signs and symptoms) or through expanded suspicions of a common cause or "exposure." Relevant screening laboratory tests of the cases are then followed up with confirmatory diagnostic testing. The more homogenous the clinical presentation, the more likely a common source of exposure can be identified. A Lyme disease case, one of the most rapidly increasing incidence rates of vectorborne diseases in the USA, is defined for surveillance purposes by the presence of a rash (erythema migrans), clinical signs (musculoskeletal, cardiovascular, neurologic), and laboratory determination of the presence of *Borrelia burgdorferi* in consideration of exposure to areas with infected ticks (Bacon et al., 2008). In addition to clinical and laboratory criteria for defining a case, epidemiologic criteria may be utilized as was with the surveillance case definition of Severe Acute Respiratory Syndrome (SARS). Epidemiologic criteria for SARS included one or more of the following exposures in the 10 days before onset of symptoms: Travel to a foreign or domestic location with documented or suspected recent transmission of SARS or close contact with a person with mild-to-moderate or severe respiratory illness and with history of travel in the 10 days before onset of symptoms to a foreign or domestic location with documented or suspected recent transmission of SARS (CDC, 2005).

Surveillance methodology for collecting data on confirmed or possible cases and other relating information can be accomplished through field surveys, reports of notifiable conditions from laboratories and health care providers to public health authorities, or review of existing databases or records. Table 3 describes selected surveillance systems and their target conditions. Data and trends from surveillance systems aid in planning for community- and population-based responses to emerging health problems. Data from the FoodNet consumption survey provided baseline comparisons in the general public of eating items (chicken and peanut butter) to help isolate the outbreak strain and source of a multistate outbreak of *Salmonella* infections associated with peanut butter and peanut butter-containing products (Medus et al., 2009).

Surveillance can be active or passive. The surveillance strategy selected depends upon the definition of the case, the objectives of the surveillance, and how information about risk factors for the condition is collected and also should consider the national health priorities for surveillance (Table 4). Regardless of the surveillance method used, medical and public health system resources should be prepared for action if a surveillance system identifies:

- A number of cases of an illness meeting a specific definition are larger than expected
- Unusual severe diseases or routes of transmission
- Unusual geographic presentation, seasonal occurrence, or absence of normal vector or
- Higher attack rates in persons with normal levels of exposure

It is important to note that surveillance systems or surveillance activities are not intended to support case management or referral services when cases are identified.

Active Surveillance

Active surveillance is the systematic, active searching for all possible events in real time using routine prospective collection of information about specific health problems and their risk factors. Cases are identified from laboratory results, admissions records to hospitals or emergency departments, radiology reports, outpatient facilities, or doctor's office's logs or billing records of presenting complaints. Active surveillance involves the process of screening, namely, locating cases with signs and symptoms that meet well-defined criteria related to a diagnosis, or proxies of human cases. Active surveillance is directed at determining if changing risk factors or more toxigenic strains are emerging which may impact communities and health care settings and to attempt to prevent through rapid case identification the spread

Table 3 Examples of surveillance systems

Surveillance system	Purpose	Website
Behavioral Risk Factor Surveillance System (BRFSS)	On-going telephone health survey system, tracking health conditions and risk behaviors in the USA yearly since 1984.	www.cdc.gov/brfss
Foodborne Diseases Active Surveillance Network (FoodNet)	The principal foodborne disease component of CDC's Emerging Infections Program (EIP) using active surveillance of 650 clinical laboratories that test stool samples in the ten FoodNet sites	www.cdc.gov/foodnet
Illinois environmental public health tracking	Surveillance of environmental hazards, exposure to environmental hazards, and human health effects potentially related to these exposures	www.idph.state.il.us/about/epi/epht.htm
International clearinghouse for birth defects surveillance and research	Brings together birth defect programs from around the world with the aim of conducting worldwide surveillance and research to prevent birth defects and to ameliorate their consequences	www.icbdsr.org
National child abuse and neglect data system	Compiles case-level data on as child-specific records for each report of alleged child maltreatment for which a completed investigation or assessment from a local child protective service agency has been made during the reporting period. Data collected annually from states since 1993	http://www.childwelfare.gov
National Electronic Injury Surveillance System (NEISS)	Recording of an injury associated with consumer products derived from emergency visits to a probability sample of hospitals in the USA and its territories and includes patient information	www.cpsc.gov/library/neiss.html
World Health Organization (WHO) STEPwise approach to Surveillance (STEPS)	Provides a methodology for obtaining core data on the established risk factors that determine the major chronic disease burden with a special focus on stroke	www.who.int/chp/steps/en
Surveillance, Epidemiology, and End Results (SEER)	Source of information on cancer incidence, martality and survival in the USA since 1973	www.seer.cancer.gov

Table 4 Disease syndromes targeted for surveillance and possible etiologies

Disease syndrome	Possible etiology
Gastrointestinal illness	Cholera, salmonella, shigella; Food poisoning due to: *S. aureus, B.cereus, E.coli*, ricin toxin, etc.
Hepatitis illness	Hepatitis A, yellow fever, alflatoxin, many chemical poisonings
Influenza-like illness	Influenza, RSV, rhinoviruses. Early stages of pulmonary anthrax, plague, and tularemia
Encephalitis	Eastern equine, Venezuelan equine, western equine, West Nile virus
Neuro-toxic	Botulism, shellfish toxin, chlorinated hydrocarbons, organophosphates, organic mercury, sarin, VX nerve agent, BZ, cyanide
Pulmonary disease	Pulmonary forms of anthrax, plague, tularemia, glanders, hantavirus, and chlorine gas
Rash illness	Cutaneous anthrax, smallpox, T2 mycotoxins, and mustard agents
Sepsis	Crimean-congo, ebola, lass, and marburg hemorrhagic fevers
Systemic disease	Brucellosis, typhoid, bubonic plague, Q fever, rift valley fever, tularemia
Radiation	Exposure to radioactive chemicals, X-rays, or other radiation source

of transmissible disease which has a high potential for serious illness or death such as *Clostridium difficile* or West Nile Virus (WVN) (Lindsey et al., 2008; Rabatsky-Ehr et al., 2008). Active surveillance for a condition similar to WNV involves collecting weekly information on the presence of this arbovirus in humans, animals, and mosquitos. Compiled data by state health departments are communicated to the CDC through a web-based system based upon reports from: (1) health care providers and clinical laboratories regarding human cases of WNV disease, (2) WNV presumption blood donors from blood collection agencies, (3) the testing of dead birds, (4) veterinarians to collect reports of WNV infection in nonhuman mammals, and (5) mosquitoes (Lindsey et al., 2008). Although typically identified as an essential component of public health practice for the control of transmissible diseases, the value of surveillance for noninfectious health problems is increasingly utilized in health services settings. For example, surveillance is an intervention utilized by nurses in the prevention of falls through the documentation of risk factors (e.g., physical impairments, cognitive impairments, inability to walk independently, incontinence, and use of certain medications such as diazepam, etc.) at admission and then monitoring these risk factors through the collection and monitoring clinical information throughout the course of the hospital stay. However, as with any active surveillance activities, the cost of the system needs to be considered relative to the resultant cost savings from the control or prevention of the outcome under surveillance (Klaucke et al., 1988; Shever et al., 2008). Thus, increasing the effectiveness of nursing intervention for surveillance for fall prevention may result in higher costs if more nursing staff would be required.

Two types of active surveillance are enhanced surveillance and syndrome surveillance. Enhanced surveillance is a type of active surveillance involving the prospective detection and simultaneous aggressive follow-up of reports of newly identified persons meeting the case definition of the disease to investigate. Enhanced surveillance: (1) focuses on the collection of accurate risk factor information, (2) guides prevention efforts, and (3) ensures referral to appropriate treatment

Table 5 Sample national goal for surveillance and surveillance systems, United States (U.S.D.H.H.S., 2002)

	Increase the number of States with an asthma surveillance system for tracking asthma
24–8.	cases, illness, and disability

Target: 25 states
Baseline: 19 States had a surveillance system for tracking asthma cases, illness, and disability in 2003
Target setting method: 32% improvement
Data source: Behavioral Risk Factor Surveillance System (BRFSS), CDC

for cases and their contacts. This type of surveillance is commonly activated when clusters of disease are identified or reported emerge and rapid response by public health agencies is likely (Leuchner et al., 2008).

The early identification of epidemics of contagious diseases commonly relies on the presentation of syndrome clusters is termed syndromic surveillance (Table 5). A syndrome is the grouping of nonspecific general conditions commonly representing the early symptoms of a disease. Chief complaints of selected conditions of public health concern, upon presentation during the registration process, most commonly to the emergency room. The chief complaints are then scored or coded, typically by a software package, to be assigned and grouped to syndrome category. This is of particular importance as the detecting of these clusters of symptoms can provide an early warning of a major epidemic of transmissible diseases or bio-chemical-radiological terror attack. Thus, syndrome surveillance is viewed as a type of active surveillance. The identification of certain syndromes would trigger reporting to public health officials. Data for the identification of syndromes through active surveillance can come from emergency rooms, STD programs, lead poising prevention programs, vital records, immunization programs, ambulance calls, pharmacy medication sales of prescription and over the counter medications, and linked demographic, outpatient pharmacy claims, physician and facility claims. Syndromic surveillance can be used to estimate the burden of disease in a community, recognizing that only a limited number of persons may come in contact with the health care system to be identified. The source of the disease could be human, exposures, or from environmental sources (*Cryptosporidium* contamination of water). Because it is a type of active surveillance, it may be a more rapid and hence efficient and effective means of providing data to prioritize the direction of field investigations as to a potential cause. It is estimated that for every flu-like illness presenting in an emergency room, 60 illnesses may occur among residents; every visit for diarrheal illness may represent 251 illnesses in the community (Metzger et al., 2004).

Passive Surveillance

Passive surveillance requires that the case has already been identified through diagnosis and/or coding or databases (see Boxed Example 2). Both infectious and noninfectious conditions can be identified through passive surveillance depending if the need to identify the condition and the validity of the signs and symptoms predicting

Boxed Example 2 The Practice of Surveillance in a Health Plan (Source: Shatin et al., 2004)

Problem: The prevalence of Hepatitis C virus (HC) had increased over twofold between 1975 and 1998, particularly among individuals of working age. This presents an opportunity for managed care plans to adopt surveillance strategies to identify HCV positive individuals for the purpose of implementing effective treatment strategies.

Case Definition: At least one outpatient claim with a Current Procedural Terminology-4 (CPT-4) for one or more criteria: (1) hepatitis C antibody test (CPT-4 86803), (2) hepatitis panel (CPT-4 80059) including hepatitis A, B, and C antibody tests; (3) hepatitis C, confirmatory test (CPT-4 86804); or (4) HCV RNA test (CPT-4 87520, 87521, 87522). A physician, health facility, or pharmacy claim with at least one primary or secondary ICD-9 diagnosis for HCV (070.44 or 020.54) or at least one prescription for interferon in combination with ribavirin.

Surveillance Strategy: Longitudinally link computerized claims with enrollment files containing patient demographics, with patient-specific identifiers eliminated.

Surveillance Results: The prevalence of HCV was 6.7% among those who were tested. The likelihood of HCV was higher among males (OR = 1.8) and older (≥25 years, OR = 32.0). Less than 35% of those identified with chronic HCV received treatment. Follow-up testing was more likely for those on combination therapy than compared with those on interferon monotherapy (OR = 6.2).

Managerial Epidemiology Interpretation: The continuous surveillance of health plan members can identify early those at high risk for HCV. Aggressive follow-up for treatment among those testing positive should be promoted by the health care manager.

the condition is not urgent. The National Notifiable Diseases Surveillance System (see chapter "Health Risks from the Environment: Challenges to Health Services Delivery") is an example of passive surveillance. States provide weekly reports of notifiable disease to the Centers for Disease Control and Prevention. The specific diseases and conditions that are notifiable are determined by the states and territories and reported information includes: the date identified, the location of the diagnosis, demographics of the case, and data specifically related to the disease/condition.

Passive surveillance can be conducted using existing datasets when the data on cases within it have been validated. For example, population-based surveillance of HRQoL is conducted as a means of promoting the health and quality of life of US residents and monitoring progress toward two *Healthy People 2010* goals, (1) increase the quality and years of healthy life and (2) eliminate disparities

(Zahran et al., 2005). The HRQoL data used are from validated items collected through the Behavioral Risk Factor Surveillance System using the measures of self-rated health and within the preceding 30 days, number of physically unhealthy days, number of mentally unhealthy days, and days of activity limitation. Passive surveillance can also be conducted through mapping strategies including those using global positioning systems coupled with geographic information systems form a new epidemiologic technique called geographic surveillance. As cases occur, they are assigned a coordinate for mapping purposes. The use of spatial statistics associated with these graphical techniques adds a new dimension of identifying significantly elevated numbers of cases in geographic areas that could be useful in identifying both infectious and noninfectious cases (Blumenstock et al., 2000; Roche et al., 2002). Various spatial statistics also determine if attribute values form a clustered, uniform, or random pattern across a region. Cluster analysis determining the location of the center of the data, the shape or orientation of the data, and the dispersion of the data may be evaluated using spatial statistical software such as ArcGIS (ESRI, Inc., Redlands, CA) and Spatial Statistics Toolbox for Matlab 2.0 (MathWorks, Inc. Natick, MA).

Evaluating the Quality of a Surveillance System

The quality of a surveillance system is measured in terms of seven dimensions, its: sensitivity, representativeness, timeliness, simplicity, flexibility, acceptability, and PPV (Klaucke et al., 1988). These criteria apply regardless of the health condition is transmissible, chronic, or another health problem (e.g., abuse). *Sensitivity* is the ability to accurately identify cases both in terms of diagnostic accuracy as well as the total count of the cases and their severity. Hence, sensitivity is essential to establishing the validity of the measurement of the phenomena under surveillance (see also chapter "Measurement Issues in the Use of Epidemiologic Data"). To assess if the criterion of sensitivity is met, the following questions should be asked: (1) Are reporting laboratories following appropriate protocols, including quality assurance, for testing? (2) Are providers following guidelines for the clinical spectrum for the definition of cases? (3) Can potential cases access the health care system to come to diagnostic attention, or will cases have to be identified through field surveys (e.g., contacting exposed persons by telephone)? Sensitivity of the system is also a function of the timeliness and completeness of reporting *Representativeness* is the assurance that all possible sources of data from which a case could be ascertained are funneled in to the surveillance system (e.g., for sexually transmitted disease [STD]: from STD clinics, prenatal clinics, prisons, etc.) and if these sources can accurately capture the projected incidence of the health event in the target population. *Timeliness* is defined as how quickly the cases are identified, specimens are transmitted for analysis, results transmitted to a central repository for analysis, and reports are prepared and disseminated. Increasingly, health departments are seeking to arrange for reporting through electronic means. Overhage et al. (2008) found that automated electronic laboratory reporting identified 4.4 times more cases and 7.9 days earlier compared with traditional spontaneous, paper-based methods or by postmail. Timely identification and reporting of cases, particularly within the disease-specific incubation period, is critical to not only accurately identify all cases, but also to capture information accurately about exposures, and implementation control measures quickly. Electronic reporting can also enhance the completeness of reporting to the health department and then support more focused investigation of the cases (Kit-Powell et al., 2008). *Simplicity* of the system is essential in order for staff as well as the population under surveillance and is a criterion which refers to both the structure as well as the processes. Less time is spent in staff training, formatting databases for analysis, and the timely distribution of information. Less error is generated with simple forms by increasing compliance with collecting and recording (see also chapter "Advancing Patient Safety Through the Practice of Managerial Epidemiology"). *Flexibility* is the ability to accommodate and adapt to new and different diseases or health conditions because of variations in case definition, reporting sources, testing protocols, or exposures. Automated electronic reporting systems can also meet the criteria of *simplicity* and *flexibility* with entry of information directly onto computer screens and into computer databases which can be modified with ease. *Acceptability* is the level of participation individual practitioners (health care providers and public health), health care organizations, and labs are willing to engage in regarding ascertaining cases and reporting them. Concerns regarding measures to ensure confidentiality of the case, time involved in reporting, who assumes the cost of case finding, and liability may affect reporting. The reader is advised to consult and be familiar with federal and state laws and guidelines on the collection, storage, and use of protected health information which may change over time. The Centers for Disease Control (2003) is an important source of guidance regarding the HIPAA Privacy Rule and Public Health. The *PPV* of a surveillance system (or a screening or diagnostic test) is the proportion of individuals identified as a case who actually do have the condition under surveillance (or who are positive to screening and who have the condition targeted for screening) (see also Table 4 of chapter "Measurement Issues in the Use of Epidemiologic Data"). The value of the PPV is a function of all the preceding quality elements of a surveillance system. The higher the PPV, the less likely that there are false leads in accurately characterizing an epidemic and more efficient deployment of resources in control measures.

Surveillance in Monitoring Progress in Disease Control

Surveillance is most effective when augmented with other surveillance activities being implemented such as electronic laboratory reporting, geographical information systems (GIS), animal health monitoring, ambulance runs, poison control data, and over-the-counter drug surveillance systems (Overhage et al., 2008). Incidence surveillance for HIV infection has been adopted as a component of the existing national HIV/AIDS reporting system which covers 22 states. The ability to identify new from long-standing cases of HIV-infection aids in determining if there has been a shift in population subgroups at risk because of changes in risk factor patterns and if disparities in health care or access to health care. The new system confirmed that the majority of new cases (72%) continued to be among men having sex with men. The HIV incident surveillance system has identified an increasing disparity in the incidence of HIV. The rate among black males 13–29 years was found to be 7.1 times higher than comparable age white males. Among black females, the incidence rate was 14 times the rate in white females (Prejean et al., 2008). These data stress the need for both more preventive efforts as well as improving access to care for high risk groups. Syndromic surveillance has been found particularly useful in detecting and monitoring annual outbreaks of influenza, norovirus, and rotavirus (Balter et al., 2005). Syndromic surveillance systems in "high-profile" urban areas can also provide a reassurance during heightened terror or other security alert situations to provide reassurance to the public that a certain condition or exposure (e.g., anthrax) is not present. Chronic disease surveillance in the USA utilizes 92 indicators from nine data sources (Pelletier et al., 2005). With increased data capacities and cross-walks among data systems, the use of multiple indicators in surveillance to monitor progress in achieving disease control is desirable.

Challenges Encountered with Surveillance Systems

The main challenge in implementing and maintaining a surveillance system is the cost. Cost categories include: personnel, operating costs, transportation, laboratory materials and supplies, intervention costs, communications costs, and capital equipment. The Centers for Disease Control and Prevention has developed a spreadsheet-based software, *SurvCost*, for estimating the cost resources involved operating a surveillance system. The program files and system specifications for use are available at: http://www.cdc.gov/idsr/survcost.htm.

Because of the cost, surveillance systems typically maintain the minimum amount of information required for addressing the targeted health problem and detailed clinical information may not be available. Individual-level socioeconomic information is also seldom included and population subgroups at greatest risk may not be identified. The inclusion of area-based socioeconomic indicators could provide increased sensitivity to surveillance of health disparities (Subramanian et al., 2006).

Lastly, a limitation of surveillance is that most systems rely on reporting or passive surveillance. The delay in reporting may not be sufficiently sensitive to detect a disease outbreak as a diagnosis may take days to weeks. Knowledge of the type of surveillance systems upon which decisions are made may aid in planning the timing of the deployment of system health care resources when surge capacity is needed. To address all these challenges, the next generation of surveillance systems for notifiable disease called the National Electronic Disease Surveillance System (NEDSS) will integrate the various reporting sources (labs, public) with clinical databases from hospitals, clinics, emergency rooms that are secured by Health Level Seven American National Standards Institute (HL7) security protocols for protected health information as well as an interface of automated grouping software (for syndromes), statistical and geospatial analysis (see Fig. 3). HL7 covers how messaging transactions regarding patient information to various data repositories are transmitted, authenticated, and determined to be complete and accurate (Edwards, 2008). This new system architecture will facilitate real-time surveillance and the early detection of outbreaks. The eventual integration of databases from outside the hospital setting, such as from pharmacies, is critical. Lack of access to health care and/or lack of health care insurance may prompt individuals to self-care/medications (e.g., purchase of over-the-counter antidiarrheals, cold remedies at pharmacies) or seek no care thereby missing and underestimating emerging diseases in some communities. The early detection of outbreaks through the integration of administrative data, public health data, laboratory data, and public/provider reporting through surveillance is an important strategy not only for preventing widespread disease outbreaks but also for combating infectious disease resistance to antibiotics through implementing control measures earlier when the first signs of increased statistical trends in diseases of public health importance emerge.

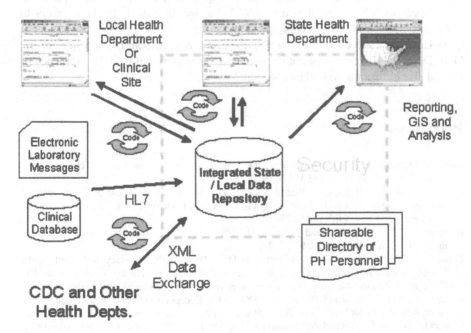

Fig. 3 Systems architecture of the National Electronic Disease Surveillance System (NEDSS) (Source: Centers for Disease Control and Prevention, http://www.cdc.gov/NEDSS (2008))

Summary

With costs of health care, impending health manpower shortages, and the increased prevalence of chronic conditions, fewer resources may be available in the near future for disease and health problem treatment. Screening and surveillance as measures for promoting population health will become increasingly important, not only in public health, but also in every health services delivery setting as well as for payors in the USA and worldwide. The availability of many large publicly available data sets as well as the increasing use of electronic health records in the delivery of care will make surveillance of populations served a standard of care for managerial epidemiologic practice. Although different in purposes and methodologies, screening and surveillance provide opportunities for potentially more cost-effective means of promoting health in populations served, particularly if the health care organization is serving populations at high risk for chronic conditions.

Discussion Questions

Q.1. Using epidemiological measures, prioritize what population subgroups should be targeted in a screening program for cancers of the following anatomic areas: breast, cervix, colorectal, prostate, and skin (including melanoma).
Q.2. If you were conducting a health screening in a Native American population, what conditions would you target? What would potentially be barriers to participation in this screening program?
Q.3. How can a surveillance system be utilized to reduce health care disparities?
Q.4. Describe the impacts of not being able to accurately estimate the incidence of a disease from a surveillance system.

References

Bacon, R.M., Kugeler, K.J., and Mead, P.S., 2008, Surveillance for Lyme disease—United States, 1992–2006, *Surveill. Summ. M.M.W.R.* **57**:1–9.
Balter, S., Weiss, D., Hanson, H., Reddy, V., Das, D., and Heffernan, R., 2005, Three years of emergency department gastrointestinal syndromic surveillance in New York City: What have we found? *M.M.W.R.* **54(Suppl.)**:175–180.
Blumenstock, J., Fagliano, J., and Bresnitz, E., 2000, The Dover Township childhood cancer investigation, *New Jersey Med.* **97**:25–30.
Centers for Disease Control and Prevention (CDC), 2003, HIPAA Privacy Rule and public health: guidance from CDC and the U.S. Department of Health and Human Services, *M.M.W.R.* **52(Suppl)**:1–19 available from: http://www.cdc.gov/mmwr/PDF/wk/mm52SU01.pdf.
Centers for Disease Control and Prevention (CDC), 2008, Epilepsy surveillance among adults – 19 states, Behavioral Risk Factor Surveillance System, 2005, *Survell. Summ., M.M.W.R.* **57**:No. SS-6.
Centers for Disease Control and Prevention (CDC), 2005, *Public Health Guidance for Community-Level Preparedness and Response to Severe Acute Respiratory Syndrome (SARS) Version 2* available from http://www.cdc.gov/ncidod/sars/reporting.htm.

Chowdhury, P.P., Balluz, L., Murphy, W., Wen, X., Zhong, Y., Okorno, C., Bartoli, B., Garvin, B., Town, M., Giles, W., and Mokdad, A., 2007, Surveillance of certain health behaviors among states and selected local areas - United States, 2005, *Surveill. Summ. M.M.W.R.* **56**:1–8.

Crosbie, A., Eichner, J., and Moore, W., 2008, Body mass index screening and volunteer bias, *Ann. Epidemiol.* **18**:602–604.

Cummiskey, J., Mavinkurve, M., Paneth-Pollak, R., Borrelli, J., Kowalski, A., Blank, S., and Branson, B., 2008, False-positive oral fluid rapid HIV tests—New York City, 2005–2008, *M.M.W.R.* **57**:660–665.

Edwards, W., 2008, Standards development and HIM: HL&'s IT standards work and its uses in health information management, *J.A.H.I.M.A.* **79**:58–59.

Frankenburg, W.K., Dodds, J., Archer, P., Shapiro, H., and Bresnick, B., 1992, The Denver II: a major revision and restandardization of the Denver Developmental Screening Test, *Pediatrics* **89**:91–97.

Kit-Powell, A., Hamilton, J.J., Hopkins, R.S., and DePasquale, J.M., 2008, Potential effects of electronic laboratory reporting on improving timeliness of infectious disease notification— Florida, 2002–2006, *M.M.W.R.* **57**:1325–1328.

Klaucke, D.N., Buehler, J.W., Thacker, S.B., Parrish, R.G., Trowbridge, F.L., Berkelman, R.L., and the Surveillance Coordination Group, 1988, Guidelines for evaluating surveillance systems, *M.M.W.R.* **37(S-5)**:1–18.

Kriege, M., Brekelmans, C.T.M., Boetes, C., Besnard, P.E., Zonderland, H.M., Obdeijn, I.M., Manoliu, R.A., Kok, T., Peterse, H., Tilanus-Linthorst, M.M.A., Muller, S.H., Meijer, S., Oosterwijk, J.C., Beex, L.V.A.M., ollenaar, R.A.E.M., deKoning, H.J., Rutgers, E.J.T., and Klijn, J.G.M. for the Magnetic Resonance Imaging Screening Study Group, 2004, Efficacy of MRI and mammography for breast-cancer screening in women with a familial or genetic predisposition, *New Engl. J. Med.* **351**:427–437.

Leuchner, L., Lindstrom, H., Burstein, G.R., Mulhern, K.E., Rocchio, E.M., Johnson, G., and Smith, P., 2008, Use of enhanced surveillance for hepatitis C virus infection to detect a cluster among young injection-drug users—New York, November 2004-April 2007, *M.M.W.R.* **57**:517–521.

Lindsey, N.P., Lehman, J.A., Staples, J.E., Komar, N., Zielinski-Gutierrez, E., Hayes, E.B., Nasci, R.S., Fischer, M., and Duffy, M., 2008, West Nile Virus activity—United States, 2007, *M.M.W.R.* **57**:720–732.

Medus, C., Meyer, S., Smith, K., Miller, B., Viger, K., Forstner, M., Brandt, E., Nowicki, S., Salehi, E., Phan, Q., Kinney, A., Cartter, M., Flint, J., Bancroft, J., Adams, Hyytia-Treesm, E., Theobald, L., Talkington, D., Humphrys, M., Bopp, C., Gerner-Smidt, P., Barton Behravesh, C., Williams, I.T., Sodha, S., Langer, A., Schwenson, C., Angulo, F., Tauxe, R., Date, K., Cavallaro, E., and Kim, C., 2009, Multistate outbreak of Salmonella infections associated with peanut butter and peanut butter-containing products—United States, 2008–2009, *M.M.W.R.* **58(Early Release)**:1–6.

Metzger, K.B., Hajat, A., Crawford, M., and Mstashari, F., 2004, How many illnesses does one emergency department visit represent? Using a population-based telephone survey to estimate the syndromic multiplier, *M.M.W.R.* **53(Suppl)**:106–111.

Neovius, M.G., Linné, Y.M., Barkeling, B.S., and Rossner, S.O., 2004, Sensitivity and specificity of classification systems for fatness in adolescents, *Am. J. Clin. Nutr.* **80**:597– 603.

Overhage, J.M., Grannis, S., and McDonald, C.J., 2008, A comparison of the completeness and timeliness of automated electronic laboratory reporting and spontaneous reporting of notifiable conditions, *Am. J. Pub. Health* **98**:344–350.

Pelletier, A.R., Siegel, P.Z., Baptiste, M.S., and Maylahn, C., 2005, Revisions to chronic disease surveillance indicators, United States, 2004, *Prev. Chronic Dis.* Available from: URL: http:// www.cdc.gov/pcd/issues/2005/jul/05_0003.htm.

Piriyawat, P., Šmajsová, M., Smith, M.A., Pallegar, S., Al-Wabil, A., Garcia, N.M., Risser, J.M., Moyé, L.A., and Morgenstern, L.B., 2002, Comparison of active and passive surveillance for cerebrovascular disease: The Brain Attack Surveillance in Corpus Christi (BASIC) Project, *Am. J. Epidemiol.* **156**:1062–1069.

Prejean, J., Song, R., An, Q., and Hall, H.I., 2008, Subpopulation estimates from the HIV Incidence Surveillance System—United States, 2006, *M.M.W.R.* **57**:985–989.

Rabatsky-Ehr, T., Mlynarski, D., Mshar, P., and Hadler, J., 2008, Surveillance for community-associated *Clostridium difficile* – Connecticut, 2006, *M.M.W.R.* **57**:340–343.

Radloff, L.S., 1977, The CES-D scale: A self-report depression scale for research in the general population, Appl. Psychologic. Measure. **1**:385–401.

Roche, L.M., Skinner, R., and Weinstein, R.B., 2002, Use of a geographic information system to identify and characterize areas with high proportions of distant stage breast cancer, *J. Pub. Health Manage. Pract.* **8**:26–32.

Shatin, D., Schech, S.D., Patel, K. and McHutchinson, J.G., 2004, Population-based hepatitis C surveillance and treatment in a national managed care organization, *Am. J. Managed Care* **10**:250–256.

Shever, L.L., Titler, M.G., Kerr, P., Win, R., Kim, T., and Picone, D.M., 2008, The effect of high nursing surveillance on hospital cost, *J. Nurs. Scholarship* **40**:161–169.

Subramanian, S.V., Chen, J.T., Rehkopf, D.H., Waterman, P.D., and Krieger, N., 2006, Comparing individual- and area-based socioeconomic measures for the surveillance of health disparities: a multilevel analysis of Massachusetts births, 1989–1991, *Am. J. Epidemiol.* **164**:823–834.

Terry, M.B., Neugut, A.I., Schwartz, S., and Susser, E., 2000, Risk factors for a causal intermediate and an endpoint: reconciling differences, *Am. J. Epidemiol.* **151**:339–345.

Therrell, B., Forey, F., Eaton, R., Frazier, D., Hoffman, G., Boyle, C., Green, D., Devine, O., and Hannon, H., 2008, Impact of expanded newborn screening—United States, 2006, *M.M.W.R.* **57**:1012–1015.

U.S. Department of Health and Human Services, 2000, *Healthy People 2010: Understanding and Improving Health*, 2nd ed., U.S. Government Printing Office, Washington, DC.

U.S. Preventive Services Task Force, 2008, *The Guide to Clinical Preventive Services*, (February 21, 2009), http://www.ahrq.gov/clinic/pocketgd.htm.

Wright, V.C., Chang, J, Jeng, G., and Macaluso, M., 2008, Assisted reproductive technology surveillance–United States, 2005, *Surveill. Summ. M.M.W.R.* **57**:1–23.

Zahran, H.S., Kobau, R., Moriarty, D.G., Zack, M.M., Holt, J., and Donehoo, R., 2005, Health-related quality of life surveillance--United States, 1993–2002, *Surveill. Summ. M.M.W.R.* **54**:1–35.

Zauber, A.G., Lansdorp-Vogelaar, I., Knudsen, A.B., Wilschut, J., van Ballegooijen, M., and Kuntz, K.M., 2008, Evaluating test strategies for colorectal cancer screening: a decision analysis for the U.S. Preventive Services Task Force, *Ann Intern Med.* **149**:659–669.

Chapter 6
Strategic Planning and Its Epidemiological Basis

Learning Outcomes

After completing this chapter, you will be able to:

1. Develop a mission statement for a health care organization based upon its population served.
2. Identify sources of epidemiologic data which can be used for strategic planning in a health care organization.
3. Apply the steps in the strategic planning process to favorably position a health care organization within the next 5 years.
4. Utilize epidemiologic methods to project the demand for health care services in a community.

Keyterms Capacity building • Market Mission • Stakeholders

Organizations that have as a mission the delivery of health care services cannot isolate themselves from the environments that surround them, particularly the population and other organizational entities, both public and private. According to Jaeger (2001), "strategic planning offers organizations a tool for analyzing the impact of changing trends and environmental conditions. It equips health care managers with a systematic process for setting future direction, developing effective strategies, and ensuring that the organization's structure and systems are compatible with long-term survival and success." Relevance of the mission is another consideration organizations must continue to address otherwise they face obsolescence. The rate of change in the health care environment renders an inflexible organization the possibility of failure. For these reasons, strategic planning is essential to any health care organization regardless of level of service provided. This chapter introduces the elements of strategic planning important for the health care manager and its epidemiological basis.

D.M. Oleske (ed.), *Epidemiology and the Delivery of Health Care Services: Method and Applications*,
DOI 10.1007/978-1-4419-0164-4_6, © Springer Science+Business Media, LLC 2009

What Is Strategic Planning?

Planning, in the epidemiological sense, is the process of addressing the health needs of a population in a geographically defined area through an assessment of the population's health and risk factors and organizations' capacity of promoting health and addressing health care needs. Planning establishes goals, objectives, priorities, and strategies for a particular setting. To establish a goal, planning requires a baseline measurement, informed decisions regarding a goal, a time frame for achieving the goal, and the ability to measure progress toward achieving the goal. Planning as a framework for the development of strategies takes into account the influence of social, behavioral, regulatory, organizational, technological developments, and environmental impacts upon health problems for the purpose of identifying priorities for interventions. Thus, resources, such as manpower can be more effectively deployed and technology acquired.

Strategic planning helps establish an organization's position relative to others in a competitive environment in making decisions about those resources. According to Jaeger (2001), it is "a systematic process that involves a series designed to define a situation or problem, develop strategies, and implement solutions." In the process of strategic planning, the members of the organization gain focus in the process of gathering data, making decisions, thereby aiding in the redirection of any cultural change required to achieve the stated goals.

Epidemiological Basis of Planning

The epidemiological basis of strategic planning according to Jaeger (2001) is: "to influence health positively by anticipating and responding to changes in needs and health status among population targeted for service." Knowledge of how populations change over time, in terms of size, demographic characteristics is also essential in beginning the strategic planning process. As population factors change, the types of health care services needed and the factors which influence utilization of these services change. Population size, regardless of age composition, is the most basic predictor of future health needs and services. The specific impact of population change is a function of the absolute numbers and relative proportion in the various age-gender subgroups (see chapter "An Epidemiologic Framework for the Delivery of Health Care Services," Fig. 2). The impacts are both in terms of the health needs profile of the population and the resultant estimated impact upon the health system. Because of this, organizations need to "employ a process, such as strategic planning, to maintain awareness of demographic changes and altered disease patterns" (Jaeger, 2001). If organizations are not appropriately responsive, that may not be responding appropriately to new health needs and service demands and risk obsolescence resulting in financial collapse.

The initial application of epidemiology in the planning process is to use or compute rate measures to quantify the frequency of events in population units (e.g., per 10,000 population) to judge trends in need. Prevalence data are the most useful epidemiologic measure in this regards because it reflects the total number of cases with a condition, new and continuing, in a specific time period and population, who are most likely in need for some form of health services. Subsequent to identifying need, epidemiological rate measures aid in planning health care utilization trends in relationship to identified needs. Utilization prevalence data are a proxy measure of need when disease rates are not available and aid in planning and assessing capacity of the health care organization or system to address the need (Fig. 1). Figure 1 illustrates the high need for emergency services for abdominal pain among all age groups. Planning from an epidemiologic perspective would seek to identify risk factors for this condition, particularly for those 18-29 years of age in order to address potential areas of unmet needs.

To illustrate how prevalence rates can be used in planning services, data from Table 1 are used to estimate the number of magnetic resonance imaging (MRI) procedures. To obtain the number of MRIs in a time period for this age group, the MRI rate in each specific age group is multiplied by the population in that same age group by a factor of 10. (Note: Convention dictates the same number of decimals to the right in the age-specific rate measures across strata or levels of a variable. The factor of 10 applied in each strata must be the same.) The number of MRIs utilized on average during 2004–2005 by individuals in the 45–64-year age group is computed as follows:

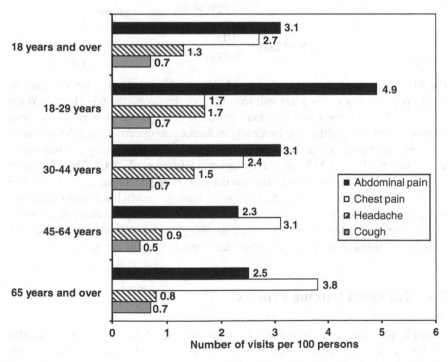

Fig. 1 Reasons for emergency department visits, U.S., 2006 (National Center for Health Statistics, 2009)

Table 1 Hospital discharges with at least one magnetic resonance imaging procedure in nonfederal short-stay hospitals, both sexes, by age group, United States, average annual 1994–1995 and 2004–2005 (National Center for Health Statistics, 2007)[a]

Age group (years)	MRI per 10,000 hospital discharges, 1994–1995	MRI per 10,000 hospital discharges, 2004–2005	Avg. US pop. 1994–1995	Avg. US pop. 2004–2005	No. of MRI 1994–1995	No. of MRI 2004–2005	1994–1995 to 2004–2005 % change in No. of MRI
45–64	12.0	10.8	52,056,080	71,767,767	62,467	77,509	24.1
65–74	24.5	23.7	18,827,940	18,551,643	46,128	43,967	4.7
75+	29.2	37.1	14,722,114	17,990,407	42,989	66,744	55.3
Total			85,606,134	108,309,817	151,584	188,221	24.2

[a] Utilization rates and population numbers have been averaged between the 2 successive years

$$\text{Rate} = \frac{\text{Events}_{g,t}}{\text{Population}_{g,t}} \times \text{Factor of } 10$$

Where g = age group and t = time period

$$\text{No. of MRI}_{45-64\,\text{years},\,2004-2005} = \frac{\text{MRI utilization rate}_{45-64\,\text{years},\,2004-2005}}{10,000}$$

$$\times \text{Population}_{45-64\,\text{years},\,2004-2005}$$

$$77,509\text{MRIs} = \frac{10.8}{10,000} \times 71,767,767$$

The MRI utilization rate as a measure of health need illustrates to planners that: the elderly population age 75+ years will require more resources, the 65–74-year-old age group may be a relatively healthy cohort, but those in the 45–64-year group following them may not be as healthy. The increasing incidence rate of certain neurological disorders in older persons, such as Alzheimer's and Parkinson's diseases, may also be prompting the increased use of MRIs to aid in diagnosis (Hebert et al., 2003; Van Den Eeden et al., 2003). Given epidemiologic data and the increasing population in the 45–64-year age group (baby boomers), and the anticipated increase in MRI utilization rates with increasing age, health planners should begin to consider the construction of additional facilities, new technologies, and the credentials, hiring and training of manpower (technicians and nurses) to handle the anticipated future needs for MRI services.

The Strategic Planning Process

Strategic planning is a systematic process conducted on a regular basis that involves a series of steps designed to position an organization to respond to a situation or problem, develop strategies, or to implement solutions. Epidemiological data provide on-going information regarding if new situations or problems arise in the geographic area of the organization as well as worldwide trends (e.g., increase in medical tourism). The strategic planning model assumes the organization has a vision and mission. The vision is a statement of the aspiration of an organization, namely where it sees itself, as defined by some criteria, in the future. The mission statement "provides a sense of purposefulness and direction for members of the organization (Gordon, 2002)." The mission statement defines the population served, the problem the organization intended to address, and the organization's response to the problem. The problems or responses cited in the mission statement represent, in rank order, the organization's priorities. The mission statement also informs external constituencies, including stakeholders.

The strategic planning process is based upon an epidemiologic framework asking the questions:

- *Who* is the organization? (current state, strengths, and weaknesses)
- *Where* does the organization want to be? (its vision)
- *Why* is the organization relevant to the market? (its mission)
- *How* will it get there? (resources)
- *When* can the organizations goals be achieved? (timing of final goal and supporting goals regularly evaluated)

The initiation of the strategic planning process cycle may be as short as every 3 years to as long as 5 or 10 years although the plan should be reviewed at least annually. The epidemiologic framework described in chapter "An Epidemiologic Framework for the Delivery of Health Care Services" and the sources of data described in chapter "Measurement Issues in the Use of Epidemiologic Data" are fundamental to the success of the strategic planning and are involved in most steps of the process. The steps and related tasks of the strategic planning process are schematically summarized as an iterative cycle in Fig. 2.

Step 1. Plan the Planning and Ensure Favorable Conditions for Effective Strategic Planning

The strategic planning process involves time, effort, and other resources, such as the acquisition of data and the staff designated for their compilation, analysis, summarization, and results dissemination. Because of this it should only be launched when favorable conditions or cultural expectations exist to give energy to the process and credibility, such as in the case of a newly filled President/Chief Executive Officer position within an organization. When initiating strategic planning, leadership must emphasize the on-going process of the activity and that it is not an isolated event.

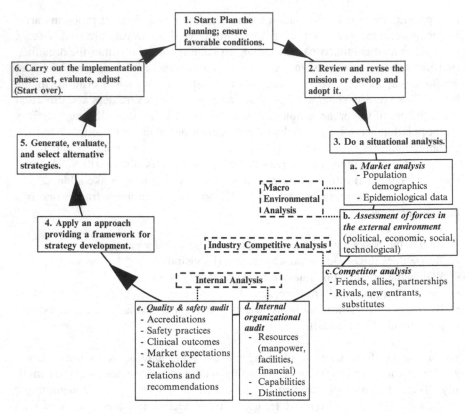

Fig. 2   Strategic planning process for health care organizations (Adapted from Jaeger, 2001)

Step 2. Review and Update the Organization's Mission Statement and Revise It as Necessary to Ensure That It Remains Relevant to the Organization's Future. If No Written Statement of Mission Exists, Develop and Adopt One

Upon convening the resources to conduct the strategic planning process and establishing that the conditions are favorable for proceeding, the features of the organization and its priorities should be embodied within the mission statement. The mission statement "provides a sense of purposefulness and direction for members of the organization (Gordon, 2002)." The mission statement defines the population served, the problem the organization (or other health service provider) intends to address, and the organization's response to the problem. The problems or responses cited in the mission statement represent, in rank order, the organization's priorities. The mission statement also serves to inform external constituencies, including stakeholders.

Table 2 Key elements of a mission statement (Adapted from Jaeger, 2001)

Identification of the organization
Specification of the population targeted for service (based upon geography, level of prevention
   service, disease type, other)
The health-related needs or problems the organization intends to address
How the organization will respond to the health needs or problems of the population targeted
   for the service
How the organization will relate to key stakeholder and their values in promoting stakeholder
   relationships
Features that distinguish the organization

Elements of a mission statement are summarized in Table 2. Statements of an organization's values, beliefs, and cultural orientation are often displayed on the same page as its mission statement to illustrate the responsibilities employees have in decision-making, commitment, and in action to support the mission. Thus, the values guiding the strategic planning process represent the "who" in the epidemiological context.

An excellent example of a mission statement is that of Rush University Medical Center which is in the top tier of academic medical centers nationwide and has Magnet designation by the American Nurses Credentialing Center:

> The Mission of Rush University Medical Center is to provide the very best care for our patients. Our education and research endeavors, community service programs and relationships with other hospitals are dedicated to enhancing excellence in patient care for the diverse communities of the Chicago area, now and in the future (available at http:// www.rush.edu).

This mission statement clearly identifies the priority importance of patient care with underpinnings of education, research, and community service. The population targeted for this organization's services is the Chicago area. This organization values excellence in patient care as part of its cultural orientation and clearly stated in its home page.

Since the strategic planning process typically is undertaken at the very minimum only every few years, the organization must ensure that it will be able to commit to and support the mission over that time period. Changing markets, competition, technologies, and leadership should prompt the organization to engage in the strategic planning process sooner or more often. Therefore, the mission of the organization should be examined and reaffirmed or modified each time the strategic planning process is initiated. Additionally, it is recommended that the mission statement be reviewed and reaffirmed annually. Only the parent organization can have a mission or mission statement. Subunits within the organization that have the same geographic or patient or client population have "a statement of purpose." These statements are in effect the subordinate unit's mission and must align with the parent organization.

Step 3. Do a Situational Analysis That Encompasses Assessments of Elements of the Organization's External and Internal Environments as Well as an Evaluation of the Impact of the Organization's Efforts

The situational analysis is the comprehensive assessment of the status of internal operations and forces of the external environment impacting the health care organization. The situational analysis involves the following components:

1. Macro-environmental forces identified and assessed as either a threat or an opportunity.
2. Industry competitive forces assessed regarding the relative threat upon the organization.
3. Internal analysis of the organization relative to its strengths and weaknesses. Resources, capabilities, and core competencies (present and needed) are identified.

Each component of this analysis is focused on a comprehensive assemblage and evaluation of specific data from a market analysis, assessment of forces in the external environment, competitor analysis, internal organizational audit, and quality audit. The tasks within each of these three components of the situational analysis follows.

Macro-Environmental Forces Identification and Analysis

Task A: Market Assessment

A "market" is the set of the population who have an actual or potential interest in a product or service. The market analysis is a planning task which is oriented to characterizing the current and future population served by an organization. Included in the market analysis is an examination of demographic, health, disease, and disability trends of the population subgroups which are actual or potential markets (see chapter "An Epidemiologic Framework for the Delivery of Health Care Services"). Using an epidemiologic framework, the questions to be answered in the task are: What are the important health problems? What are important risk factors? What is their magnitude and trend over time? What populations and population subgroups are affected by the problems and risk factors? Epidemiologic measures used in this task to evaluate an organization's market are: disease and health problem mortality, incidence, and prevalence rates data and other markers of health needs in populations including fertility patterns, birth rates, years of potential life lost by condition, and prevalence of personal (e.g., high cholesterol), health system (e.g., vaccination levels), and environmental (e.g., prevalence of lead in homes) risk factors. Vital statistics from the state health department, data from the US Census, and data from the Center for Disease Control and Prevention's Behavioral Risk Factor Surveillance Survey for the market area assessed should be obtained as part of this task. The record number of births in 2006, the continuing high birth rate in teens, and the increasing percentage of pre-term and low birthweight babies across all age groups of mothers signal the potential of heightened future demands for health care services and the imperative to plan accordingly (Martin et al., 2009). Health service utilization data, such as those displayed in Table 1, are useful in this task as proxy markers of health care need. Utilization available for population units as small as communities when not available can be extrapolated by applying national rate measures to the population size of the service market or be obtained by a survey. The Center for Studying Health System Change through its Community Tracking Study (CTS) provides periodic survey data from 60 community areas (http://www.hschange.org). Household survey data cover topics such as health care access, utilization, insurance, perceptions of care quality. Physician survey data include topics pertaining to quality of care, access to care, and care practices. Regardless of epidemiologic measures used, they should be bench-marked relative to state, national, and international health goals (see *Healthy People 2010*, http://www.healthypeople.gov for US; see *Millennium Development Goals*, http://www.who.int/mdg/goals/en/index.html of the World Health Organization) using appropriate adjustment methodologies, at least for age and gender when making the comparisons. The answers derived from the analyses associated with this task are intended to lead to trend identification. These data then guide the organization to consider increasing, decreasing, or initiating new services in anticipation of changing health care needs as well as the consequences to the organization in terms of resources required relative to any benefits change(s) may yield.

Task B: Assessment of Forces in the External Environment

Given the information from Task A, the assessment of the external forces impacting a population aids in understanding if the health care organization (which can be a hospital, dental practice, health department, home care service, etc.) can successfully respond to any anticipated capacity changes in the market. This task involves gathering data according to the categories put forth by Bryson (1988) represented in the acronym PEST which refers to the *p*olitical, *e*conomic, *s*ocial, and *t*echnical forces in the external macro-environment. The intent of data from this task is to determine threats and opportunities to the organization and respond to each of these categories such any challenges become opportunities. For example, knowing that the Centers for Medicare and Medicaid Services will not reimburse for certain conditions arising out of a hospitalization episode may compel an organization to strategically increase its RN-patient ratio by hiring RN case managers or nurse practitioners as an additional layer of managing a unit's patient population to prevent the occurrence of these adverse conditions. Assessment of the external environment, particularly policy documents will also provide direction on potential new types of manpower the organization should plan for. An example may be a requirement implied by the Centers for Medicare and Medicaid Services (2008) for an organization to have a recovery audit coordinator whose responsibilities could include determining the congruence of the claims for services delivered between the facility and the provider. The only requirement from federal regulations may be that this is an "educated" person, but the organization may require an RHIA (Registered Health Information Administrator) or RHIT (Registered Health Information Technologist) credential for this purpose.

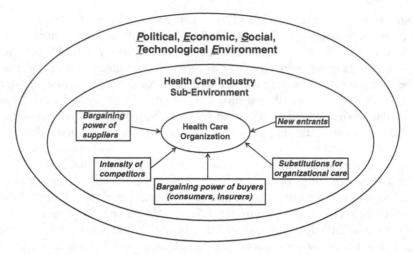

Fig. 3 The macro-environmental sphere forces impacting health care organizations

The external macro-environment impacting an organization can be further segmented into the subenvironment which is industry-specific (Fig. 3). For the health care industry sector subenvironment, buyers of health care and suppliers exert bargaining positions which not only influence the organization's price, but also its quality and efficiency. Substitutions for the organization's care practices may emerge if price, access, or consumer preferences change such is the case for alternative health clinics or "medical spas." The intensity of marketing or strategic positioning by existing competitors may intensify as the market changes such that all health care organizations may be competing for the same service lines associated with more favorable reimbursement levels (e.g., interventional radiology). New rivals may aim to compete for segments of a health care organization such as the emergence of specialty hospitals competing for the same favorable reimbursement sought by a general medical-surgical hospital.

Industry Competitive Force Analysis

Task C: Competitive Assessment

According to Jaeger (2001), a "competitive analysis assesses an organization's position in the marketplace relative to other organizations, some of which may compete for the same customers or valued resources or otherwise interfere with an organization's ability to serve its selected markets." This task first requires that the organization identify its competitors. This may be difficult as some specific service offerings (e.g., orthopedic surgery services) within an organization may vie against service lines within another similar organization or against another organization which is designed to only offer that service (e.g., an orthopedic hospital).

An organization then evaluates how it is valued and utilized relative to others in a population-based market of users and potential users by geographic unit through an analysis of market share. Market share is the percentage of the total number of users in a given geographic area who are served by an organization and is represented in the following generalized form for computation:

Given

	Total utilization (No. of persons)	No. zip code X1 users (market share %)	No. zip code X2 users (market share %)
Organization A	1,000	800 (50.0)	200 (12.5)
Organization B	2,000	600 (37.5)	600 (37.5)
Organization C	3,000	200 (12.5)	800 (50.0)
Totals		1,600	1,600

$$\text{Market share of Org. A in zip code X1} = \frac{\text{No. of users of Org}}{\text{No. of users in zip code X1}} \times 100\%$$

$$= 800 / 1,600 \times 100\% = 50.0\%$$

In this example, Organization A has the dominant market share of the users in zip code area X1 whereas it has the lowest market share in zip code area X2. Organization A should consider strategies to keep its dominance where it has the greatest market share and consider if resources would warrant favorable yield for increasing market share in zip code area X2. The challenge in computing market share is determining the residence of the users whereby users are assigned by zip code residence to the market regardless of the organization "used." Another challenge is determining the geographic area considered the market (or population base of users and potential users) of a health care organization. Urban geographic areas with many providers of the same or similar types may each possess very small market share of a service with the exception of the immediate surrounding area, unless that organization is a referral center. Typically, the market share of an organization is greatest in the geographic area immediately surrounding it. Market share is an indicator of the relative competitive position of an organization relative to other similar organizations serving customers/patients in the same market area. Market share is an important indicator of competitive position for all health care organizations, systems, and even payors. Organizations with larger market shares are assumed to be more preferred by providers and consumers in the geographic service areas and hence considered more stable given their dominant market presence. However, they may also employ monopolistic practices or not embrace innovation. Those with lower market share are more vulnerable to exit the market. Exiting a market may give rise to opportunity, such as being the first hospital in a metropolitan area to conduct operations in a new suburban development (see "Metro Health Hospital - Taking Health Care to a Better Place" http://www.metrohealth.net/locations/hospital). Porell et al. (2006) found that home health agencies (HHAs) with greater Medicare beneficiary market shares in their market area "were less likely to contract in their service area (OR = 0.92) or exit the market (OR = 0.95), but they were also less likely to expand their service area (OR = 0.96)." This may suggest that competitive success may be due to less visit-intensive patient practice styles (i.e., more efficiency) or taking on niche markets (e.g., home intravenous [IV] infusion services). The authors also found that while the larger HHAs were more stable, they were less likely to expand their Medicare patient volumes and competitive market position. The concept of market share can be applied to potentially adverse market circumstances such as the percentage market share of uncompensated care expenses in a metropolitan statistical area (MSA) which could affect the strategic position and viability of voluntary and nonvoluntary safety net hospitals (Bazzoli et al., 2006). Many public and proprietary sources are available to determine hospital market share such as the data supplied in this Hospital Discharge database made available by the Illinois Department of Public Health (http://app.idph.state.il.us/emsrpt/hospitalization.asp) from uniform information collected by the Illinois Hospital Association on virtually all hospitalizations within the state. Potential limitations of such databases are the timeliness of the information (may be greater than 1-year-old before publicly available), the proportion of service organizations participating in the database, the quality of the information collected, and local variations in medical practice styles regarding diagnosis labeling and referral for service utilization.

Competitive analysis also yields information on potential strategies used by competitors such as joint ventures, mergers, and affiliations to ensure the adequacy of resources for organizational effectiveness and maintenance. An assessment of the competitor's strengths and weaknesses on common criteria used in the internal assessment should be performed when feasible. The task can also provide guidance in the use of nondirectly competitive strategies (e.g., purchase of a new primary care group). For competitor analysis where only one or two hospitals or major health systems operate in a market area or for countries which have a national health system or subsystems, the performance relative to national or international goals such as one of the 8 United Nations (2000) Millenium Goals, "Improve maternal health" with the target: "Reduce by three-quarters, between 1990 and 2015, the maternal mortality ratio") serves as the indicator of competitiveness.

Internal Analysis

Task D: Internal Organizational Audit

The internal organization audit is "an assessment of the resource under and organization's control (or in the case of a health system, available for application to the system's mission) (Jaeger, 2001)." Using an epidemiological framework, the internal audit determines the ratios of the general categories of manpower, technology, and facilities to the population of users and potential users of its services. The most critical of these resources will be the category of health manpower. Anticipated areas and types of manpower shortages can be found through reports and data available from the Health Resources and Services Administration (http://datawarehouse.hrsa.

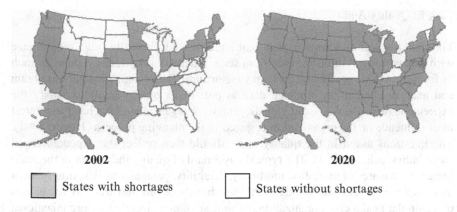

Fig. 4 States with projected shortages of registered nurses, 2000 and 2020 (Bureau of Health Professions, Health Resources and Services Administration, 2002), http://bhpr.hrsa.gov/health-workforce/reports/nurseed/1.htm (December 30, 2008)

gov/, December 20, 2008). Shortages in most every category of health manpower are anticipated, in particular, registered nurses and physician intensivists (USDHHS, HRSA, 2006) (Fig. 4). Schools of medicine and nursing are not putting out the capacity required for a growing and aging population. In addition to the numbers of health manpower needed, an assessment of the core competencies of these is required. What is the desired composition of specialists? Generalists or cross-trained personnel? What are the credentials required now and in the future of health manpower? The role of an organization's division of human resources is central in this task as they should be the repository of an organization's knowledge and skill competencies of its workforce, provide the necessary training to support retention and safe practice, and compile data on retention and vacancy rates of various categories of personnel. The impacts and strategies for restructuring employment situations (e.g., benefits, working hours, etc.) and changing health care delivery roles and models (e.g., increase mid-level providers, promote self-care management) by all health care organizations should be considered. The strategic planning for the competency of its workforce is a key element in yielding a sustainable competitive advantage by a health care organization.

Other more specific questions which need to be answered in the internal audit are as follows:

- Is the equipment current and safe? Are staff appropriately trained and credentialed for use of the equipment?
- Are the technologies "leading-edge"?
- What is the relative financial strength of the organization (e.g., determined by bond ratings)?
- How old is the physical plant?
- What is the reputation or brand strength of the organization?

The latter question may be answered from a population-based survey within the market area(s) of the organization.

Task E: Quality Audit

The *quality audit* may involve data that are collected internally (e.g., compliance with care pathways) or utilize data from state, federal or proprietary databases such as from the University Health System Consortium. The organization should obtain and analyze clinical performance data as part of its quality audit to satisfy the expectation of stakeholders, individuals, groups, or organizations that have an interest in or influence on the organization engaged in the planning process (Jaeger, 2001). The questions asked in the quality audit should then reflect the expectations of these individuals (Table 3). The typical dashboard of quality indicators in the audit includes measures of mortality, morbidity, disability, pain, and satisfaction (patient and employees). The quality data are then benchmarked and trended relative to other similar health care organizations of similar volume, location, or organizational type and/or industry standards. Industry standard quality data can be obtained from the Centers for Medicare and Medicaid Services (http://www.cms.gov) for hospitals and skilled care facilities or the National Committee for Quality Assurance's (http://www.ncqa.org) Healthcare Effectiveness Data and Information Set (HEDIS) used to measure performance of various dimensions of care delivered by health plans among others. Improving quality is not only a fundamental strategy to promote patient safety, but it is also a means of improving organizational image, and provider and patient relations. Quality performance becomes a differentiator in the

Table 3 Questions to address in the quality audit task of the situational analysis of the strategic planning process (Adapted from: Jaeger, 2001)

- What does quality mean to the stakeholders and constituents of the organization: the members of the governing board of the organization, the staff (at all levels), those who it serves, those who it seeks to serve?
- What infrastructure is in place to support the activities of on-going quality initiatives (e.g., electronic health record, clinical decision support systems, use of evidence-based clinical pathways, quality improvement office, process engineers)?
- What mechanisms are in place to continuously monitor the quality of health care, including processes and outcomes of care (such as committees monitoring customer satisfaction)?
- How are quality and patient safety initiatives interrelated within the organization? Is there duplication of effort? Is one team covering all areas?
- Does the organization meet the performance standards commonly utilized by other similar service organizations (e.g., Joint Commission on Accreditation of Healthcare Organizations, Commission for Accreditation of Rehabilitation Facilities, College of American Pathologists)?
- Is there epidemiological evidence that the health outcomes of the populations served is improving (by decreasing morbidity, mortality, disability, or pain)?
- What gaps in service quality do customers (internal and external) experience when using services or systems?
- Does the organization have the capability to provide and/or improve quality, and if not, what does it lack?
- How do quality initiatives within an organization link to, support, or are complementary to patient safety initiatives?
- Can any deficiencies or gaps identified through the quality audit be realistically addressed within the strategic planning period?

market if sustained by the provider at a level at or above industry standards. It also provides a long-term competitive advantage to which the population in a market area may respond to through increased utilization of the providers services.

Step 4. Apply an Approach for Defining the Key Issues, Focusing the Attention of the Organization, and Establishing the Framework for the Next Step of Strategy Development

In this step, the organization's leadership will develop a vision for success, reframe goals and objectives, and focus on the key issues that may be barriers to success using the Epidemiologic Model of the Delivery of Health Care Services (Fig. 1 of chapter "An Epidemiologic Framework for the Delivery of Health Care Services") as the framework. The vision is a statement of aspiration indicating "where" the organization is headed. The situational analysis lays the foundation for the formulation of the organization's goals and objectives. The goals and objectives relating to the organization are proposed in this step with the intent of achieving consensus about their relevance to the future success of the organization. According to Jaeger (2001), a goal is "a broad statement indicating general direction toward a desired future. Objectives are more specific statements that indicate in measurable terms what is to be accomplished and when." The goal can also be reconstructed as a vision statement if framed in inspirational terms. The goal can also be formulated into a strategic goal of constructed using a set of specific, measurable, long-range statements of a position the organization strives to achieve. In this format, the strategic goal becomes the organization's strategic intent and answers "when" the organization will attain its vision. Goals are the means by which an organization fulfills its mission (the "what") and moves toward the achievement of its vision. Objectives should be meaningful to the health care organization, promote the health and safety of the population served, be realistic, and attainable within the timeframe specified by the strategic planning process and "consistent with the organization's responsibilities and authority, and compatible with its goals and values (Jaeger, 2001)." Epidemiological data are obtained and used that can set and measure goals and objectives and guide in the formulation of strategic initiatives. For example, there has been a marked increase in the treated incidence of serious mental disorders, particularly in the 18–64-year age group, possibly in part due to increased awareness of the ability to treat these conditions (NCHS, 2007; Smith et al., 2008). Psychiatric disorders have been known to be associated with increased health care utilization and type of insurance coverage affects type of health care utilization for mental health services (Mark et al., 2007; Trivedi et al., 2008). Compared with adults without a chronic condition, adults who have both major depression and a chronic condition are more likely to utilize emergency room services (1 + emergency room visits in 12 months, odds ratio[OR] = 1.94; 95% confidence interval of OR = 1.55, 2.45) (Egede, 2007). The strategic development of community partnerships or outreach teams by a hospital may aid in reducing use of inpatient services by persons with psychiatric disorders, who often have long lengths of stay and are without health insurance (Commander et al., 2005). The framework for relating the components of this step is displayed in Table 1. It is important to remember that "action plans" for each of the objectives are as an important element of the planning process as the formulation of a vision statement otherwise the planning process is not an iterative process.

A tool for summarizing the key issues and facts identified in this step is a SWOT analysis, an assessment of an organization's *strengths*, *weaknesses*, *opportunities*, and *threats*. This analysis begins by summarizing *opportunities* and *threats* to the organization from the macro-environment (Fig. 5) and then followed by an inventory of its internal *strengths* and *weaknesses* from an internal audit (Fig. 6). The SWOT also provides information about an organization's current position in the market.

Sample Opportunities and Threats Worksheet
for a Health Care Organization

Instructions:
Complete sections A-D below by identifying which elements or forces/trends are within it. Then identify each as a(n): opportunity (**O**), threat (**T**) or a combination of opportunity/threat (**O/T**).

A. Current/Future Market(s): Clearly describe the current population (or patients, customers, potential customers) that the organization is serving as well as the population it intends to serve in the future. Specify size, geographic base, demographic and epidemiological trends and risk factors that are relevant to the health needs of the market(s).

B. Key Stakeholders: List the key stakeholders that influence your organization (such as accrediting bodies and funding sources); briefly summarize the expectations of these stakeholders relative to your organization.

C. Competitors and Allies: Identify both current or potential competitors, current or potential allies and their market share; briefly indicate the factors that affect the nature of the relationship with these and estimate the probability of a change (positive or negative).

D. Environmental Forces and Trends: List the PESTs—political, economic, social, and technological trends (local, national, and global) —that will affect the market(s) and its health needs as well as the ability of the organization to respond to needs. Examples: changing birth rates and family/household structures, attitudes toward self management versus governmental responsibility for health care, probability of technological improvements and anticipated treatment break-throughs, passage of new health insurance provisions to cover indigent care or based upon provider performance.

Fig. 5 Sample opportunities and threats worksheet for a health care organization (Adapted from Jaeger, 2001)

Sample Internal Organizational Audit Worksheet to Identify Strengths and Weaknesses of a
Health Care Organization

Instructions:
1. In column A, summarize the status or current level of each resource with key performance indicator data.
2. In column B, summarize strengths related to each resource category as well as weaknesses. Be specific and identify what health goal(s) of population(s) served cannot be achieved or what quality expectation(s) cannot be achieved at current or projected future resource levels.
3. In column C, indicate the ideal future level and the key characteristics of each category designed that will be required within 3-5 years using the same metrics specified in column A.

A.	B.	C.
Current status	Strengths and weaknesses	Desired future state Vision statement:_____
(Where are we now?)	Related to achievement of health goals and quality expectations. *(How are we doing?)*	
Today's date:_____		Target date:_____

Staff:

Financial
resources:

Facilities:

Systems/technology
for planning,
information,
and control:

Market assets:

Fig. 6 Sample worksheet for recording an organization's strength and weaknesses (Adapted from Jaeger, 2001)

The analysis of the market should consider both the local, national, as well as global market. For example, is the organization losing some of its elective procedure volume to other nations which can boast hospital accreditation standards comparable to those in the USA? Is the organization in a state which it can parlay its low cost of services along with high quality outcomes relative to other states and hence attract business from other states? The conclusions drawn from the SWOT analysis can provide the template for generating ideas for strategies to achieve organizational goals and objectives aligned to with its capabilities relative to environmental challenges.

Step 5. Generate, Evaluate, and Select Alternative Strategies for Achieving Organizational Goals and Objectives or the Best Alignment of the Organization with the Opportunities in Its Environment

For each objective formulated in Step 4, alternative strategies and associated actions are developed in this step. Epidemiologic data should also be utilized in evaluating the alternative strategies and actions because populations of users are being served and populations of potential users are targeted for services. Various approaches exist to selecting strategies to move the organization toward its vision of success, but creative thinking and idea-generating approaches for developing new strategies are recommended (Hall, 1995). These include brainstorming, visual displaying (posting every idea), rearranging, force fitting (two or more ideas), and substituting (what other process, who else). Regardless of the approach used for selecting a strategy, the organization should strive for those which are innovative. Drucker (1998) offers four internal areas of potential for innovation within a company: unexpected occurrences, incongruities, process needs, and industry and market changes. Sources outside the company that offer opportunity for innovation that he cites are: demographic changes, changes in perception, new knowledge, and new technologies. Epidemiologic data can be used to take advantage of a competitor's weaknesses, particularly in identifying unmet needs of the population (e.g., not addressing a high prevalence of obesity in a market) not addressed by the competitor and providing opportunities (e.g., diet and nutrition counseling) for meeting those health care needs. Once the strategies have been identified that are consistent with objectives, resources are the main factor in the selection of strategies for implementation to move the organization in the desired direction. According to Jaeger (2001), "...when resources are plentiful, multiple strategies may be selected. In the more usual scenario of scarce resources, a limited number of alternatives can be selected and some order of priority may be assigned." Thus, all the more need for a careful, thorough situation analysis and access to the best possible data, particularly population-based data, will yield a critical and accurate SWOT analysis of the organization and its competitive position in the market. A scheme of the interrelationship of the organization's vision to its action plans is detailed in Table 4.

Step 6. Carry Out the Implementation Phase of Strategic Planning, Detailing Operational Action Plans and Budgets, Monitoring Impact, and Making Midcourse Adjustments as Necessary

This step involves "translating decisions about strategic directions into plans that specify the organization's programs, tactics for attracting customers and promoting the organization's products and services, and the application of resource to support the implementation efforts" (Jaeger, 2001). During this step, it is important to

Table 4 Interrelationship of vision to action plans generated from the strategic planning process over time

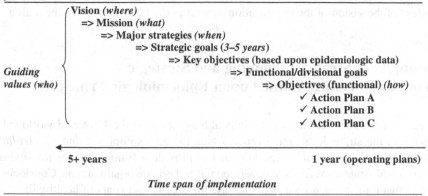

```
                    ⌜ Vision (where)
                    |    => Mission (what)
                    |        => Major strategies (when)
                    |            => Strategic goals (3–5 years)
                    |                => Key objectives (based upon epidemiologic data)
  Guiding           ⟨                    => Functional/divisional goals
  values (who)      |                        => Objectives (functional) (how)
                    |                            ✓ Action Plan A
                    |                            ✓ Action Plan B
                    ⌞                            ✓ Action Plan C
```

5+ years   1 year (operating plans)

Time span of implementation

continue a focus on implementing strategies which are not only innovative, but also are population-based and address known risk factors. Epidemiologic data are used in this step to evaluate and adjust a strategy. Implementation, in order to be effective, requires continuous monitoring (the macro- and internal-environments and competitors) and providing feedback as described in chapter "Epidemiological Study Designs for Evaluating Health Services, Programs, and Systems" (see also Fig. 1 of chapter "Epidemiological Study Designs for Evaluating Health Services, Programs, and Systems") relative to the consensus goals and measurable objectives specified in Step 4. The tactics used to implement the strategies may need to be adjusted to achieve the desired outcomes. Jaeger (2001) proposes that the answers to two questions are necessary to judge if the planning process resulted in effective strategic initiatives:

1. "Were the recommended tactics or actions carried out?
2. If yes, did they accomplish the stated objectives [goals]?"

Ideally, for any health care organization, all strategic initiatives should lead to improving the health of the population served as measured by epidemiologic data. Since continuous change is expected in health care and its external environment, the organization should be prepared to make appropriate mid-course adjustments in tactics if necessary. The strategic planning document for the nation, *Healthy People 2010*, was developed in consideration of evidence-based objectives to be achieved with a 10-year time frame. The document underwent a midcourse review for the purposes of determining the accuracy and relevance of the objectives. The review involved not only federal agencies but also other scientific experts. Comments from the public were considered as well. From the review, changes were made to objectives and subobjectives in terms of wording, deletion or addition objective and subobjectives, and revising baseline and target numbers as new epidemiological data became available. The organization should also be prepared to reinitiate the planning process quickly at the next level beyond the operating plans, particularly when progress toward the objectives has been achieved. Following this process in year-long increments is advised so as to realize and prospectively and therefore accurately document resulting changes. Any revisions to a plan should also be made in the context of the vision of the organization as well as the health goals for the nation.

Examples of Strategic Planning and Strategic Planning Documents Based upon Epidemiologic Principles

Both private organizations and public health agencies, in the USA and worldwide engage in the strategic planning process (see Boxed Examples 1 and 2). *Healthy People 2010* is the national plan intended to provide a framework for improving the health of Americans for both governmental and private organizations. Considered within that framework are goals to increase the quality and years of healthy life and to eliminate disparities. The national plan is reformulated every 10 years. However, for a health care organization, the velocity of change demands shorter planning intervals. Consistent with the strategic planning process described above, the planning process for the development of *Healthy People 2020* included invited public comment early on in the formulation of objectives (http://www.healthypeople. gov/hp2020/, December 31, 2008). Emerging issues in prevention and preparedness along with new knowledge of risk factors will be incorporated in the revised national plan.

States have adopted various forms of planning. The Illinois Department of Public Health has adopted the IPLAN Data systems for assessment of local health needs in Illinois jurisdictions (http://app.idph.state.il.us/, December 31, 2008). The planning process is every 5 years and is one of the requirements for Local Health Department Certification under Illinois Administrative Code for Public Health Practice Standards. State plans are another example of strategic planning efforts. The document, *Heart Disease and Stroke in Illinois: Now Is the Time for Public Health Action, 2007–2012 State Plan* (Illinois Department of Public Health [IDPH], 2007a), is a statewide plan targeting a specific set of health problems, cardiovascular disease and stroke, identified through extensive epidemiologic evidence as a major concern to the state of Illinois in terms of disability, death, and cost. Multiple stakeholders, private and public, were involved in the development of this plan which was led by the IDPH. Key features of this plan include the dissemination efforts of progress toward achieving goals and recommendations specific to the state as well as to those relevant to local and community areas.

Included in any planning effort should be the goal of capacity building. Capacity building is planning strategy aimed at promoting sustainability of positive change. In health care, this refers to an initiative by a community or organization to support and/or develop competencies, infrastructure, and resources necessary to promote favorable health and health outcomes in populations served. The Capacity Building Branch within the Centers for Disease Control and Prevention's Division of HIV/AIDS Prevention provides and coordinates capacity building assistance and related resources to improve the delivery and effectiveness of HIV prevention for high-risk populations. Capacity planning can also aid in reducing quality-related errors and treatment delays in hospital care by enhancing bed capacity (Walley et al., 2006).

The Nursing Agenda for Michigan 2005–2010 (http://www.michigan.gov/documents/nurse1_151632_7.pdf, December 31, 2008) is an example of a strategic planning document concerning capacity building for health manpower. The Agenda emanated from the policy document, Michigan Healthy People 2010. It was identified in Michigan Healthy People that the goals could not be achieved without an adequate supply of health manpower, particularly registered nurses. The position of Chief Nurse Executive was created by Governor Jennifer Granholm to provide leadership for the formation of a coalition and support to the coalition in the development of the Agenda. A coalition of 30 nursing organizations in the State of Michigan was the primary stakeholder in the development of this strategic plan. The Chief Nurse Executive regularly reports to legislators on progress in achieving the objectives associated with the Agenda and aids in the development of policies and legislation as well for this purpose.

Summary

Epidemiologic data are essential in the formulation of a strategic plan as well as in the evaluation of the attainment of objectives and action plans stated therein. The strategic plan, in order to be effective, needs to be viewed as a living document. It should be reviewed on a regular basis, even quarterly, to determine objectives that are relevant, not relevant, or those that need to be modified. During the review process, it should be determined what additional epidemiologic data are needed, what is realistic to be collected, how the data should be assessed, and most importantly whether the data will require any actions to modify the strategic position of the organization. Lastly, it is important for an organization in the planning process not to perceive an unrealistic view of its capabilities and to be prepared for the unexpected, quickly readjusting strategies or redoing a plan should unexpected events occur either within the organization or external to it. It is for this reason that the majority of effort in the strategic planning process should focus on the formulation of plans using sound epidemiological data because of the need for a health care organization to have a population-based perspective to achieve optimal strategic position in an ever-changing market with a third of an organization's effort devoted to implementation such that the strategic process is: plan, plan, plan...execute!

Discussion Questions

Q.1. Develop a mission statement for a health care service delivery organization that has identified a growing population of aged persons within its geographic area and the organization expects that a large number of these will develop Alzheimer's disease (see Table 3).

Q.2. In order to develop a strategic plan for a health care organization, what types of epidemiological data are needed?

Q.3. Identify at least one important trend from the political, social, economic, and technological environments that will affect the epidemiology of a health problem. Provide examples of organizational strategies for responding to the changes.

Q.4. Select a health care condition which is observed to have recent increasing hospital utilization rates. Determine the impact of a continued impact on hospitalization trends in the community served by the hospital of your choice. If you were the CEO of this hospital, how would you address the impact in your strategic planning process?

Boxed Example 1 Strategic Planning to Eliminate Tuberculosis

Problem: According to the Centers for Disease Control and Prevention (CDC), the incidence of tuberculosis (TB) declined in the US to a rate of 4.4 cases per 100,000 in 2007. However, TB still poses a concern owing to the fact that the incidence of foreign-born TB cases is 9.7 times higher than US-born persons and the rate for US-born blacks nearly eight times US-born whites. The complexity of the disease is also increasing as drug resistant TB cases are on the rise along with HIV-associated TB cases (CDC, 2008).

Methods: The strategic planning process of the Centers for Disease Control and Prevention (CDC, 1989), Division of Tuberculosis Elimination (DTBE) set forth the following two goals:

- Domestic – Elimination of tuberculosis (TB) in the USA (defined as less than 1 case per million population); and
- Global – Contribute to reductions in global TB incidence and mortality (by 50% each compared with 1990 baseline, based on the Global Plan to Stop TB 2006–2015 (http://www.stoptb.org/global plan]).

Results: The planning process identified the following core functions (or strategies) of DTBE to support priority areas of concern directed at achieving the goals:

1. Conduct routine surveillance (including drug susceptibility surveillance) and periodic surveys.
2. Provide funding and technical assistance to state and local programs for case finding, contact investigation, and completion of treatment, including support for care and treatment with assistance.
3. Guide preparedness and outbreak responses.
4. Conduct program evaluation.
5. Provide laboratory diagnostic services and help build laboratory capacity.
6. Conduct critical, programmatically relevant operational research to develop and evaluate new tools and interventions for diagnosis, treatment, prevention, and control of TB
7. Provide data management, statistical, and information technology support.

(continued)

Boxed Example 1 (continued)

8. Support intramural services.
9. Obtain external expert consultation and advice to ensure DTBE research and program activities are responsive to emergent public health concerns.
10. Develop and evaluate evidence-based training and educational materials, policies, and guidelines to ensure program and health care competency in TB prevention, control, diagnosis, treatment, and laboratory capacity.
11. Develop education, risk, and media communications (web- and print-based) to aid in preparedness and public awareness of TB prevention and control issues.
12. Cultivate relevant external partnerships.

Managerial Epidemiological Interpretation: The health care manager should be aware of and support national and international goals regarding the elimination of TB. In practice, this support is demonstrated by: revising organizational policies and procedures as necessary to be congruent with CDC guidelines for TB prevention and control; providing training to staff to ensure competency in the prevention, control, diagnosis, and treatment of TB; and, ensuring that rapid reporting to the local health department occurs when cases are identified.

Boxed Example 2 Strategic Planning by a Cancer Control Organization

Problem: The highest proportion of individuals presenting with late state colorectal cancer in the state are Blacks. An organization whose mission is the control of the cancer problem in a state wishes to develop a strategic plan to address this problem.

Methods and Data: The state's tumor registry was the source of information on cancer incidence data for the colon and rectum. Mortality data were obtained from the state's vital statistics section of the state department of public health. The state's department of public health compiled the Behavioral Risk Factor Surveillance Survey data on colorectal screening. Staff from the state public health department computed the age-adjusted incidence and mortality rates.

Results: In Illinois, the incidence rates of colon and rectum cancer for Non-Hispanic Blacks (NHB) have increased between 1990 and 2004 whereas the rates for Non-Hispanic Whites (NHW) have decreased. The colon and rectal cancer mortality rates have decreased, but as compared with both NHW males and females, NHBs of both genders still have on average a higher rate. Early detection is known to effectively decrease mortality from colon cancer.Age Adjusted* Rate (per 100,000) Trends in Invasive Cancer Colon and Rectum Incidence and Mortality, by Race and Gender, Illinois (Source: Illinois Department of Public Health, 2007b)

(continued)

Boxed Example 2 (continued)

Rate type	Year	Total non-Hispanic whites	Non-Hispanic white males	Non-Hispanic white females	Total non-Hispanic blacks	Non-Hispanic black males	Non-Hispanic black females
Incidence							
	2004	55.8	66.2	47.8	65.6	76.9	57.9
	2000	60.6	73.9	50.7	66.3	80.7	57.0
	1995	58.2	70.0	50.3	66.0	80.7	57.0
	1990	61.5	75.2	52.3	64.1	75.8	56.8
Mortality							
	2004	19.6	24.1	16.6	29.6	36.3	25.3
	2000	22.9	27.7	19.5	32.1	40.0	27.1
	1995	24.7	31.1	20.7	31.6	40.8	26.3
	1990	27.3	35.1	22.1	39.8	48.8	34.3

*Age –adjusted to the 2000 US standard million population

Strategic Planning Process

Assessment of Conditions

The problem was examined by key committees within the organization to obtain a comprehensive view of the situation. The Early Detection Committee and the Cancer Incidence and End Results Committee (CIER) concurred on targeting the African American population with colorectal cancer on early detection awareness and screening. These two Committees reviewed the data sources. The Prevention and Public Affairs Committees reviewed national nutrition data and school policies. The CIER Committee was charged with goal setting the goal for the planning process.

Establishment of Goal

The CIER Committee after reviewing the data established the goal:

By 2008, 50% of people aged 50+ years in the state will have received colorectal screening following American Cancer Society Guidelines* as measured by the preferred test of Fecal Occult Blood Test.

State Baseline 2001: 21.8%
National Baseline 2001: 23.4%"

Boxed Example 2 (continued)

Establishment of Continued Progress

Committee consensus based upon prevalence rate changes prior to baseline year expected within the next strategic planning review (7 years) and the following goal additional was established:

> By 2015, 75% of people aged 50 + years in the state will have received colorectal screening following American Cancer Society Guidelines* as measured by the preferred test of Fecal Occult Blood Test.

Data Source for Tracking Progress

The establishment of a goal requires that valid and reliable data be available to evaluate progress to achieving the goal. The Committees identified the following data source for tracking progress: *Behavioral Risk Factor Surveillance System Public Use Data Tape, 2001, National Center for Chronic Disease Prevention and Health Promotion*, Centers for Disease Control and Prevention, 2002.

Strategies for Intervention

The planning process requires that realistic strategies be employed to achieve the goal. Education and colorectal screening programs targeted at high population density African American communities in five areas of state using culturally sensitive messages and strategies. The need for environmental modification (safe playgrounds, change in nutritional content of vending machines, etc.) for younger children who are at risk for obesity and physical inactivity, etiologic factors for colorectal cancer.

Evaluation

The Committees on Early Detection Prevention, CIER, and Public Affairs will review the data annually regarding progress to achieving goal and adjust strategies as necessary.

---

* A fecal occult blood test within the past year.

Boxed Example 2 (continued)

Managerial Epidemiology Interpretation: Managers should work with the communications department and local stores with pharmacies to promote distribution of Fecal Occult Blood Test to the target audience of Blacks 50+ years of age. Simultaneously, working with physicians to receive referrals for positive results and follow these up with further testing closes the loop on the screening process.

References

Bazzoli, G.J., Lindrooth, R.C., Kang, R., and Hasnain-Wynia, R., 2006, The influence of health policy and market factors on the hospital safety net, *HSR: Health Serv. Res.* **41**:1159–1180.

Bryson, J.M., 1988, *Strategic Planning for Public and Nonprofit Organizations*, Jossey-Bass, San Francisco, CA.

Centers for Disease Control and Prevention, 1989, A strategic plan for the elimination of tuberculosis in the United States, *M.M.W.R.* **38(Suppl. 3)**:1–25.

Centers for Disease Control and Prevention, 2008, Trends in tuberculosis—United States, 2007, *M.M.W.R.* **57(Suppl. 3)**:281–285.

Centers for Medicare and Medicaid Services, 2008, *The Medicare Recovery Audit Contractor (RAC) Program: An Evaluation of the 3-Year Demonstration* (March 3, 2009) http://www.cms.hhs.gov/RAC/Downloads/RAC%20Evaluation%20Report.pdf.

Commander, M., Sashidharan, S., Rana, T., Ratnayake, T., 2005, North Birmingham assertive outreach evaluation: patient characteristics and clinical outcomes, *Soc. Psychiatry Psychiatr. Epidemiol.* **40**:988–993.

Drucker, P.F., 1998, The discipline of innovation, *Harv. Bus. Rev.* **76**:149–157.

Egede, L.E., 2007, Major depression in individuals with chronic medical disorders: prevalence, correlates and association with health resource utilization, lost productivity and functional disability, *Gen. Hosp. Psychiatry* **29**:409–416.

Gordon, J.R., 2002, *Organizational Behavior: A Diagnostic Approach*, 7th ed., Prentice-Hall, Upper Saddle River, NJ.

Hall, D., 1995, *Jump Start Your Brain*, Warner Books, New York.

Hebert, L.E., Scherr, P.A., Bienias, J.L., Bennett, D.A., and Evans, D.A., 2003, Alzheimer disease in the US population: prevalence estimates using the 2000 census, *Arch. Neurol.* **60**:1119–1122.

Illinois Department of Public Health, 2007a, *Heart Disease and Stroke in Illinois: Now Is the Time for Public Health Action, 2007–2012 State Plan*, State of Illinois, Springfield, IL.

Illinois Department of Public Health, 2007b, *Illinois Cancer Statistics Review, 1986–2004*. Epidemiologic Report Series 07:03, IDPH, Springfield, IL.

Jaeger, F.J., 2001, Strategic planning: an essential management tool for health care organizations and its epidemiological basis. In *Epidemiology and the Delivery of Health Care Services: Methods and Applications*, 2nd ed. (D.M. Oleske, ed.), Plenum, New York.

Mark, T.L., Levit, K.R., Buck, J.A., Coffey, R.M., and Vandivort-Warren, R., 2007, Mental health treatment expenditure trends, 1986–2003, *Psychiatr Serv.* **58**:1041–1048.

Martin, J.A., Hamilton, B.E., Sutton, P.D., Ventura, S.J., Menacker, F., Kirmeyer, S., and Mathews, T.J., 2009, Births: final data for 2006, *National Vital Statistics Report* **57**:1–27.

National Center for Health Statistics, 2009, *Health, United States, 2008, With Chartbook*, Hyattsville, MD.

Porell, F.W., Liu, K., and Brungo, D.P., 2006, Agency and market area factors affecting home health agency supply changes, *HSR: Health Serv. Res.* **41**:1847–1875.

Smith, R.P., Larkin, G.L., and Southwick, S.M., 2008, Trends in U.S. emergency department visits for anxiety-related mental health conditions, 1992–2001, *J. Clin. Psychiatry* **69**:286–294.

Trivedi, A.N., Swaminathan, S., Mor, V., 2008, Insurance parity and the use of outpatient mental health care following a psychiatric hospitalization, *J.A.M.A.* **300**:2879–2885.

United Nations, 2000, *United Nations Millennium Declaration* (July 4, 2009) http://www.un.org/millennium/declaration/ares552e.pdf.

U.S. Dept. of Health and Human Services, Health Resources and Services Administration, 2006, *Report to Congress, The Critical Care Workforce: A Study of the Supply and Demand for Critical Care Physicians*, Requested by: Senate Report 108–81, Senate Report 109–103 and House Report 109–143 (December 30, 2008), ftp://ftp.hrsa.gov/bhpr/nationalcenter/criticalcare.pdf

Van Den Eeden, S.K., Tanner, C.M., Bernstein, A.L., Fross, R.D., Leimpeter, A., Bloch, D.A., and Nelson, L.M., 2003, Incidence of Parkinson's Disease: variation by age, gender, and race/ethnicity, *Am. J. Epidemiol.* **157**:1015–1022.

Walley, P., Silvester, K., and Steyn, R., 2006, Managing variation in demand: lessons from the UK National Health Service, *J. Healthcare Manag.* **51**:309–322.

Chapter 7
The Role of Managerial Epidemiology in Infection Prevention and Control

Learning Outcomes

After completing this chapter, you will be able to:

1. Understand the roles and responsibilities of health care managers in infection prevention and control in health care organizations.
2. Apply epidemiologic principles to manage an outbreak of a transmissible disease in a health care setting.
3. Develop a strategy for infection prevention in a health care setting.

Keyterms Case-fatality rate • Epidemic • Health care-associated infection • Immunity • Incubation period • Outbreak • Pandemic • Pathogenicity • Virulence

Introduction

Infectious and parasitic diseases are the second leading cause of mortality worldwide, following mortality from cardiovascular disease (Fig. 1). Within the category of infectious and parasitic diseases in 2002, there were 31.1 million deaths worldwide from infectious diseases, with 2.7 million of those deaths due to HIV/AIDS, followed by diarrheal diseases, tuberculosis (TB), and malaria. The persistence of infectious diseases, epidemics, and infectious disease outbreaks is attributable to a number of factors including: crowding and migration (e.g., tuberculosis), international travel (e.g., Severe Acute Respiratory Syndrome, SARS), global commerce, resistance promoted by the widespread use of antimicrobials (e.g., increased use and resistance to fluroquinolones and increased rate and severity of *Clostridium difficile*-related disease, changes in medical practice requiring more invasive procedures and more aggressive procedures (e.g., increased bloodborne catheter infections), changes in the environment (e.g., flooding and increased fecal-oral disease, vector-borne disease, and rodent-borne disease), and changes in social and behavioral factors

D.M. Oleske (ed.), *Epidemiology and the Delivery of Health Care Services:*   181
Methods and Applications,
DOI 10.1007/978-1-4419-0164-4_7, © Springer Science+Business Media, LLC 2009

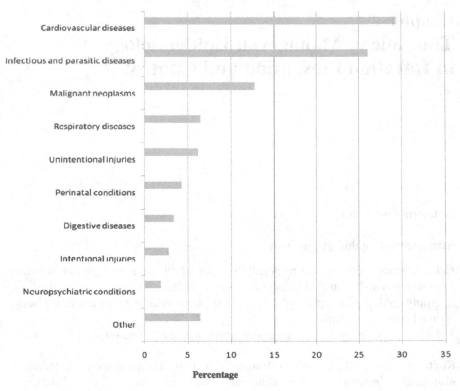

Fig. 1 Percentage distribution of mortality by condition, World, 2002 (Source: World Health Organization, 2004)

(e.g., exchange of sex for drugs) (Ahern et al., 2005; Lienhardt, 2001; McDonald et al., 2005; Newman et al., 2004; Olsen et al., 2003).

Health care-acquired infections contribute to increased lengths of hospital stays, readmission to hospitals, the potential for litigation, and affects the quality of life among individuals in skilled care facilities and hospices. The recognition of the impact of infectious conditions acquired in the hospital has reached national legislative attention because of its impact on federal health care spending. In the Deficit Reduction Act (DRA) of 2005, Section 5001(c) required the Secretary to identify, by October 1, 2007, at least two conditions that are (a) high cost or high volume or both, (b) result in the assignment of a case to a DRG that has a higher payment when present as a secondary diagnosis, and (c) could reasonably have been prevented through the application of evidence-based guidelines. For discharges occurring on or after October 1, 2008, hospitals will not receive additional payment for cases in which one of the selected Hospital-Acquired Conditions (HAC) was not present on admission and the case would be paid as though the secondary diagnosis was not present. Section 5001(c) provides that the Centers for Medicare and Medicaid Services (CMS) can revise the list of conditions from time to time. In the final FY 2008 IPPS rule, CMS identified three infectious HAC subject to this rule:

catheter-associated urinary tract infections, vascular catheter-associated blood stream infection, and surgical site infection (mediastinitis after coronary artery by-pass graft [CABG] surgery). Conditions being considered for fiscal year 2009 are ventilator-associated pneumonia and *Staphylococcus aureus* septicemia. This legislation will signal the era of intense focus on infection prevention and control and prevention efforts in health care facilities. The use and application of epidemiologic data and principles are fundamental to the success of these efforts.

Prevention of infection can span a wide variety of topics from animal to food to environment. The purpose of this chapter is to provide an introduction to the principles and practices of infectious disease epidemiology as they may be applied in health care services delivery settings.

Infectious Disease Concepts

There are five elements involved in the emergence of an infectious disease. These elements are: (1) characteristics of the infectious agent, (2) reservoir of the agent, (3) mode of transmission, (4) portal of entry/exit of the agent, and (5) the characteristics of the susceptible host.

Infectious Agent

An infectious agent is characterized in terms of its biological classification, incubation period, and manifestation in the host.

Biological agents relevant to human diseases are classified as viruses, bacteria, fungi, and parasites. Most human diseases caused by biological agents are due to bacteria or viruses. Biological agents are classified according to the presence or absence of specific traits. Bacteria are classified based on the mechanism of movement and features of the cell wall. Viruses are classified based on the type of nucleic acid and its size, shape, and mode of replication. Table 1 illustrates the major categories of microbial agents and their commonly associated disease. To determine whether a biological agent is causative in a disease, it must be isolated and identified in the host.

Each infectious agent has a unique incubation period. The incubation period is the time from the introduction of the agent into the host to the onset of the signs and symptoms of the disease. The incubation time is determined from a histogram of the onset of the signs and symptoms of illness by time unit. Commonly, the median or peak of the distribution from the histogram is the referent time unit from which to trace back in time the possible exposure source as ascertained from interviews of ill persons (Fig. 1). The incubation period may be hours, days, weeks, months, or even years. For example, microbial agents that cause food poisoning typically have an incubation period of 24–72 h; microbial agents that cause respiratory infections typically have an incubation period of 7–10 days. A group of subacute degenerative diseases such as bovine spongiform encephalopathy or "mad cow

Table 1 Common transmissible diseases according to medically important classification and associated biological agent

Classification	Transmissible disease	Biological agent
Bacterial disease: Bacteria with gram-positive cell wall structure	Tuberculosis	*Mycobacterium*
Bacteria disease: Bacteria with gram-negative cell wall structure	Gonorrhea	*Neisseria gonorrhoeae*
Bacterial disease: Bacteria with no cell walls	Pneumonia	*Mycoplasma pneumoniae*
Helminthiases	Trichinellosis	*Trichinella spiralis*
Mycoses	Ringworm	*Trichophyton*
Pediculosis, acariasis, other	Head lice	*Pediculus capitis*
Prion	Creutzfeldt-Jakob disease	Proteinaceous infectious particles
Protozoal disease	Trichomoniasis	*Trichomonas vaginalis*
Viral disease: Virus-DNA	Cervical cancer	Human papillomaviruses, Types 16 and 18
Viral disease Virus-RNA	Acquired Immunodeficiency Syndrome (AIDS)	Human immunodeficiency virus (HIV)

disease," kuru, and Creutzfeldt-Jakob disease can be from 15 months to over 30 years depending upon the route of exposure (Heymann, 2008).

Manifestation in the host is described in terms of the agent's pathogenicity and virulence. Pathogenicity is the ability of the organism to alter normal cellular and physiological processes. Virulence is the invasive ability of an organism to produce clinically manifest disease because of damage to tissues. Virulence is another term used when describing the potential for an agent to cause morbidity and mortality. It can also be epidemiologically characterized in terms of the case-fatality rate (see Boxed Example 1). Noroviruses are highly virulent because they are highly contagious and quickly spread from person to person and "few as 100 virus particles thought to be sufficient to cause infection (http://www.cdc.gov)," but have low pathogenicity because symptoms last between 24 and 60 h and recovery is usually complete with no evidence of the emergence of any serious long-term adverse health problems.

The accurate identification of an infectious agent requires the following steps to ensure the integrity of the specimen: select the appropriate body area for collection of the clinical specimen(s) for testing; select an appropriate method of collection

---

Boxed Example 1 Interpreting the SARS Case Fatality Rate (Source: Karlberg et al., 2004)*

Problem: Severe Acute Respiratory Syndrome (SARS) is a novel coronavirus presenting with high fever (>38°Celsius/100.4°F) and coughing or breathing difficulty. Transmission is from person to person through direct contact with

(continued)

Boxed Example 1 (continued)

the secretions or droplets of suspect or probable cases with SARS. It is not well-established if susceptibility varies by age, gender or race.

Methods: Cases of SARS were determined by treating physicians according to patient clinical signs, a chest X-ray, and appropriate diagnostic tests or autopsy reports. The case-fatality rate is the number of persons dying from a particular disease in a specific period who were diagnosed with the disease within that same time period multiplied by 100 or 100%. Mortality data were from 42 Hong Kong Government hospitals from the period early March to September 22, 2004.

Data and Results: The case fatality rate for males was $170/776 \times 100\% = 21.9\%$. The case fatality rate for females was $129/979 \times 100\% = 13.2\%$. The difference between the two groups was $p < 0.0001$. The crude relative risk of death among males was 1.66 (21.9%/13.2%).

Managerial Epidemiology Interpretation: Males are more severely affected by SARS than females experience a risk of dying that is 1.66 times greater than females. Health care managers need to understand that some population subgroups may be at higher risk than others. Resource allocation for prevention efforts (e.g., workplace exposures, smoking cessation) or more thorough diagnosis (e.g., symptoms/signs overlooked in females) should be considered.

(e.g., oral swab, spinal puncture, etc.); a sufficient quantity of material to be tested; preparation of the sample for transport (e.g., icing) including proper labeling for patient identification number; date and time of collection of the specimen; and a timely and safe transport of the specimen to the laboratory. If multiple specimens are to be taken from the same patient or if the same type of specimen is to be obtained from multiple patients, prepare and secure one specimen at a time to avoid cross-contamination, change gloves between samples and patients, avoid splashing, spilling, or aerosolizing samples. Proper frequent disinfection of the work area, immediately cleaning up spills, and ensuring that biosafety cabinets/areas are available for specimen storage while awaiting transport to the laboratory. It is also important for the health care manager to ensure the facilities and equipment for proper specimen collection are readily available and that services are organized in a manner to ensure the timely and safe delivery of the specimen(s) (e.g., tube system, refrigerated transport services).

Reservoir of Infectious Agent

A reservoir is where the agent lives, grows, and multiplies. Reservoirs can be living (human, animal, arthropod, plant) or a substance (soil, water) or some combination thereof. The agent depends on the conditions of the reservoir to survive and be transmitted to a susceptible host. Human reservoirs can be clinical cases or carriers. Clinical cases are those persons who manifest signs and/or symptoms of the disease. Carriers are individuals who are a source of the infection by harboring a specific infectious agent, but they themselves do not manifest any signs or symptoms of the disease. An individual may be a carrier during the incubatory, convalescent, or postconvalescent phases of a disease. Also a carrier may be asymptomatic during the entire course of the infection. The carrier state may be temporary, transient, or long term (chronic carrier) (Heymann, 2008).

Transmission of Infectious Disease

Transmission is the mechanism by which an infectious agent is spread from a source to a susceptible host. The modes of transmission are: (1) direct or contact, (2) indirect, and (3) airborne.

Direct or contact transmission involves physical contact, commonly through person-to-person, such as through biting, kissing, touching, sexual intercourse or through direct projection of droplet spray onto the mucous membranes from coughing, singing, spitting, sneezing, or close (within 3 ft) talking. Direct exposure of the susceptible host to an infectious agent can also occur from an animal bite, to contaminated soil, or transplacentally. Food and water are the most common vehicles for the transmission of infectious agents.

Indirect transmission is through vehicle-borne or vector-borne methods and is a means for transporting the infectious agent into the susceptible host. Vehicles for infectious disease transmission include but are not limited to inanimate objects or materials such as soiled bedding or clothes, door handles, eating utensils, objects of personal care (toothbrushes, shavers), water, milk, surgical instruments, wound dressings, or biological substances (e.g., transplanted organs, blood transfusion, etc.). Vector-borne transmission may be mechanical or biological. Mechanical transmission is the physical transmission of an infectious agent, which is not an essential element in its life cycle. Flies can transmit *Salmonella* on their appendages from contaminated feces to food, representing mechanical transmission. Biological transmission occurs when a vector harbors a pathogen within its body and delivers the pathogen to a host in an interactive manner, such as through propagation, a bite. Malaria is caused by the biological transmission from the bite of a female *Anopheles* mosquito infected with *Plasmodium falciparum*, a protozoan parasite into a susceptible host.

Some infections, such as Trachoma, can be transmitted by multiple mechanisms, including direct contact with ocular or nasopharyngeal discharges, indirectly through contact with fomites (contaminated objects) from infected people, or through vector-borne mechanical transmission by flies (Heymann, 2008). Knowing how a disease is transmitted aids in understanding how to break the cycle of infection and control its spread. Table 2 displays selected infectious diseases and the recommended associated transmission precautions.

Table 2 Selected infectious problems, type of transmission and transmission precautions

Infectious problem	Type of transmission	Transmission precautions
Acquired immunodeficiency syndrome (AIDS)	Sexual contact, percutaneous, permucosal, perinatal	Standard
Hepatitis B, Viral	Blood, blood products, saliva, cerebrospinal fluid, peritoneal, pleural, pericardial and synovial fluid, amniotic fluid, semen and vaginal secretions, other body fluid containing blood, unfixed or transplanted tissues and organs	Standard
Measles (rubeola)	Airborne by droplet spread, direct contact with nasal or throat secretions of infected persons	Airborne
Salmonella species	Person-to-person fecal oral or ingested of organisms in food or contaminated by feces of infected animal or person	Standard
Meningitis		
Aseptic	Direct contact, including respiratory droplets from nose and throat of infected persons	Standard, Contact for infants and young children
Bacterial		Standard
Small pox	Respiratory tract (droplet spread), skin inoculation, conjunctiva	Airborne, Contact

Portal of Exit/Portal of Entry of Infectious Agent

The portal of exit is where the infectious agent leaves the host. The portal of entry is the way the organism enters the host and invades the tissue. The portals of entry/exit are: gastrointestinal, genitourinary, respiratory, and integumentary (skin, mucous membranes). Often, the portal of exit is the same as the portal of entry. Staphylococcal disease in the community, a common bacterial skin lesion, manifests itself as folliculitis, carbuncles, abscesses, or infected lacerations, and is transmitted through contact with the person who has a draining or purulent lesion.

Host Susceptibility

Host susceptibility is not having sufficient resistance to protect against acquiring disease from an infectious agent if exposed to it. Susceptibility depends on age, genetic factors, general health and immunity. Decreasing age, especially before 11 years of age when the immune system reaches maturity, and increasing age, especially over 65 years, each are associated with increased susceptibility. General health is influenced by nutrition and the presence of comorbidities, with better health associated with a lower likelihood of developing infectious disease. HIV is a major risk factor for the progression from latent TB infection to TB disease.

Immunity is a biological defense primarily provided by two categories of circulating white blood cells: lymphocytes which produce antibodies (a humoral immunity secreting antibodies) or a through a cell-mediated immunity (detecting and destroying antigens or destruction of foreign cells), and monoctyes (a phago-cytic response) which have a specific action on the microorganism or on its toxin. Immunity can be characterized as passive (natural or artificial) or active (natural or artificial). Passive natural immunity is the transplacental transfer of antibodies from mother to fetus. Passive artificial immunity is the inoculation of specific protective antibodies in globulin preparations. Passive artificial immunity has a short-term efficacy (less than 6 months). Active immunity is provided through a humoral mechanism can be natural, as in the case of acquiring an infection (with or without clinical manifestations of disease), or artificial in which the agent itself in a killed or modified form (via a vaccine) is injected to stimulate protective antibodies.

Epidemics

The occurrence of a disease in excess of what is expected is called an epidemic. The existence of an epidemic is determined in different manners depending upon epide-miologic data on the frequency of its natural occurrence and seasonal variation. Influenza epidemics are defined as rates occurring in excess of one standard deviation above historical trends. Epidemics occurring where the frequency of a disease is expected to be low are determined through a graphical method or the construction of an epidemic curve. A point source epidemic curve follows a bell-shaped distribution of a histogram plotting the number of cases occurring on each date when a case became ill. The peak of the histogram represents the date where the median number of cases became ill. Knowing the suspect infection agent and tracing the incubation time from the date associated with the peak of the histogram an estimate of the time of exposure to the agent can be obtained. A propagated epidemic curve is illustrated by a histogram of the onset of the disease demonstrating repeated peaks of occurrence (Fig. 2a). Epidemics can also be cyclic, recurring according to certain time periods. Influenza and pneumonia-associated deaths typically occur as a cyclic epidemic, with the epidemic threshold exceeded during winter months (Fig. 2b). Epidemics can occur in any setting, in the community or in any setting where populations are in congregate settings (hospitals, prisons, skilled care facilities, schools, etc.). A pan-demic is an epidemic that is an epidemic manifest world-wide. The severity of pandemic disease can vary over the phases of its course. Miller et al. (2009) describe the signature features of past pandemics, including a shift in the virus sub-type, a shift toward increased mortality in younger age groups, multiple successive lethal waves, and high susceptibility of populations resulting in increased transmissibility. Depending upon the features of the pandemic including its potential for animal-human transmission and the extent of countries and regions involved, the World Health Organization (2009) proposed a scheme of phases guiding the deployment of different levels of resources, interventions, and communications for disease control. The determination of an epidemic or pandemic requires the mobilization of many

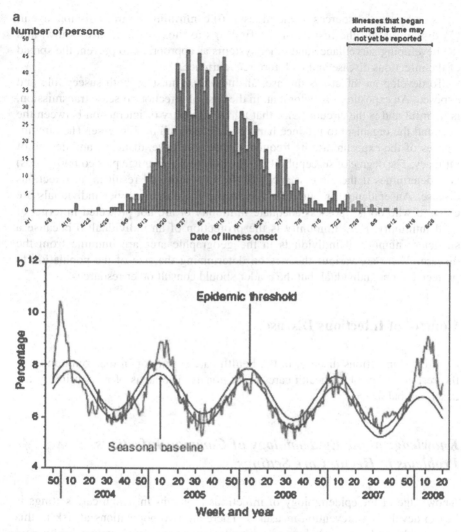

Fig. 2 (a) Propagated epidemic curve – Outbreak of Salmonella. From National Center for Zoonotic, Vector-Borne, and Enteric Diseases, http://www.cdc.gov/salmonella/saintpaul/epidemic_curve. html (2008). (b) Cyclic epidemic (Source: Centers for Disease Control and Prevention, 2008)

resources within the organization, locally, and even nationally to monitor the progress of an epidemic and to institute appropriate control and prevention measures.

An outbreak is an epidemic confined to a particular geographical area, such as a community, or organizational entity (e.g., school, hospital, jail). Outbreaks and epidemics require the same investigative process to investigate the cause and control the disease spread. The steps in this process are: (1) defining the case, (2) collecting information in the field regarding the signs and symptoms of case to determine who is ill and who is not ill, (3) collecting risk factor information, (4) analyzing the data graphically and statistically to identify associations between exposure and disease, (5) obtaining specimens for laboratory confirmation from cases and potential sources of the illness, (6) confirming the transmissible agent, (7) disseminating the results of the findings to those who need to know, and (8) developing surveillance and other systems as appropriate to prevent the spread of the infectious disease and its future reoccurrence.

To develop an infectious disease, an individual must be both susceptible and exposed. An exposure is a factor that, in the case of infectious disease transmission, is harmful and is the circumstance that allows for entry or interaction between the host and the organism to produce harmful effects or clinical disease. The circumstances of the exposure are its frequency, duration, dose, distance, and degree of intimacy. The degree of susceptibility of the host (e.g., older age plus comorbidities) also determines if the circumstances of the exposure will result in an infectious disease. An epidemic or outbreak may occur if a large number individuals are exposed who do not possess adequate immunity or are not protected in terms of herd immunity. Herd immunity is the protection of an individual(s) because a sufficient number of individuals in the geographic area are immune from the disease. There are various theories on determining the size of the population to protect any one individual, but the reader should consult other resources.

Control of Infectious Disease

Control of infectious disease, in the health care setting or in the community, is the responsibility of all health care professionals. The areas of responsibility are described below.

Knowledge of the Epidemiology of Common Infectious Problems in Health Care Settings

Knowledge of the epidemiology of infectious problems in health care settings is key to developing prevention measures. There are two populations at risk in this framework, health care workers and patients. Infectious diseases that health care workers are at greatest risk for are:

Hepatitis B, Hepatitis C, and HIV via blood/body fluid exposure and influenza other respiratory conditions transmitted through airborne exposures. Table 3 summarizes the epidemiology of Hepatitis B as an example of the core knowledge that a health care manager should possess when confronted with either planning for or responding to an outbreak or epidemic.

Patients are also at risk for a variety of transmissible diseases in any health care setting. Risk of infectious disease transmission varies by health care setting (Siegel et al., 2007). It is also important to protect patients from diseases transmitted by health care workers. Hence, health care facilities should have policies and procedures in place regarding when workers have become exposed and/or are ill with transmissible diseases (e.g., remain home if have a fever above 101°F). Policies may involve

Table 3 Epidemiology of acute Viral Hepatitis B

Agent:	Hepatitis B virus (HBV) a hepadnavirus, partially double-stranded DNA virus
Classification codes:	ICD-9 070.3; ICD-10 B16
Signs and symptoms:	Jaundice (70%), fatigue, abdominal pain, loss of appetite, nausea, vomiting, joint pain (30% have no signs or symptoms)
Incidence rates (US, 2006):	Overall: trend declining (81% since 1990); 1.6 per 100,000; Race/ethnicity highest among blacks: 2.3 per 100,000; Highest age group: 25–44 years (3.1 per 100,000); Highest rates in the South; Male to female ratio 1.8:1
Clinical course:	40% of cases hospitalized; 0.8% died; increased rate of hospitalization with increasing age
Reservoir:	Man
Mode of transmission:	Infected blood or blood products or any other body fluids containing blood or unfixed tissues or organs
Risk groups:	• Sex contacts with infected persons
	• Men who have sex with men
	• Diagnosis of a sexually transmitted disease
	• Individuals having sex with multiple partners
	• Household contacts of chronically infected persons
	• Infants born to infected mothers
	• Infants/children of immigrants from areas with high rates of HBV infection (Southeast Asia, China, Korea, Indonesia, and the Philippines; the Middle East, except Israel; South and Western Pacific islands; the interior Amazon River basin; Haiti and the Dominican Republic)
	• IV drug users
	• Health care and public safety workers with exposure to blood
	• Hemodialysis patients

ICD = International Classification of Disease

active screening of employees to protect patients against this risk. Screening may include: measles and hepatitis B titre levels and skin testing for latent TB infection. Guidelines for targeted tuberculin testing of health care providers are available through the Centers for Disease Control and Prevention (CDC, 2005). The magnitude and type risk to infectious disease of patients in health care settings varies according to the specific patient population (e.g., adult, pediatric, geriatric, etc.), types of exposures to devices, and types of invasive procedures performed.

In *hospitals*, there are three areas of concern for transmission risk. Intensive care units (ICU) care for patients with life threatening diseases and trauma who are treated with invasive technology often with extended antibiotic use and long stays. ICU patients are at risk for multidrug resistant organisms and various *Candida* species. Over 20% of hospital-acquired infections are likely to arise in ICUs. Burn unit patients are susceptible to infection in proportion to the amount of total body surface exposed. Prevalent organisms in burn units include methicillin-resistant *Staphylococcus aureus* (MRSA), vancomycin-resistant enterococci (VRE), gram-negative bacteria, and various *Candida and Aspergillus* species. Pediatric unit patients are at risk of transmission of community-acquired infections because these patients do not have fully developed immune systems, are low birthweight, have incomplete immunization series, or because of seasonal epidemics occurring in the community. Organisms common in pediatric units include: *Bordetella pertussis* [pertussis], respiratory viral infections including those caused by respiratory syncytial viruses (RSV), influenza viruses, parainfluenza virus, human metapneumovirus, adenoviruses, rubeola [measles], varicella [chicken-pox], and rotaviral enteritis (Boxed Example 2).

Long term care facilities (LTC) (skilled nursing facilities, in-patient rehabilitation centers, in-patient behavioral health centers, assisted breathing centers, homes for the developmentally disabled, hospices) are a source of risk for transmissible disease because their residents may have limitations in or impaired mobility or cognition, share common areas for extended periods of time, and/or have chronic illnesses. The rate of health care-acquired infections has been reported to range from 3 to 7 per 1,000 resident-care days in the more rigorous studies (Siegel et al., 2007). In LTC facilities, transmissible organisms of concern are: various viruses (e.g., influenza virus,

---

Boxed Example 2   Catheter-related Bloodstream Infection:Effectiveness of an Intervention

Problem: In intensive care units, catheter-related bloodstream infections are common and potentially lethal.

Methods: A cohort study compared infection rates before, during, and up to 18 months after implementation of study intervention. The Michigan Health and Hospital Association (MHA) promoted hospital involvement to use interventions (hand washing, full-barrier precautions during the insertion of central venous catheters, cleaning the skin with chlorhexidine, avoiding the femoral site, and removing unnecessary catheters) as part of a statewide safety initiative in ICUs (the MHA Keystone: ICU Project). The National Nosocomial Infections Surveillance System definition of catheter-related blood-stream infection was used which included clinical signs and/or cultures of blood or other infection sites.

Data and Results (Sources: Pronovost et al., 2006; Goeschel et al., 2006):

Study period	Incidence-rate ratio (IRR) (95% CI)	p-value
Baseline	1.00	
During implementation	0.76 (0.57–1.01)	0.063
After implementation		
0–3 months	0.62 (0.47–0.81)	0.001
7–9 months	0.47 (0.34–0.65)	<0.001
16–18 months	0.34 (0.23–0.50)	<0.001

Managerial Epidemiology Interpretation: A risk ratio less than 1.0 indicates that the outcome is less likely the study period than in the baseline period. The significant (a p-value of less than 0.001) "protective (or reduction)" effect (IRR = 0.34) of intervention reducing catheter-related bloodstream infections persisted as long as 18 months after the introduction of the intervention (incidence rate ratio of 0.34, 95% CI: 0.23–0.50, $p < 0.001$).

rhinovirus, adenovirus [conjunctivitis], norovirus) and bacteria, including group A streptococcus, *B. pertussis*, nonsusceptible *S. pneumoniae*, various other multidrug resistant organisms, and *Clostridium difficile*.

In *ambulatory care settings*, the risk of disease transmission is largely influenced by seasonal epidemic trends in the community as well as the types of patient populations served and their treatments. Transmission of bloodborne pathogens (Hepatitis B, Hepatitis C, HIV/AIDS) and transmission of airborne pathogens (M. tuberculosis, measles, rubella varicella-zoster virus) have been reported in ambulatory settings. M. tuberculosis and measles transmission have been most frequently reported in emergency departments, where measles virus transmission has been most frequently reported in physician offices (Siegel et al., 2007). Another common source of transmissible disease in ambulatory settings are contaminated equipment, and failure to use safe injection practices or aseptic technique. Cohorting patients presenting to ambulatory care settings (e.g., a well-child area and sick-child area in a waiting room, negative pressure rooms in the emergency department for persons suspected of serious airborne disease transmission) is a strategy for minimizing the chances of health care-acquired infectious.

In *nontraditional settings* for health care delivery, health care may be provided such as workplaces with occupational health clinics, adult day care centers, assisted living facilities, homeless shelters, jails and prisons, and school clinics. Each setting faces unique challenges and organisms because of the patient populations served (e.g., HIV/AIDS and TB in incarcerated populations and homeless shelters) requiring the health care management to seek guidance from local health authorities.

Reporting

Ideally, all health care facilities should have dedicated infection control professional (ICP) whose primary responsibility is the prevention of infection. The ICP is responsible for having the knowledge of which infectious diseases must be reported by state legislation or regulation to the local or state health department. In the absence of an ICP, the designated manager is responsible for the reporting. The general categories of conditions reported are communicable diseases, sexually transmitted diseases, TB, and vaccine preventable disease. Notifiable diseases vary somewhat by state although all states require reporting of diseases subject to quarantine (cholera, plague, and yellow fever) according to the World Health Organization's International Health Regulations. The responsibility for reporting diseases to the local health authority depends upon the requirements set forth by that authority. A report to the local health authority in whose jurisdiction the reporter is located is required by any person having knowledge of a known or suspected case or carrier of communicable disease or a death caused by a communicable disease determined notifiable by the local health authority. Among those required to report include: physicians, nurses, nurse aides, dentists, laboratory personnel, school personnel, long-term care personnel, day care personnel, and college/university personnel. Health care providers may disclose individually identifiable health information for use in public health to public health authorities without individual consent without violating HIPAA regulation. The specific data required for reporting includes patient information (name, address, date of birth, gender, race, ethnicity) and testing information (name of test and test result). The Centers for Disease and Control website should be consulted for the latest listing of notifiable diseases in the USA which is revised periodically depending upon the emergence of new pathogens or a decline or elimination of an existing pathogen (Table 4). Even under the best of circumstances, it may take 2–3 weeks to confirm a patient's illness was part of an outbreak because of the time to contact the health system, the timing of the collection of the specimen, clinical laboratory identification of the agent, shipping time of the specimen to the public health lab, and confirmation by the public lab. Thus, cases

Table 4 Notifiable communicable diseases in the United States, 2008 (Source: Centers for Disease Control and Prevention, 2008)

Acquired immunodeficiency syndrome (AIDS)	Novel influenza A virus infection
Anthrax	Pertussis
Arboviral neuroinvasive and nonneuroinvasive diseases (e.g., St. Louis encephalitis, West Nile virus disease)	Plague
Botulism	Poliomyelitis, paralytic and nonparalytic
Brucellosis	Psittacosis
Chlamydia trachomatis, genital infection	Q Fever
Cholera	Rabies, animal and human
Coccidioidomycosis	Rocky Mountain spotted fever
Cryptosporidiosis	Rubella, including congenital syndrome
Cyclosporiasis	Salmonellosis
Diptheria	Severe Acute Respiratory Syndrome-associated Coronavirus (SARS-CoV) disease
Ehrlichiosis/Anaplasmosis	Shiga toxin-producing *Escherichia coli* (STEC)
Giardiasis	Shigellosis
Gonorrhea	Smallpox
Haemophilus influenza, invasive disease	Streptococcal disease, invasive, Group A or toxic-shock syndrome
Hepatitis A, acute	*Streptococcus pneumoniae*, drug resistant invasive disease or nondrug resistant invasive disease in children less than 5 years of age
Hansen disease (leprosy)	Syphilis, including congenital
Hantavirus pulmonary syndrome	Tetanus
Hemolytic uremic syndrome, postdiarrheal	Toxic-shock syndrome (other than Streptococcal)
Hepatitis, viral, acute and chronic (Hepatitis A, Hepatitis B, Hepatitis C)	Trichinellosis (Trichinosis)
HIV Infection (adult or pediatric)	Tuberculosis

(continued)

Table 4 (continued)

Influenza-associated pediatric mortality	Tularemia
Legionellosis	Typhoid fever
Listeriosis	Vancomycin intermediate or resistant *Staphylococcus aureus*
Lyme disease	Syphilis
Malaria	Varicella (morbidity or mortality)
Measles	Vibriosis
Meningococcal disease	Yellow fever
Mumps	

enumerated by signs and symptoms while an outbreak of a disease is occurring should be considered preliminary until confirmed by laboratory findings.

Surveillance

Surveillance is the systematic collection of data pertaining to defined cases or behaviors related to a disease (infectious in this discussion), analysis, evaluation, and the dissemination of results to those who are in a position to initiate control measures. To prevent outbreaks, local health authorities rely on communicable disease reported to surveillance systems. Data collection may range from computerized reports of syndromes, compilation of reports from systematic field studies/or surveys, adverse events (e.g., needle stick injury), or environmental factors (surveillance of dead birds in association with West Nile disease) (Patnaik et al., 2007). A more detailed discussion of surveillance systems is in chapter "Screening and Surveillance for Promoting Population Health." Health care workers need to be active in surveillance efforts through participation in the reporting and utilization of data from surveillance systems to plan and evaluate control efforts.

Vaccines

Vaccination is the conferring of active immunity through the administration of an antigen that is not pathogenic. The principle of vaccination is to stimulate the antibody (B-cell) response and cell-mediated response (T-cell) such that the immune system will mount an immediate, sustained and sufficiently powerful attack against exposure to the pathogen invading the host. Vaccination should have long-term, lasting protection. Table 5 lists diseases that are preventable through available vaccines.

However, there are limitations to the value of existing vaccinations. The protective effective of the vaccination may take longer than the time between exposure and onset of disease, many vaccines require multiple doses to achieve a protective immune response, not all persons mount an immune response subsequent to the vaccination, and finally, persons with impaired immunity either

Table 5   Vaccine preventable diseases

Anthrax	Pertussis (Whooping Cough)
Cervical cancer	Pneumococcal infection
Diptheria	Poliomyelitis (Polio)
Hepatitis A	Rabies
Hepatitis B	Rotavirus
Haemophilus influenzae type b (Hib)	Rubella (German Measles)
Human Papillomavirus (HPV)	Shingles (Herpes Zoster)
Influenza (Flu)	Smallpox
Japanese Encephalitis (JE)	Tetanus (Lockjaw)
Lyme disease	Tuberculosis (TB)
Measles	Typhoid fever
Meningococcal infection	Varicella (Chickenpox)
Monkeypox	Yellow Fever
Mumps	

cannot generate an immune response to the vaccine or may experience side effects to the vaccine. Vaccines, as with any therapeutic product, may have side effects. Most side effects may be minor (injection site swelling, fever, malaise). Major side effects may include allergic reactions because of the medium the vaccine was grown in (egg or tissue culture) or additives or the disease itself from the administration of a live virus.

There are recommended vaccinations and vaccination schedules not only for children, but also for adults and health care workers (Centers for Disease Control and Prevention, 2007; Centers for Disease Control and Prevention, 2009a, b). The purpose of immunization of health care workers is not only to protect themselves, but also to promote patient safety by "doing no harm," that is, not being a potential source of hospital-acquired infection. Immunization of health care workers additionally contributes to providing herd immunity. Herd immunity is the protection from an infectious agent afforded to a population as a whole because large numbers of its members are immune to an infectious problem and do not harbor it. Following current recommendations for vaccination is a responsibility of all health care providers as it is one aspect of promoting patient safety. The major cost savings to health care organizations are to promote the wide-spread coverage of influenza vaccination among its employees. The prevalence of employees obtaining influenza vaccination will be an important component of hospital infection prevention and control programs to meet new CMS (2007) Guidelines. In 2003, the prevalence of health care workers who received influenza vaccination was only 40%.

Passive antibody administration conferring rapid immunity through humoral mechanisms (e.g., Anthrax vaccination), regardless of the immunity level of the individual, has been proposed as a specific defense against biological weapons and would be useful to health care workers, first responders, and military personnel who are at risk for exposure to biological weapons (Casadevall, 2002). However, the cost of the development and administration of such vaccinations is questionable if readily available drug therapy is available.

Managerial Responsibilities in the Control of Infectious Diseases

Health care managers are responsible for coordinating the general effort of the prevention and control of transmissible diseases in health care organization. Areas of responsibility are described below.

Administrative Controls

Administrative controls are the development and use of policies, procedures, and protocols regarding the prevention and rapid detection, isolation, treatment, and spread of infectious disease within a health care facility. Administrative controls are aimed at the environment as well as employee and patient behaviors. Evidence from the recent literature, epidemiologic principles of infectious disease, national priorities, and accreditation agency criteria, state, or local regulations should guide in the development of administration controls. The Joint Commission on Accreditation of Healthcare Organizations (2008) has targeted selected infections and infection prevention and control activities to be included in its *2008 National Patient Safety Goals*. These are displayed in Table 6. The increasing costs associated with hospital-acquired infection have prompted the implementation of federal standards aimed at hospital responsibilities for infection prevention and control practices. The CMS Guidelines mandate hospitals to have active programs for the prevention, control, and investigations of infections and communicable diseases. The Guidelines further require that an infection prevention and control officer or officers are designated in writing, a log of all incidents related to infections

Table 6 2008 National patient safety goals pertaining to infection prevention and control (Source: Joint Commission for Accreditation of Healthcare Organizations, 2008)

Goal 7 Reduce the risk of health care-associated infections

  7A Comply with current World Health Organization (WHO) Hand Hygiene Guidelines or Centers for Disease Control and Prevention (CDC) hand hygiene guidelines [Ambulatory, Assisted Living, Behavioral Health Care, Critical Access Hospital, Disease-Specific Care, Home Care, Hospital, Lab, Long Term Care, Office-Based Surgery]

  7B Manage as sentinel events all identified cases of unanticipated death or major permanent loss of function associated with a health care-associated infection [Ambulatory, Assisted Living, Behavioral Health Care, Critical Access Hospital, Disease-Specific Care, Home Care, Hospital, Lab, Long Term Care, Office-Based Surgery]

Goal 10 Reduce the risk of influenza and pneumococcal disease in institutionalized older adults

  10A Develop and implement a protocol for administration and documentation of the flu vaccine [Assisted Living, Disease-Specific Care, Long-Term Care]

  10B Develop and implement a protocol for administration and documentation of the pneumococcus vaccine [Assisted Living, Disease-Specific Care, Long-Term Care]

  10C Develop and implement a protocol to identify new cases of influenza and to manage an outbreak [Assisted Living, Disease-Specific Care, Long-Term Care]

and communicable disease among both patients and staff, the CEO, medical staff, and nursing director assume the responsibility for addressing problems identified by infection prevention and control officer(s) in quality assurance and training programs, and that corrective action plans are in place for problems identified by the infection prevention and control officer(s) (CMS, 2007).

Increasingly, the use of evidence-based guidelines and protocols is used to improve outcomes and/or prevent infections (Hauck et al., 2004; Pronovost et al., 2006). The Michigan Health and Hospital Association Keystone ICU Project promoted the use of evidence-based protocol by a hospital's ICU implementation team which had the goals of eliminating bloodstream infections and ventilator-associated pneumonia. The Project had many successful outcomes including patient lives, hospital days, and health care dollars saved (see Boxed Example 2) (Michigan Health and Hospital Association, 2008).

Employee risk assessment and education are administrative control measures. The first step is to classify all employees according to risk of exposure to bloodborne pathogens or airborne disease transmission. Volunteers and students should also be assessed of their risk. Risk assessment for bloodborne disease is according to three levels: Level I, individuals at highest risk because they work with blood or blood products, sharps, perform invasive tasks, or work with equipment which may be contaminated with blood or bodily fluids (e.g., lab technician, nurse); Level II individuals are at medium exposure due to limited contact with patients, blood, or body fluids (e.g., dietary workers); and, Level III individuals have no direct patient contact and no contact with contaminated items such as sharps (e.g., accounting personnel). The next steps involve the communication of the risk to the affected persons, monitoring the exposures, and offering exposure reduction plans to employees (e.g., on site availability of Hepatitis B vaccine series) and training on risk reduction and infection prevention and control practices at orientation and annually.

Administrative controls also include the establishment of an infection prevention and control program and credentials of its personnel should follow the practice standards adopted by the Boards of the Association for Professionals in Infection Control and Epidemiology, Inc. (APIC) (http://www.apic.org). APIC promotes guidelines, based upon epidemiologic principles, for the development and staffing for infection control programs within health care organizations. Criteria for staffing include a consideration of number of occupied beds (average daily census), complexity of health system, patient population, and diagnostic and therapeutic interventions used in the setting (O'Boyle et al., 2002). Elements of an infection prevention and control program are listed in Table 7. Even if the health care facility has an infection prevention and control program, it is the responsibility of each employee to be engaged in the control of transmissible disease. Management responsibilities regarding infection prevention and control are displayed in Table 8.

Other administrative controls involve patient placement (e.g., cohorting ill patients in waiting rooms or air pressure negative rooms), transportation procedures (specimen and patient), handling of laundry, management of solid waste disposal, handling of dietary materials, and the management of visitors.

Table 7 Elements of an infection prevention and control program

1. Establish authority of infection prevention and control, organizational position, reporting relationships, and staffing
2. Construct an exposure matrix for all employee job classifications
3. Plan, develop, implement, and operate method(s) for infection surveillance:
   a. Targeted (e.g., high risk patients: immobile, ICU)
   b. Active (e.g., encourage or require reporting of needle stick injuries, culturing for a specific organism, Staphylococci)
   c. Passive (e.g., monitor microbiological reports of Assisted Breathing Unit)
   d. Periodic (e.g., rotating sampling of reports or specimens among wards)
4. Develop policies and procedures in accordance with regulatory bodies, credentialing bodies, the current literature, and the types of exposures anticipated among the health care workforce
5. Establish mechanisms and procedures for communicable disease reporting, within organization and to local health authority
6. Conduct preemployment testing and mandatory immunizations
7. Conduct education for all new employees and annually thereafter on latest CDC recommendations for infection prevention and control
8. Conduct periodic employee screenings (e.g., for tuberculosis)
9. Provide recommended immunizations for employees (hepatitis B, influenza)
10. Provide treatment for workplace exposures if indicated (e.g., chemotherapy for post HIV/AIDS exposure)
11. Provide support for personnel employee health (e.g., smoking cessation programs, asthma awareness)
12. Disseminate feedback to staff on organizational progress in infection prevention and control

Table 8 Healthcare manager responsibilities regarding infection prevention and control

Prevention

1. Classify work activity and exposure levels for all job titles
2. Develop policies and procedures for workplace exposure control
3. Provide training an education in infection prevention and control
4. Develop procedures to ensure and monitor compliance to infection prevention and control policies and procedures
5. Provide access to Hepatitis B vaccination
6. Establish an annual influenza vaccination program that includes at least staff and licensed independent practitioners
   - Provide access to influenza vaccinations on-site
   - Education staff and licensed independent practitioners about flu vaccination, diagnosis and transmission, and impact of diagnosis and nonvaccination control measures (e.g., cohorting of patients, protect sneezes and coughs, prevent hand mucous membrane contact)
   - Annually evaluate vaccination rates and reasons for nonparticipation in the organization's immunization program
   - Implement enhancements to the program to increase participation

Workplace environment

1. Provide for safe needles and sharps disposal
2. Install hand washing facilities and redundant systems for hand hygiene (e.g., alcohol-based hand sanitizers)

(continued)

Table 8 (continued)

3. Supply approved cleaning, disinfecting, sterilizing equipment materials
4. Fit and provide personal protective equipment and training in its use
5. Arrange for safe disposal of biological waste
6. Maintain proper airflow in isolation rooms
7. Ensure timely and protected transport of biological specimens within and out of facility

Medical response to individual exposure

1. Provide baseline assessment and appropriate laboratory testing at time of exposure
2. Secure documentation of exposure circumstances (work tasks, protective equipment, exposure source, and features)
3. Arrange for follow-up assessments, testing, and treatment for symptomatic disease emerging related to exposure
4. Institute workplace restrictions or duty-reassignment for workers highly susceptible to transmissible disease depending upon employee's physician

General operations

1. Report exposure and subsequent exposure-related disease to OSHA and as appropriate to local health authority
2. Communicate with local authorities in the event of intentional exposure of employees or patients to biologic agents (e.g., evidence of aerosolized anthrax in health care facilities)
3. Communicate with employees and/or patients in the event of accidental or intentional exposure of employees or patients to biological agents (e.g., contaminated surgical equipment)

Engineering Controls

Engineering controls are modifications to the environment or devices that remove the hazard or reduce the exposure in the workplace. Examples are: sharps containers that are leak-proof and puncture resistant, needle-less intravenous connections, mouth-to-mouth, resuscitation mouthpieces, and nitrile gloves. Structural features such as certified biological safety cabinets and laminar flow rooms are engineering measures aimed at infection prevention and control. Cost-effectiveness analysis guides the manager in selecting engineering measures which are typically more expensive control options than either the use of administrative controls or personal protective equipment (PPE).

Personal Protective Equipment

Health care managers must assure that PPE is available to employees as appropriate, in addition to administrative controls. PPE consists of items to protect patients and staff from exposures during work tasks. In particular, PPE is designed to reduce the risk of a health care worker's exposure through the skin, mucous membranes, or respiratory system. Examples of PPE include gloves, gowns, masks, eyeglasses, face shields, shoe covers, goggles, and respirators. The sequence of donning and removing PPE is extremely important an infection prevention process and the recommended sequences are displayed in Fig. 3.

a   **Example of Safe Donning of Personal Protective
          Equipment (PPE)**

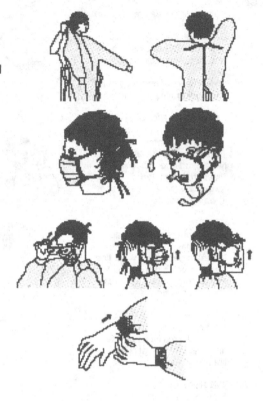

GOWN
- Fully cover torso from
  neck to knees, arms to
  end of wrist, and wrap
  around the back
- Fasten in back at neck and
  waist

MASK OR RESPIRATOR
- Secure ties or elastic band
  at middle of head and
  neck
- Fit flexible band to nose
  bridge
- Fit snug to face and below
  chin
- Fit-check respirator

GOGGLES/FACE SHIELD
- Put on face and adjust to
  fit

GLOVES
- Use non-sterile for
  isolation
- Select according to hand
  size
- Extend to cover wrist of
  isolation gown

SAFE WORK PRACTICES
- Keep hands away from face
- Work from clean to dirty
- Limit surfaces touched
- Change when torn or heavily contaminated
- Perform hand hygiene

Fig. 3 (a) Sequence for donning personal protective equipment (PPE)

Managing Disease Outbreaks   484

There are circumstances, despite the most comprehensive administrative efforts, that   485
a disease outbreak or epidemic will occur in a health care facility. An epidemic is   486
the occurrence of cases of a condition occurring in excess of what would be expected   487

b   REMOVING PERSONAL PROTECTIVE (PPE)
                              EQUIPMENT

Remove PPE at doorway before leaving patient room or in
anteroom

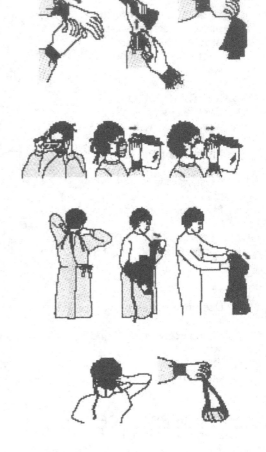

GLOVES
  ▪ Outside of gloves are
     contaminated!
  ▪ Grasp outside of glove with
     opposite gloved hand; peel off
  ▪ Hold removed glove in gloved
     hand
  ▪ Slide fingers of ungloved hand
     under remaining glove at wrist

GOGGLES/FACE SHIELD
  ▪ Outside of goggles or face
     shield are contaminated!
  ▪ To remove, handle by "clean"
     head band or ear pieces
  ▪ Place in designated
     receptacle for reprocessing or
     in waste container

GOWN
  ▪ Gown front and sleeves are
     contaminated!
  ▪ Unfasten neck, then waist ties
  ▪ Remove gown using a peeling
     motion; pull gown from each
     shoulder toward the same
     hand
  ▪ Gown will turn inside out
  ▪ Hold removed gown away
     from body, roll into a bundle
     and discard into waste or
     linen receptacle

MASK OR RESPIRATOR
  ▪ Front of mask/respirator is
     contaminated – DO NOT
     TOUCH!
  ▪ Grasp ONLY bottom then top
     ties/elastics and remove
  ▪ Discard in waste container

HAND HYGIENE
Perform hand hygiene immediately
after removing all PPE!

Fig. 3 (b) Sequence for removing PPE (From: Centers for Disease Control and Prevention, 2007)

during the same time interval during the same season of the year. A disease outbreak
is the occurrence of cases of disease in excess of what would normally be expected
in a short-time period in a defined population, community, geographical area, or
season. An outbreak may occur in a restricted geographical area, or extend over
several countries within the same few days, weeks, or years. According to the World
Health Organization (2007), "A single case of a communicable disease long absent

from a population, or caused by an agent (e.g., bacterium or virus) not previously recognized in that community or area, or the emergence of a previously unknown disease, may also constitute an outbreak and should be reported and investigated." The actual number of cases constituting an epidemic depends upon the infectious agent and the circumstances of the case presentation. Two cases of botulism occurring among patrons of a restaurant may be considered an epidemic. An epidemic may arise for several reasons, including: (1) an increase in the number of susceptible persons; (2) the emergence of a new organism; (3) changes in the environment; (4) changes in human behavior; (5) new media for the growth of organisms; (6) the migration of infected persons, animals, birds, or insects into an area; (7) change in the virulence of an organism; (8) inadequate immunization levels in a population; (9) improper sanitation or sanitary practices; or, (10) the intentional introduction of an infectious agent. A clue, if the epidemic is due to the intentional introduction of an infectious agent, is when a case is found to have developed the disease not through usual route of transmission or reservoir. For example, the development of anthrax in the respiratory system is not consistent with the common mode of transmission, namely direct contact with the tissues of animals dying of the disease.

Health care settings are susceptible to epidemics and outbreaks. In theses setting, both the patient population and health care employees are at risk including because of the closeness of contact, the immunocompromised state of many patients from diseases, inadequate vaccination levels. During the SARS epidemic, there were a large number of health care workers documented as having acquired the disease from exposure to patients. The health care organization must be proactive and reactive, responding in a quick manner to decrease further infectious disease spread. This requires an organized effort by the organization.

In the event an outbreak occurs in a health care facility, the role of the health care manager is to initiate an organized strategy for its control. The action steps then taken by the manager would include the deployment of the personnel and resources to: (1) define the case; (2) screen all persons potentially exposed with laboratory studies to define the magnitude of the outbreak; (3) characterize the demographics of the cases, place of onset of disease, and time of onset of signs and symptoms; (4) isolate the infected cases and the source, if known; (5) disinfect portals of exit; (6) break identified chains of entry; (7) defend portals of entry; (8) arrange for the immunization and/or treatment of other susceptible persons, if indicated; (9) promote the investigation of risk factors (optimally using a case-control design); and (10) establish and maintain surveillance that serves to identify the potential for future outbreaks and gauges the efficacy of control measures. Of these steps, rapid detection is probably the most important and a responsibility of all health care professionals in the facility.

Health Care Manager Responsibilities in Infection Prevention

Health care managers in practice should support the use of a combination of control measures, both in terms of organizational structure as well as policies and procedures.

The mandated use of "Standard Precautions" in a health care setting is an example of a combination of control measures. Standard precautions emphasize administrative controls and the use of PPE. The epidemiologic principle behind this is twofold. First, excluding sweat, all body fluids, secretions, excretions, mucous membranes, and nonintact skin are presumed to be potentially infectious so that contact with these portals of exit and bodily fluids should be avoided. Second, health care settings often have a high prevalence of patients who are immunocompromised and therefore Standard Precautions should be used in the care of all patients (Table 9). Although for most communicable diseases, Standard Precautions are recommended, there are also Airborne, Contact, and Droplet Precautions which may be indicated for selected infections and conditions (Siegel et al., 2007). The U.S. Department of Labor, Occupational Health and Safety Administration (OSHA) provides information

Table 9 Recommendations for application of standard precautions for the care of all patients in all healthcare settings (Source: Siegel et al., 2007)

Standard precautions component	Recommendations
Hand hygiene	After touching blood, body fluids, secretions, excretions, contaminated items; immediately after removing gloves; between patient contacts
Personal protective equipment (PPE):	
Gloves	For touching blood, body fluids, secretions, excretions, contaminated items; for touching mucous membranes and nonintact skin
Gown	During procedure and patient-care activities when contact of clothing/exposed skin with blood/body fluids, secretions, and excretions is anticipated
Mask, eye protection (goggles), face shield[a]	During procedures and patient-care activities likely to generate splashes or sprays of blood, body fluids, secretions, especially suctioning, endotracheal intubation
Soiled patient-care equipment	Handle in a manner that prevents transfer of microorganisms to other and to the environment; wear gloves if visibly contaminated; perform hand hygiene
Environment control	Develop procedures for routine care, cleaning, and disinfection of environmental surfaces, especially frequently touched surfaces in patient-care areas
Textiles and laundry	Handle in a manner that prevents transfer of microorganisms to others and to the environment
Needles and other sharps	Do not recap, bend, break, or hand-manipulate used needles; if recapping is required, use a one-handed scoop technique only; use safety features when available; place used sharps in puncture-resistant container
Patient resuscitation	Use mouthpiece, resuscitation bag, other ventilation devices to prevent contact with mouth and oral secretions

(continued)

Table 9 (continued)

Standard precautions component	Recommendations
Patient placement	Prioritize for single-patient room if patient is at increased risk of transmission, is likely to contaminate the environment, does not maintain appropriate hygiene, or is at increased risk of acquiring infection or developing adverse outcome following infection
Respiratory hygiene/cough etiquette (source containment of infectious respiratory secretions in symptomatic patients, beginning at initial point of encounter e.g., triage and reception areas in emergency departments and physician offices)	Instruct symptomatic persons to cover mouth/nose when sneezing/coughing; use tissues and dispose in no-touch receptacle; observe hand hygiene after soiling of hands with respiratory secretions; wear surgical mask if tolerated or maintain spatial separation, >3 feet possible

[a]During aerosol-generating procedures on patients with suspected or proven infection transmitted by highly pathogenic respiratory aerosols (e.g., SARS, tuberculosis), wear a fit-tested N95 or higher respirator in addition to gloves, gown, and face/eye protection

on assessing the risk of various exposures to biological agents (e.g., anthrax) and procedures for clean-up of the workplace after contamination http://www.osha.gov/SLTC/biologicalagents/index.html.

Outbreak, Hazard, and Communicable Disease Rate Communication

Communication is an essential management responsibility. Hazard communication involves not only written policies and procedures, but also communication in terms of signage and training. Warning labels affixed to biohazardous waste containers, refrigerators, and biohazardous waste bags identified by red color as signage on patients' doors are examples of hazard communication. Training given to employees on their risk level to bloodborne disease and other occupational exposures at orientation and annual retraining is another form of communication. Communication in the event of outbreaks is essential not only to employees, but also to patients and the community. The World Health Organization (WHO, 2005) identified a list of best practices in communicating with the public during outbreaks which apply in any culture, political system, or developmental state of a nation. According to the WHO, the communications of the existence of an outbreak should include the following elements: trust-building; announcing early; transparency (candid, easily understood, complete, accurate); an understanding of the public's beliefs, opinions and knowledge about risks; and, a preparedness plan. It is felt that greater cooperation by the public in participating with control measures will result with effective communication.

There is growing interest by public groups for information regarding the morbidity and mortality rates of infectious diseases in health care facilities.

The Consumers Union (2007) is one of several new organizations taking web-based action to promote the reporting of hospital infection rates, and hence consumer awareness, as a means of reducing the likelihood of hospital infection. Recognizing the need for greater transparency of communication, governmental agencies are also responding to consumers' interest in quality data. The Hospital Compare web-based quality tool provides information of selected conditions and procedures related to hospital-acquired infection (http://www.hospitalcompare.hhs.gov). The Michigan Quality Improvement Consortium publishes annual reports on procedures and preventive practices among members in Michigan health plans, commercial and Medicaid participants. Reports of indicators include: immunizations, appropriate testing for childhood pharyngitis, and *Chlamydia* screening (http://www.mqic.org). Health care managers need to understand the computation of the epidemiologic measures and data collection procedures of reports published by private and public organizations to prepare appropriate responses to members of the community's need for communication and information. Internet social media websites (e.g., Facebook, Twitter) and Really Simple Syndication (RSS) web feeds along with blogs are used with increasing frequency to transmit critical updates to as many people as possible news and information pertaining to emerging outbreaks and epidemics.

Summary

Infection prevention is a continuing priority in health care services. Not only is there the potential for litigation for health care-acquired infections (HAI), but the direct and indirect costs associated with the treatment of HAI's including risks of lost reimbursement, compel health care managers to scrutinize each step of the health care delivery process to ensure safeguards for infection prevention. Tasks as simple as the regular cleansing of public surfaces in health care institutions to monitoring the health of employees, volunteers, and students in the setting. Knowledge of the epidemiology of transmissible diseases common in health care settings is fundamental to the development, implementation, and evaluation of any infection prevention program.

Discussion Questions

Q.1. Compare and contrast the case-fatality rate from SARS described in Boxed Example 1 to the case-fatality rates of three other infectious diseases (e.g., AIDS, Ebola, etc.). Comment on the challenges in specifying the definitions of the numerator and the denominator used in calculating each rate.

Q.2. Outline an alternate study design to evaluate the effectiveness of intervention to reduced bloodborne catheter infection than the one described in Boxed Example 2.

Q.3. Propose alternative methods to those described in Boxed Example 3 for improving health care worker compliance to participation in an influenza vaccination program.

Q.4. You are an administrator of a nursing program offered through a university with residence halls. You find out that many of the nursing students have called in sick to their instructors of their clinical rotations. The students have reported

---

Boxed Example 3 Improving Influenza Vaccination Coverage in Health Care Workers (Source: Kimura et al., 2005)

Problem: In 2003, influenza vaccination coverage was only 40% among health care workers (HCW). HCW can transmit influenza to patients. CMS (2007) is mandating infection prevention and control programs that include both patient and employee populations.

Methods: A controlled study in 70 southern California nursing homes during the 2002–2003 influenza season. Nursing homes were selected by convenience sample and were assigned to one of four groups: (1) group A ($n = 25$), which conducted no interventions; (2) group B ($n = 15$), which conducted an educational campaign; (3) group C ($n = 15$), which held [influenza] Vaccine Days; and (4) group D ($n = 15$), which conducted both an educational campaign and held Vaccine Days.

Data and Results: The control group (group A) had 27% vaccination coverage. Vaccine Days when implemented in combination with the educational campaign (group D) had 53% coverage; adjusted odds ratio [AOR] = 3.54; 95% confidence interval [CI] = 2.17–5.72) and when implemented alone (group C) (45%; AOR = 2.28; CI = 1.30–3.98). The educational campaign alone (group B) had a vaccination coverage of 34% (AOR = 1.31; CI = 0.76–2.25).

Managerial Epidemiologic Interpretation: The control group in an intervention study is the referent. The higher AOR for the educational campaign alone was not significantly different from the control group because the 95% CI contained 1.0. The Vaccine Days intervention alone was effective in increasing the prevalence of vaccination coverage because the CI lower limit (1.30) was greater than 1.0. Vaccine days offered in combination with an educational campaign yielded a significantly higher coverage than the control group (AOR = 3.54) and was the most effective strategy. Considering the national prevalence of health care worker (HCW) influenza vaccination coverage rate is 40% in 2003, a multi-component intervention will be necessary to increase the rate in HCWs.

to their instructors a variety of gastrointestinal problems including acute-onset vomiting, watery nonbloody diarrhea with abdominal cramps, and nausea. How would you respond to this situation?

References

Ahern, M., Kovats, R.S., Wilkinson, P., Few, R., and Matthies, F., 2005, Global health impacts of floods: epidemiologic evidence, *Epidemiol. Rev.* **27**:36–46.

Casadevall, A., 2002, Passive antibody administration (immediate immunity) as a specific defense against biological weapons, *Emerging Infectious Dis.* **8**:833–841.

Centers for Disease Control and Prevention, 2009a, Recommended immunization schedules for persons aged 0 through 18 years—United States, Errata: *M.M.W.R.* 2009;**57**:1419.

Centers for Disease Control and Prevention, 2009b, Recommended adult immunization schedule—United States, 2009, *M.M.W.R.* **57**:Q1–Q4.

Centers for Disease Control and Prevention, 2008, Prevention and control of influenza: recommendations of the Advisory Committee on Immunization Practices (ACIP), 2008, *M.M.W.R.* **57(No. RR-7)**:1–45.

Centers for Disease Control and Prevention, 2007, Healthcare personnel vaccination recommendations (January 17, 2009), http://www.cdc.gov/vaccines/pubs/pinkbook/downloads/appendices/appdx-full-a.pdf

Centers for Medicare and Medicaid Services (CMS), 2007, *Interpretive Guidelines for 42 CFR 482.42, Hospital Condition of Participation: Infection prevention and control*, Department of Health and Human Services, CMS, Baltimore, MD.

Consumers Union, 2007, Fighting Deadly Hospital Infections Maryland and Virginia: Major differences found among hospitals within each state in preventing infections http://www.consumersunion.org/pdf/MDVAInfections.pdf,Yonkers, NY.

Goeschel, C.A., Bourgault A., Palleschi M., Posa P., Harrison D., Tacia L.L., Adamczyk M.A., Falkenberg D., Barbret, L., Clark, P., Heck, K., O'Neil, M., Pitts, V., Schumacher, K., Sidor, D., Thompson, M., Wahl, E., and Bosen, D.M., 2006, Nursing lessons from the MHA keystone ICU project: developing and implementing an innovative approach to patient safety, *Crit. Care Nurs. Clin. North Am.* **18**:481–492.

Hauck, L.D., Adler, L.M., and Mulla, Z.D., 2004, Clinical pathway care improves outcomes among patients hospitalized for community-acquired pneumonia, *Ann. Epidemiol.* **14**:669–675.

Heymann, D.L. (ed.), 2008, *Control of Communicable Diseases Manual*, 19th ed., American Public Health Association, Washington, DC.

Joint Commission on Accreditation of Healthcare Organizations, 2008, *2008 National Patient Safety Goals*, JCAHO, Oakbrook Terrace, IL.

Karlberg, J., Chong, D.S.Y., and Lai, W.Y.Y., 2004, Do men have a higher case fatality rate of severe acute respiratory syndrome than women do? *Am. J. Epidemiol.* **159**:229–231.

Kimura, A.C., Higa, J.I., Nguyen, C., Vugia, D.J., Dysart, M., Ellingson, L., Chelstrom, L., Thurn, J., Nichol, K.L., Poland, G.A., Dean, J., Lees, K.A., and Fishbein, D.B., 2005, Interventions to increase influenza vaccination of health-care workers—California and Minnesota, *M.M.W.R.* **54**:196–199.

Lienhardt, C., 2001, From exposure to disease: the role of environmental factors in susceptibility to and development of tuberculosis, *Epidemiol. Rev.* **23**:288–300.

McDonald, L.C., Killgore, G.E., Thompson, A., Owens, R.C., Kazakova, S.V., Sambol, S.P., Johnson, S., and Gerding, D.N., 2005, An epidemic, toxin gene—variant strain of *Clostridium difficile*, *N. Engl. J. Med.* **353**:2433–2441.

Michigan Health and Hospital Association, 2008, Keystone: ICU, http://www.mha.org/mha_app/keystone/icu_overview.jsp

Miller, M.A., Vibound, C., Balinska, M., and Simonsen, L., 2009, The signature features of influenza pandemics—implications for policy, *New Engl. J. Med.* **360**:2595–2598.

Newman, P.A., Rhodes, F., and Weiss, R.E., 2004, Correlates of sex trading among drug-using men who have sex with men, *Am. J. Pub. Health* **94**:1998–2003.

O'Boyle, C., Jackson, M., and Henly, S.J., 2002, Staffing requirements for infection control programs in US health care facilities: Delphi project, *Am. J. Infect. Control* **30**:321–333.

Olsen, S.J., Chang, H.L., Cheung, T.Y., Tang, A.F., Fisk, T.L., Ooi, S.P., Kuo, H.W., Jiang, D.D., Chen, K.T., Lando, J., Hsu, K.H., Chen, T.J., and Dowell, S.F., 2003, Transmission of the severe acute respiratory syndrome on aircraft, *N. Engl. J. Med.* **349**:2416–2422.

Patnaik, J.L., Juliusson, L., and Vogt, R.L., 2007, Environmental predictors of human West Nile virus infections, Colorado, *Emerg. Infect Dis.* **13**:1788–1790.

Pronovost, P., Needham, D., Berenholtz, S., Sinopoli, D., Chu, H., Cosgrove, S., Sexton, B., Hyzy, R., Welsh, R., Roth, G., Bander, J., Kepros, J., and Goeschel, C., 2006, An intervention to decrease catheter-related bloodstream infections in the ICU, *New Engl. J. Med.* **355**:2725–2732.

Siegel, J.D., Rhinehart, E., Jackson, M., Chiarello, L., and the Healthcare Infection prevention and control Practices Advisory Committee, 2007, Guideline for Isolation Precautions: Preventing Transmission of Infectious Agents in Healthcare Settings, *http://www.cdc.gov/ncidod/dhqp/pdf/isolation2007.pdf.*

World Health Organization (WHO), 2005, *Outbreak Communication Guidelines*, WHO, Geneva, Switzerland.

World Health Organization, 2007, Disease Outbreaks, http://www.who.int/topics/disease_outbreaks/en.

World Health Organization, 2009, *WHO pandemic phase descriptions and main actions by phase* (July 5, 2009) http://www.who.int/csr/disease/influenza/GIPA3AideMemoire.pdf.

Chapter 8
Health Risks from the Environment: Challenges to Health Services Delivery

Learning Outcomes

After completing this chapter, you will be able to:

1. Conduct an assessment of the main environmental health hazards in a community and the associated vulnerable populations.
2. Identify the advantages and limitations of a risk assessment for an environmental exposure to determine the likelihood of adverse human health consequences.
3. Cite examples of health services to address health risks from the environment.

Keyterms Environment • Environmental hazard • Risk assessment

Introduction

The role of the environment in the development of disease, injury, and disability has been a fundamental concept throughout the history of epidemiology. John Snow in the investigation of the cause of the cholera focused on the role of water pumps in Central London. Housing, crowding, and sanitation were found to be factors in the development of tuberculosis (Lienhardt, 2001). Studies of migrants have been important in understanding the importance of exposure to a changing environment, particularly diet. From these types of studies many diet-disease relationships have been identified including the role of dietary factors in stomach and breast cancers (Correa et al., 1982; Nelson, 2006). Various occupational exposures, ranging from chemical (benzene) to physical (vibration), were identified impacting health in terms of mortality as well as morbidity. Epidemiologic evidence has demonstrated the role of second hand exposure in the development of health conditions (e.g., second hand smoke and lung cancer). The global burden of diseases and health problem attributable to the environment is growing. The World Health Organization (WHO) has gathered evidence demonstrating that nearly one quarter of all deaths and of the total disease burden can be attributed to the environment and among

D.M. Oleske (ed.), *Epidemiology and the Delivery of Health Care Services:*
Method and Applications,
DOI 10.1007/978-1-4419-0164-4_8, © Springer Science+Business Media, LLC 2009

children, even higher with environmental risk factors accounting for about one third of the disease burden (Prüss-Üstün, 2006).

There are many definitions of environment. From an epidemiologic perspective, environment is defined in relation to the host. At its most basic level, the barriers of the integumentary system, respiratory system, the gastrointestinal system, and placenta protect the internal human environment. External to the human system, the environment may be physical, chemical, biological, social, or economic. The environment may be fixed (a dilapidated home) or ambient (air pollution, economic conditions).

The effects of the environment upon the human system or community may be immediate or long term. There is evidence from laboratory models that toxins may affect the emergence of genetic mutations resulting in the potential for heritable disease transmitted over several generations (Jirtle and Skinner, 2007). Such models support epidemiological data on the role of environment in the persistently high rate of infant mortality among Blacks.

Human behaviors and characteristics enhance or protect against environmental exposures. Environmental exposures which lead to health problems can be low level (e.g., chronic lead exposure) to disaster level (Lin et al., 2005; Dorn et al., 2007). Mitigating of exposure can be personal or behavioral, use of personal protective equipment, and response to governmental regulations. The use of personal protective equipment by farmers diminishes exposure to pesticides applied during agricultural operations. Social support mitigates posttraumatic stress disorder among disaster victims (Feng et al., 2007). Also, demographic characteristics influence morbidity and mortality from environmental exposures. Persons at risk for death in a natural disaster are those who are elderly, females, with mental disorders or moderate physical disability, or who have been hospitalized for a nonchildbirth event (Chou et al., 2004; Daley et al., 2005). Environmental features can also enhance or mitigate risk. The risk of severe injury or death from a tornado is higher among those outdoors or in a mobile home or in an automobile (Daley et al., 2005). Living in old homes built before the 1950s when lead paint was commonly used, increases the risk of lead exposure, as well as living in homes constructed after 1950 but prior to 1978 which also contained lead but at levels considerably lower (Needleman, 2004). Lastly, changes in the environment can also affect the delivery of health services. Catastrophic fires (in California) and flooding (Hurricane Katrina) had damaged infrastructure in hospitals causing evacuation of patients.

This chapter largely focuses on environmental health issues from the definition presented by the WHO, namely, the environment is that which "addresses all the physical, chemical, and biological factors external to a person, and all the related factors impacting behaviours...This definition excludes behaviour not related to environment, as well as behaviour related to the social and cultural environment, and genetics (WHO, 2008 http://www.who.int/topics/environmental_health)." This chapter also reviews the main environmental risk factors affecting human health which have been supported with epidemiologic evidence and that have implications for health services delivery. Each environmental factor addressed herein is associated with a particular risk factor profile which is important to know in developing appropriate individual and community response plans. The resultant impact of environmental stresses and hazards and environmentally developed diseases and health problems upon health services utilization is then considered. Control measures within the purview of the health services manager are presented.

Environmental Hazards

Environmental hazards of concern from an epidemiologic framework are those which can provoke an excess number of cases beyond what would be expected by chance alone, namely, they have epidemic potential. An environmental hazard is any substance, object, process, phenomenon, or event which has the potential to cause disruption, damage to communities, or threaten the health of the public. Hazards can be natural or manmade. Hazards become of particular concern because population subgroups may be a high risk because of certain vulnerabilities. Although vulnerabilities may vary somewhat with the specific type of exposure, generally age, immunization coverage rates in a community, and access to health care are highly associated with vulnerability.

Natural Environmental Factors

Earthquakes

An earthquake is a sudden slip on a fault releasing energy in waves that travels through the earth's crust causing a shaking motion. The Richter magnitude scale is a means of comparing the size of earthquakes. An earthquake measured by the Richter scale is expressed in whole numbers and decimal fractions determined from the logarithm of the amplitude of waves recorded by seismographs adjusted for the variation in the distance between the various seismographs and the epicenter of the earthquakes. A magnitude 5.3 indicates a moderate earthquake; a strong earthquake rated as magnitude 6.3. The scale has a logarithmic basis such that each whole number increase in magnitude represents a tenfold increase in measured amplitude. These values in relation to active earthquake activity worldwide can be monitored within a seven day timeframe thereby aiding in emergency service planning at the U.S. Geological Survey's Earthquake Hazards website: http://earthquake.usgs.gov. Earthquakes, rated as low as 5.1–5.6 on the Richter scale, have been associated with multiple deaths (Ramirez and Peek-Asa, 2005).

The mortality and morbidity rates associated with earthquakes depend upon a multiplicity of factors including features of the earthquake, the terrain, population density, vulnerability of the built environment, and individual characteristics of the affected population. Individuals at increased risk of mortality from an earthquake are those who are females and the elderly or who have mental disorders, moderate physical disabilities, had been hospitalized just prior to an earthquake, have lower income, reside in rural or semirural areas, and remain in buildings (Chan et al., 2003; Ramirez and Peek-Asa, 2005). There is a tendency for risk of death to exhibit a bimodal pattern with the highest rates occurring among the youngest and oldest

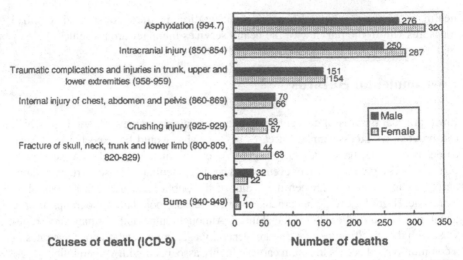

Fig. 1 Major causes of death for seismic deaths (ICD-9: E909) in the disaster area, Taiwan, 1999. The disaster area included all 13 townships in Nantou Country, and 10 out of 21 townships in Taichung Country. *Source*: Chan et al. (2003). Reprinted from Elsevier with permission

age groups (Ramirez and Peek-Asa, 2005). Figure 1 illustrates typical causes of death that may be encountered as a result of an earthquake. The distribution of the pattern of mortality indicates a need for an adequate level of trauma care staff and facilities in earthquake zones. In addition to the immediate effects of earthquakes upon the population, secondary effects need to be considered regarding how to respond in the face of disruption of infrastructure to the need for social services, sanitation, and continued management of chronic conditions.

The ideally measure to minimize morbidity and mortality from an earthquake would be a rapid response system identifying the potential of significant seismic activity. However, since accurate predictive technology is not yet available, interventions recommended are:

• Communication to residents regarding the contents of an earthquake safety backpack and its placement at the front door of one's residence
• Development and enforcement of building codes for earthquake resistant structures in earthquake zones and
• High acuity trauma facilities and adequate level of emergency department staff credentialed in trauma care within earthquake zones

Cyclones, Hurricanes, Typhoons

When winds reach 74 mph in association with a low-pressure system over water and with thunderstorm activity, then they are called hurricane, typhoon, tropical cyclone, or cyclonic storm, depending upon what regional coast the storm is approaching.

For example, such activity is called a hurricane when presenting over the North Atlantic Ocean but called a tropical cycle if forming on a coast over the Southwest Indian Ocean (Atlantic Oceanographic and Meteorological Laboratory, 2007). The risk of mortality from a cyclone can be as high as 16.5% and similar to other disasters is highest among the very young and the very old (Sommer and Mosley, 1972). The direct causes of death and injury are primarily from: blunt trauma from projectiles from the wind intensity or falling trees, drowning due to tidal surges, and electrocutions from downed power lines. Indirectly, the stresses of the storm impact preexisting medical conditions and increase the likelihood of infectious diseases because of the disruption of infrastructure, displacement of populations, damage to buildings, inadequate nutrition, and ecologic changes (Shultz et al., 2005). Response strategies aimed at minimizing morbidity and mortality from cyclones, hurricanes, and typhoons include:

- Improving the science and technology of storm forecasting
- Early warning of the community (e.g., lightening warning systems)
- Effective community evacuation plans and orders
- Family disaster plans and
- Education of the community regarding risks of the storms

Tornados

Tornados are the severest form of windstorms. Risk of death is higher among women than men and is highest among those 65+ years. The likelihood of death during a tornado varies according to location with the highest being among those who are outdoors followed by being in a mobile home than in an apartment building (Daley et al., 2005). Early warning systems, knowledge of evacuation procedures posted in public buildings, and the availability of storm shelters are key response measures. Potential health problem related to tornados is immediate as direct and indirect consequences. Direct consequences are due to flying objects and debris which can cause traumatic injuries and even death. Indirect consequences are flooding secondary to the storm effect which may result in exposure to sewage and mold which may continue to grow in buildings. Indirect consequences may also be psychological, coping with the traumatic events related to weather event.

Tsunami

A *tsunami* is a series of ocean waves generated by volcanic activity, landslides, or sudden displacements in the sea floor. A feature of a tsunami is that the wave created by the under-ocean movement may increase in height to become a fast moving wall of turbulent water several feet high (National Oceanic and Atmospheric Administration,

2008). The primary strategy for addressing health problems arising from a tsunami lies in a coordinated national effort of several federal agencies, coastal states, territorial, and Commonwealth partners to assess the risk of its occurrence, develop a warning guidance system, and a damage mitigation effort which includes an evacuation plan. Information on current tsunami risk, events, and emergency guidelines can be found at the National Tsunami Hazard Mitigation Program's website: http://nthmp. tsunami.gov/ (National Tsunami Hazard Mitigation Program, 2008).

Excessive Heat

Excessive heat can produce direct casualties by stressing the body beyond its natural cooling capabilities through pumping blood at a high rate through dilated blood vessels and sweat glands pouring water, sodium, and chloride through skin surfaces. Excessive heat is an international health problem (Kovats and Ebi, 2006). Excessive heat increases the risk of overall mortality, mortality from respiratory and cardiovascular disease. It also increases the risk of heat disorder symptoms (sunburn, heat cramps, heat exhaustion, heat stroke) and health services utilization for conditions exacerbated by heat (acute renal failure, cardiovascular disorders, epilepsy, neurological disorders, emphysema) (Semenza et al., 1999). The relative risk of heat-related deaths increases with increasing values of temperature and with age and for females higher than males among those 65+ years (Ishigami et al., 2008). The cut-point values which determine higher mortality and morbidity vary and can be as low as 20.4°C or as high as 26.3°C. A heat index (HI) is another measure used to communicate the risk of possible heat disorders. The HI is given in degrees Fahrenheit (F) with relative humidity factored in and is considered an apparent temperature or "hot it feels." A HI above 105°F is associated with an increased likelihood of excess heat-related disorders, especially with physical activity and/or continued exposure (National Oceanic and Atmospheric Administration, 2008). The epidemiologic measure triggering a concern about heat as a hazard is excess mortality or excess morbidity. Excess mortality (morbidity) is calculated as the observed number of deaths (cases) minus the expected mortality (morbidity) determined from an average of usually a preceding 2- to 5-year period (or some other referent period for morbidity) (Kovats and Ebi, 2006). A proxy measure of morbidity is the hospitalizations. Semenza et al. (1999) found in excess of hospitalizations related to acute renal failure attributable to a heat wave. Other factors enhancing the risk of heat-related disorders include air pollution (suspended matter and ozone) and stagnant or lack of air circulation as is common in urban areas. Control measures aimed at preventing mortality and morbidity from excessive heat include:

- Heat health surveillance systems
- Cooling centers
- Personal protective behavioral measures (avoid alcoholic beverages, avoid the sun, drink plenty of fluids, slow activities, dress lightly, spend time in cooling areas/centers)
- Electric fan distribution

- Public communications about the hazard and personal protective behaviors
- Working with utility companies to temporarily cease disconnection for nonpayment and
- Monitoring, outreach, relocation for high risk populations (e.g., elderly who live alone, disabled, mentally ill)

Excessive Cold

Excessive cold is as an important public health problem as excessive heat. Its effects have the greatest impact, similar to excessive heat, upon the older age groups. Excessive cold has a more profound effect in terms of increased mortality in more southern or warmer cities with the impact continuing for up to 23 days (Analitis et al., 2008). Control measures are similar to excessive heat episodes with the control substitutions of providing warming shelters and communication to the public of wind chill and other excessive cold advisories.

Man-Made Environmental Factors

Air Pollution

The major ambient air pollutants known to result in health effects are the following six substances: particulate matter ≤ 2.5 μm in aerodynamic diameter ($PM_{2.5}$), particulate matter with an average aerodynamic diameter less than 10 μm (PM_{10}), ozone (O_3), nitrogen dioxide (NO_2), carbon monoxide (CO), and sulfur dioxide (SO_2). Air pollution increases result in increases in: all-cause mortality, the symptom odds ratio asthma, rate ratios for asthma rescue inhaler use, the relative risk respiratory emergency department visits for asthma, pneumonia and chronic obstructive pulmonary disease, and an increased rate of hospitalization for elderly with congestive heart failure (Dominici et al., 2007; Peel et al., 2005; Schildcrout et al., 2006; Wellenius et al., 2005). The health effects of elevated air pollution, even short term, may persist for as long as a week afterwards elevated exposures. Mobile sources of air pollution, measured by traffic density, have been reported as the major concern (Meng et al., 2008). Control measures include:

- Air quality surveillance
- High risk individuals remaining indoors in air conditioned environments during air pollution episodes
- Public health communications to decrease motor vehicle use when high air pollution concentrations are identified
- Construction of new housing, especially in urban areas, to be air-tight and
- Environmental regulations aimed at reducing exposure to ambient agents found to affect human health (e.g., Clean Air Act Amendments of 1990)

Industrial/Occupational Exposures

Industrial and occupational health hazards to humans are numerous. Among the most well known is an accident at the Chernobyl nuclear power plant in the Ukraine which released large amounts of radionuclides subsequently found to be associated with various forms of cancer (Zablotska et al., 2008). Only those with extensive epidemiologic evaluations are considered herein. To consider each and every known chemical is beyond the scope of this text. The reader is advised to consult the major agencies whose charge is to investigate and research the potential effects of industrial and occupational hazards. These agencies are the National Institute for Occupational Health and Safety (NIOSH) (http://www.cdc.gov/niosh) and the International Agency for Research on Cancer (http://www.iarc.fr). The Occupational Health and Safety Administration (OSHA) is the federal agency responsible for the enforcement of standards which have been based upon research conducted by agencies such as NIOSH, surveys, meetings with employee and employer groups, and focus groups discussion with workers from a variety of industries throughout the nation. The authority of this agency was established under the Occupational Safety and Health Act of 1970 which stated that employers were responsible for the provision of a workplace which is safe and health for their employees. The scope of the protection focuses on hazardous conditions ranging from physical risks to carcinogens. OSHA also provides training, outreach, and education for the continuous improvement of workplace safety and health (http://www.osha.gov).

Prevention of exposure to industrial/occupational hazards can be through administrative or engineering measures. Administrative measures include the implementation of policies and procedures to protect worker health, communication of risks to workers, training of workers in situations regarding risks to health and safety (e.g., confined spaces, heights, fumes, etc.) and the provision of personal protective equipment to workers. Engineering measures would include the modification of the environment to reduce heavy lifting, noise reduction, or improving ventilation to remove exposure to fumes.

Bioterrorism

Bioterrorism is the deliberate release of bacteria, viruses, or other biological agents to cause illness or death in people, plants, or animals. These agents can be common in nature such as Salmonella or they can be rare such as anthrax. The risk of morbidity and mortality from bioterrorism varies. The highest risk agents are those easily spread or transmitted from person to person, result in high mortality, cause public panic and social disruption, and require special public health action (e.g., smallpox) (Centers for Disease Control and Prevention, 2008).

Control of morbidity and mortality from bioterrorism depends upon the preparedness of communities and the public.

War, Armed Conflicts, and Civil Disputes

War, armed conflicts, and civil disputes are unfortunately pervasive in global society.
Although all the risk factors are not well established, considered herein are the health
problems noted to arise from these man-made "disasters." Most notably associated
with war, armed conflicts, and civil disputes are traumatic injuries, primarily from
weapons or explosives assault. However, a growing number of health disorders have
emerged in association with military deployment, varying by location of deployment,
resulting in a spectrum of acute and chronic conditions including chronic multisymptom illness (from deployment in Gulf War I) and posttraumatic stress disorder and
traumatic brain injury (from bullets/shrapnel, blasts, falls, motor vehicle crashes, air/
water transport) (Blanchard et al., 2006; Schneiderman et al., 2008). The psychological
impacts of war upon active duty personnel, upon return, and the long-term impact of
military service personnel are now known as well. Military deployment, repeated and
long term, has multiple consequences upon family and social functioning to maintain
healthy living because of challenges in reintegrating into the family or community
social structure (Rentz et al., 2007). It is not within the scope of this book to provide
an epidemiologic assessment for battlefield health services. However, this section is
intended to alert health services managers of the scope of health problems when
receiving or managing victims or family members, civilians or noncivilians.

Surge capacity is a term emerging from the events related to the 9/11 terrorist
attacks. Surge capacity is the ability of a health system, particularly hospital emergency departments, to mobilize its resources to meet an increased demand for health
care services in relationship to a primary disaster event. Disasters are events which
exceed the capacities of local agencies and the events and health problems emerging
from them requires involvement from outside the communities affected. Epidemiologic
measures are proposed by Health Resources Service Administration (HRSA) to serve
as the benchmark for implementing a system which can triage, treat, and dispose
500 adult and pediatric patients per one million population who experience acute
illness or trauma requiring hospitalization from a biological, chemical, radiological,
or explosive terrorist incident. In terms of manpower, HRSA also requires that States
establish a response system that allows for the immediate deployment of 250 or more
additional patient care personnel per million population in urban areas, and 125 or
more additional personnel per million in rural areas. Health care organizations also
need to plan capacity for secondary surge related to the treatment of personnel
responding to the rescue and/or recovery of victims from the initial event. To address
the challenges that a health system would face in responding to surge, the National
Center for Injury Prevention and Control (2007) has published recommendations and
guidelines at the organizational and discipline-specific level.

Risk Assessment

There is large number of environmental agents and hazards which have been known to cause a variety of diseases and health problems (Table 1). Their ubiquity in the environment, and their varying potential for causing health effects, requires that a

Table 1 Examples of common environmentally provoked diseases and health problems and environmental etiologic agents

Disease/health problem	Etiologic agent(s)
Allergies and asthma	Air pollution, allergens
Birth defects	Certain chemicals, aspirin, cigarette smoke
Cancer (various forms)	Alcohol, asbestos, benzene, cigarette smoke, ionizing radiation, sunlight (ultraviolet radiation), 4-Nitrobiphenyl, alpha-naphthylamine, methyl chloromethyl ether, 3,3'-Dichlorobenzidine (and its salts), bis-Chloromethyl ether, beta-Naphthylamine, benzidine, 4-Aminodiphenyl, ethyleneimine, beta-Propiolactone, 2-Acetylaminofluorene, 4-Dimethylaminoazobenzene, N-Nitrosodimethylamine, Inorganic arsenic, cadmium, coke oven emissions, 1,2-dibromo-3-chloropropane, acrylonitrile, ethylene oxide, formaldehyde, methylenedianiline, 1,3-Butadiene, methylene chloride, vinyl chloride
Dermatitis	Certain chemicals in cosmetics, detergents, dyes, fabrics, foods, paints
Emphysema	Air pollution, cigarette smoke
Goiter	Lack of iodine
Heart disease	Environmental chemicals, excess dietary fat, lack of exercise
Immune deficiency diseases	Certain chemicals and drugs
Job-related injuries and illnesses	Certain chemicals, ergonomic hazards, metal fumes, noise, vibration
Kidney disease	Excessive use of ibuprofen, naproxen, COX-2 inhibitors, aspirin
Lead caused poisoning and cognitive impairment	Paint in homes constructed before 1978, lead dust, lead fumes, lead-contaminated water, lead in gasoline
Mercury poisoning	Contaminated fish (methyl mercury)
Nervous system disorders (mood changes, memory loss, blindness, paralysis, death)	Lack of use of safety devices (seat belts, car seats, helmets) to prevent accidents
Osteoporosis	Lack of exercise, inadequate calcium intake
Pneumoconiosis	Fibers from asbestos, cotton, hemp; dust from clay, coal, graphite, iron, silica
Reproductive disorders (early puberty, fertility problems, low sperm counts, ovarian cysts, cancers of reproductive system)	Diethylstilbestrol, dioxin, excess caffeine
Tooth decay	Lack of fluoridated water
Vision problems (cataracts, eye infectious)	Excessive sunlight exposure, airborne organisms (molds, fungi, viruses)
Waterborne diseases	Bacterial contamination from human and animal wastes

system for establishing priorities and allocation of resources must be in place to manage population-based exposure to environmental agents. This process is known as *risk assessment*. Risk assessment is the process (quantitative or qualitative) of identifying how likely exposure will result in an adverse condition or in some cases beneficial. Risk could mean death, injury (physical or mental), contamination, damage to community infrastructure, displacement, disruption in or loss of essential health care and economic services, and secondary hazards (e.g., explosions during a fire). According to the US Environmental Protection Agency, there are two main types of risk assessment, ecological risk assessment, and human health risk assessment, with somewhat different approaches (http://www.epa.gov/risk/ecological-risk.htm). For the purposes of this chapter, the focus is upon human health risk assessment. The five components of risk assessment according to the US Environmental Protection Agency (http://www.epi.give/risk/health-risk.htm) are:

1. Planning and scoping, which obtains the information and data needed to complete the assessment, is considered before the field investigations and site characterization work are completed (e.g., meta-analysis of existing literature). This component may be viewed as iterative accumulation additional information and data as more is known about exposure and hazard.
2. Hazard identification, which determines the capacity of a stressor to cause adverse health effects (e.g., neurobehavioral or reproductive disorders) to humans, and if so, under all circumstances which the stressor in any amount can produce health effects.
3. Dose-response assessment, which evaluates if there is a numerical relationship between the amount, duration, and timing of exposure absorbed by the target organs(s) and the incidence and severity of health effects.
4. Exposure evaluation, which concerns the extent of human exposure, its source(s), movement of the substance through the environment, and how the uptake occurs by humans (e.g., inhalation, ingestion).
5. Risk characterization, which calculates how well the data support the conclusions about the nature and extent of risk from the stressor based upon cumulative exposure over an entire average lifetime in a defined population. This information is acquired from steps 2 to 4.

Risk assessment models commonly have their origins in animal models exposed to high concentrations of the suspect hazard under the very general assumption that over time the toxic effects shown in laboratory animals often occur in humans exposed to the same agent. However, the validity of these models when extrapolated to humans must be viewed with caution as often the laboratory animals are administered near toxic doses of a "suspect hazard" over the course of their entire life. Also, what is toxic to an animal, either because of the species tested or that the substance evaluated, may not necessarily be toxic for a human. Even when testing different species, different results may occur and in these circumstances the credibility of the investigative team may be the source relied on then for the final interpretation of the animal model. Additionally, the risk assessment model may not be relevant because a person or population must be exposed to the hazard to a degree to where the risk becomes a health concern. This is the case, particularly, with "naturally" occurring carcinogens determined from animal studies in substances such as aflatoxin B1 which is considered a carcinogen by the International Agency for Research on Cancer (http://www.iarc.fr) in peanuts and peanut products.

The biomonitoring of the substance which is the subject of the risk assessment relative to human tissues is the "gold standard." For example, a blood sample collected by venipuncture is used to measure exposure to second hand smoke whereby a serum cotinine level among nonsmokers of >0.05 ng/ml is considered exposed (Schober et al., 2008). But even among humans, there is biovariability due to age, coexisting disease, proximity to exposure, and other environmental and behavioral factors. Because it is now known that children may be a greater risk than adults, Executive Order 13045, *Protection of Children from Environmental Health Risks and Safety Risks* (1997) was issued directing all federal agencies to assess environmental health risks and safety risks of potential hazards, to which children may specifically be exposed. Scientists do recognize that animal test may not be conclusive for humans. Thus, virtually all risk assessments are clouded with some level of uncertainty for this reason. It is not known how many people are or will be exposed or susceptible to a hazard and how much of the hazard will actually remain present and a form in the environment to the level of producing an adverse health effect. Epidemiologic studies, when available, help confirm (or refute) results of animal models. But, lack of epidemiologic evidence is often the greatest limitation of risk assessments because human population data when available are generally too small to draw credible conclusions. Risk assessment can be applied in a wide variety of situations ranging from assessing the potential risk of foodborne pathogens to that of various chemicals in food from absorption from environmental pollutants such as toxic metals, PCBs and dioxins, or through the intentional use of various chemicals, such as food additives, pesticides, animal drugs and other agrochemicals, or even the risk of natural disasters. A number of risk assessments pertaining to the risks from chemicals in the industrial environment and food can be found World Health Organization's website: http://www.who.int/foodsafety/chem/en/. Another resource useful for risk assessment is the comprehensive list of toxic substances and Environmental Health WebMaps available through the Agency for Toxic Substances and Disease Registry website at http://www.atsdr.cdc.gov. Regardless of the sources of information used in risk assessment, it is important to use current information on the exposures of interest.

Although risk assessment is usually conducted in the context of its regulatory application, business leaders should be engaged in the process if their companies impact the environment and health service practitioners should understand how to assist consumers in making decisions about their risk and responding to questions or concerns arising out of the decision-making process. Risk in fact is part of our everyday lives, no matter what we do, eat, drink, or become exposed to as part of our occupations or leisure activities. Risk is a matter of degree (i.e., dose of exposure to hazard) and the conditions surrounding the exposure such that what is "risk" for one person may not be a threat to another because of the different circumstances of exposure. For example, health care practitioners may encounter questions from patients such as: "Could my miscarriage be due to something in the air or water in my home or place of work?" "Is my child's autism due to chemicals in vaccines?" Thus, knowledge of the risk and communications of it may be as an important function of a health services manager as knowledge of the risk (or true exposure to environmental hazards) as the risk and response to it may affect health services utilization or an organization's policies. The classic examples of risk assessments which had implications for organizational policies are those performed in relation to exposure to environmental tobacco smoke and various ergonomic hazards (e.g., chronic exposure to lifting heavy patients, continuous use of computer keyboards, etc.) (Bernard, 1997; Morris, 1995; Steenland, 1999). The results of these risk assessments have prompted many employers and policy makers to initiate policies, guidelines, and legislation to protect the health of the public (including employees) from these hazards.

Interventions for Addressing Risk Factors from the Environment

The conceptualization of areas for intervention according to Healthy people 2010 target to maintain a healthy environment is displayed in Fig. 2. The health care services continuum relevant to addressing environmentally related health conditions

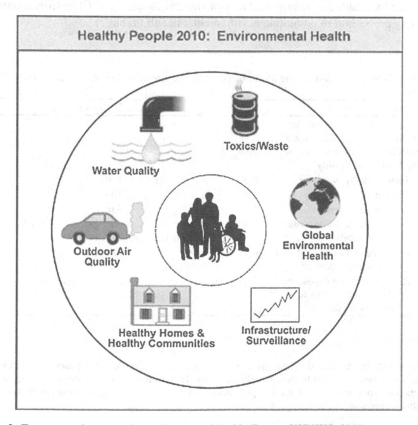

Fig. 2 Target areas for promoting environmental health (Source: USDHHS, 2000)

according to service level, primary prevention, secondary prevention, and tertiary prevention is described below.

Primary Prevention

Primary prevention should be the initial strategy of choice to protect a human population from environmental risk factors from any course. Primary prevention in this context seeks to change the social or physical environment to erect protective barriers between the environmental agent and host through laws, policies, industry, community, or individual behavior change. Examples of primary prevention are premarket evaluation of the toxicity of new chemical compounds (e.g., food additives), emission standards, dissemination of information (public education materials about reducing exposure to sunlight), accurate labeling of products (e.g., ragweed in some herbal teas), and encouraging consumers to read the label first before using any home cleaning products or pesticides. Primary prevention through education and communication of environmental risk factors to the populations receiving care through a provider and the surrounding community should be given greater priority attention by health care managers. Many of *Healthy People 2010* Objectives address primary prevention in promoting environmental health (Table 2).

Table 2 Selected *Healthy People 2010* objectives for environmental health (Source: USDHHS, 2000)

Objective	Baseline	2010 target
Increase use of alternative modes of transportation to reduce motor vehicle emissions and improve the Nation's air quality		
Trips made by bicycling	0.9%[a]	1.8%
Trips made by walking	5.4%[a]	10.8%
Trips made by transit	1.8%[a]	3.6%
Reduce per capita domestic water withdrawals	101 gallons of domestic water per capita per day[a]	90.9 gallons (10% reduction)
Eliminate elevated blood lead levels in children	4.4%[b]	0.0%
Reduce pesticide exposures that result in visits to a health care facility[d]	27,156 visits[c]	50% improvement

[a]1995
[b]1991–1994
[c]1997
[d]Pesticide exposures include those involving disinfectants, fungicides, herbicides, insecticides, moth repellants, and rodenticides, as defined by the US Environmental Protection Agency and covers approximately 93% of the US population through the American Association of Poison Control Centers surveillance system

Secondary Prevention

Secondary prevention includes the early detection of the environmentally related disease or health condition through screening to interrupt progression to a disease state. A screening test may indicate the presence of an environmentally related disease or merely a higher probability of a disease and the need for confirmatory testing. If it is performed correctly, the planning and implementation of an environmental health screening program is among the most complex health services delivery challenge. In developing the program, the health services professional must be familiar with both clinical medicine, toxicology, and the potential for environmental mitigation. In analyzing and interpreting the screening results, the health practitioner must be familiar with epidemiology and understand the applicability and limitations of environmental exposure measurements. Another useful tool for secondary prevention is the reporting of excessive levels of selected environmental toxicants in body fluids by clinical laboratories to state health departments. Such reporting allows identification of the likely source of exposure, identification of cases by geographic location, estimation if an excessive number of persons is exposed, and facilitates the probability of medical follow-up. Despite legislation and abatement efforts, there remains a large number of persons exposed to lead, a chemical substance with numerous known short-term and long-term health effects ranging from acute lead toxicity and peripheral neuropathy to cognitive deficits in children (Needleman, 2004). This supports the need for screening for lead exposure which is accomplished through assessment of blood lead levels targeting particularly children living in high risk neighborhoods. One objective within *Healthy People 2010* is to eliminate BLLs >10 μg/dl among the nation's children (U.S. Department of Health and Human Services, 2000), a benchmark measure for determining the effectiveness of a lead screening program.

Tertiary Prevention

Tertiary prevention, or medical intervention, is the least effective strategy for environmentally related health conditions. The objective of tertiary intervention is to limit harm after harm has been done, as it is exemplified with the health problem of lead poisoning. While effective treatment for lead poisoning exists, caregivers may not recognize the problem until neurological damage is profound. Unfortunately, too, the effectiveness of tertiary intervention for environmentally associated health conditions by traditional health care services may be severely limited by the resources available and the patient may return to the same hazardous environment. Fortunately, in the case of the child with lead poisoning, state resources are likely to be available to help the family reduce the lead levels in the home. Poison control centers services are another example of tertiary prevention. Poison control centers coordinate care for poison victims from point of exposure assessing the nature of the potentially hazardous exposure, transmitting information on therapies, and making referrals if appropriate. Since over 70% of poison exposure cases can be managed over the phone, Poison Control Center hotlines help reduce costly emergency room visits (American Association of Poison Control Centers (http:// www.aapcc.org). Poison control centers also are a resource for primary prevention providing education to the community regarding topics ranging from the proper handling and ventilation related to household products, bites and stings, plants, over-the-counter and prescription medications, drugs, alcohol, hydrocarbons, carbon monoxide and other types of potentially toxic fumes and gases from home, the community, as well as industrial sources.

In addition to available treatment services to address specific environmental hazards, knowledge of environmental conditions is important in ensuring the appropriate health care services are in place. Table 3 summarizes key literature on expected trends in utilization of various types of health care services in relation to types of episodes of air pollution.

Lastly, tertiary services are mobilized in the event of environmental disasters which could otherwise not have been prevented. The US Department of Homeland Security (USDHS) recommends that in addition to health care providers, families, communities, and business should have a disaster plan in place to minimize morbidity, mortality, from the immediate disaster and secondary effects from a disaster resulting from infrastructure disruption. Elements of plans for health systems are displayed in Table 4. Adequate disaster response preparedness covers policies, procedures, guidelines, resources, authority, as well as knowledge, skills, and positive attitudes of not only the members of health systems and other agencies, but also an informed public of the actions that need to be taken in preparing and skills required for preparing and responding to environmental disasters. Assistance for developing these plans can be obtained from local or state health departments or the USDHS at http://www.dhs.gov.

Table 3 Environmental factors, related conditions, and resultant health services utilization

Factor	Health condition/health service/risk level	Reference
Particulate matter (PM10)[a] (microgr/m³)	Congestive heart failure hospitalization (CHF)/hospitalization/+3.07%	Wellenius et al. (2005)
Carbon monoxide (0.55 ppm)	(CHF)/hospitalization/+3.07%	
Nitrogen dioxide (11 ppb)	(CHF)/hospitalization/+4.55%	
Sulfur dioxide (11 ppb)	(CHF)/hospitalization/+2.36%	
Particulate matter (PM10)[a] (microgr/m³)	Upper respiratory disease (URI)/ Emergency room (ER) visits/Relative risk (RR) = 1.013	Peel et al. (2005)
Ozone 25 ppb	URI/ER visits/RR = 1.024	
Carbon monoxide (1 ppm)	URI/ER visits/RR = 1.011	
Nitrogen dioxide (20 ppb)	URI/ER visits/RR = 1.016	
Carbon monoxide (1 ppm change)	Rescue inhaler use for asthma/RR = 1.06	Schildcrout et al. (2006)
Nitrogen dioxide (20 ppb change)	Rescue inhaler use for asthma/RR = 1.05	

[a]PM10: particulate matter with an aerodynamic diameter of <10 μm

Table 4 Elements of a plan for health services to prepare and respond environmental disaster

- Assessment of health and medical needs
- Health surveillance
- Adequate number and credentialed first receiver personnel
- Health and medical equipment supply adequacy
- Patient safety and patient evacuation strategy: route and method(s) of transportation
- Designated receiving hospital(s) and hospitals' bed capacity including isolation, trauma, and burn care capacity
- Establishment of advance registration system
- Food and drug preservation and distribution; medical device operation and safety
- Worker health and safety (adequacy of personal protective equipment and decontaminated sites)
- Radiological, chemical, and biological hazard containment and consultants
- Mental and behavioral health support
- Public health information and communication systems among key agencies (local health departments, Red Cross, first responders, etc.)
- Vector control
- Adequate portable water and safe disposal of solid and liquid wastes
- Veterinary services
- Victim identification and morgue services

Summary

A substantial portion of the national and international disease burden is environmentally related. The epidemiologic pattern of morbidity and mortality from environmental exposures depends upon characteristics of the host and type and intensity of environmental exposures. Knowledge of these patterns is, thus, important in planning any prevention efforts and health services to complement prevention efforts. But, because of the limitations of knowledge regarding the many and growing number environmental risk factors, prevention and screening services are not always technically feasible. This shifts the burden to tertiary health care services. Health care managers should consider adding environmental exposures to intake assessments for all levels of services, particularly for population subgroups known to be at high risk for environmental exposures (e.g., immigrants, workers from certain industries, children in poverty, urban minorities, etc.). Public health professionals in their roles as environmental monitors, inspectors, consumer educators, or health care providers may be able to significantly reduce the number of preventable environmentally related deaths. Knowledge of environmental exposures can aid health providers in not only developing more effective treatment strategies, but also guide in assisting the patient to develop personal strategies to reduce the likelihood of personal exposure to environmental hazards when returning to their homes and communities to prevent disease or health problem recurrence or exacerbation. Synergy between health services managers, environmental specialists, and the public will be vital in the implementation of preventing ill health in the work environment (which includes the health care environment), the residential environment, and the ambient environment.

Such collaboration may lead to the identification, evaluation, and subsequent modification of environmental factors that cause disease and premature mortality and disability and hence avoidable health services utilization.

Discussion Questions

Q.1. In your current employment position, how do your job responsibilities relate to the prevention of environmentally provoked diseases? How would you seek to ensure that your job responsibilities support the mission and objectives of other agencies in your community concerned with environmental health?

Q.2. What questions should be asked on a medical intake form for a clinic to ascertain a patient's risk of environmental exposures?

Boxed Example 1 Neighborhood Change and Distant Metastasis at Diagnosis of Breast Cancer

Problem: The survival rate of black women with breast cancer is significantly lower than white women. Black women present in later stages of the disease. The differences may be linked to indicators of neighborhood poverty.

Methods: Data from the Illinois State Tumor Registry were used to identify cases of breast cancer and their age, stage of diagnosis, and race/ethnicity. Residential address at the time of diagnosis was geocoded by the cancer registry to the census block level. US Census Bureau data were used to provide the neighborhood characteristics which were formed into three scales: (1) concentrated disadvantaged (percentage incomes below the poverty line, percentage of families receiving public assistance, percentage of persons unemployed, percentage of female-head of households with children), (2) concentrated affluence (percentage of families with incomes of $75,000+, percentage of adults with college education+, percentage of civilian labor force in professional/managerial occupations), and (3) concentrated immigration (percent Hispanic, percent foreign-born, percent linguistically isolated). Neighborhood change was measured by a composite score of percent change between 1990 and 2000 in owner-occupied housing value, percent of civilian labor force in professional/managerial occupations, and percent of adults with a college education or higher.

(continued)

Boxed Example 1 (continued)

Results: A multilevel logistic regression model of neighborhood upward change and distant breast cancer stage diagnosis 1994–2000 (Source: Barrett et al., 2008)

Variable	Unstandardized beta coefficient	Standard error	Odds ratio (OR)	95% CI	p-Value
Intercept	−2.55	0.03	0.08	(0.07, 0.08)	<0.001
Disadvantage	0.21	0.05	1.23	(1.12, 1.36)	<0.001
Affluence	−0.15	0.04	0.86	(0.79, 0.93)	<0.001
Immigration	0.10	0.04	1.11	(1.02, 1.21)	0.020
Neighborhood upward change	0.09	0.04	1.09	(1.01, 1.18)	0.029
Age	0.01	0.002	1.01	(1.01, 1.02)	<0.001
African American vs. Whites	0.21	0.09	1.24	(1.03, 1.48)	0.022
Hispanic vs. Whites	−0.33	0.14	0.71	(0.53, 0.95)	0.019

The OR of distant metastasis increased by 9% for each unit increased in the rate of neighborhood upward change. In the same neighborhoods, African Americans were more likely than whites to have distant metastasis, but not for Hispanics. Higher disadvantage concentration and immigration concentration were each associated with greater odds of distant metastasis.

Managerial Epidemiology Implications: Rapid upward mobility in a neighborhood represented by construction of new housing and businesses may disrupt access to care for poor older women, displacing federally qualified health centers and social support systems. Public health agencies should consider neighborhoods in transition to gentrification as temporary high risk areas for health needs (e.g., screening) especially for African Americans where poverty may make health care seeking not feasible. Transportation subsidies, mobile clinics, or outreach by mid-level providers may assist with continuity of care.

Q.3. What federal, state, and local agencies (public and private) would be involved in the event of a hurricane disaster in a community? How would these agencies interact with local health care providers? What types of epidemiologic data were collected after Hurricane Katrina to understand the health impact of this catastrophic event? (Refer to: Injury and Illness Surveillance in Hospitals and Acute-Care Facilities After Hurricanes Katrina and Rita - New Orleans Area, Louisiana, September 25-October 15, 2005 (http://www.cdc.gov/mmwr/preview/mmwrhtml/mm5502a4.htm).

Boxed Example 2   Excess Hospital Admissions During a Heat Wave

Problem: Heat waves are an international health problem. An increase in hospitalizations is expected during these episodes overall and due to heat-related conditions. Less well-known is what comorbidities arise so that appropriate staffing and resources can be available.

Methods and Data: A computerized file of discharge diagnoses from 47 non-Veterans Administration hospitals in Cook County was examined. Primary and secondary diagnoses were examined and compared between the heat wave period and comparison periods. The excess or deficit of admission during July 1995 was subtracted from the corresponding July 1994 day of the week average from the number of admissions recorded for July 1995. The 95% confidence interval (CI) was calculated based on the t-distribution for differences between independent means with unknown but equal population variances. The significance of the excess was determined by a two-tailed t-test.

Results: Selected excess in-patient admissions by primary and secondary discharge diagnosis: Underlying and/or comorbid conditions, Chicago, July, 1995 (Source: Semenza et al., 1999)

Diagnosis	ICD-9	Observed No.	Observed >65 years (% of total)	Expected No.	Excess (95% CI)	p-value
Diabetes	250	1,322	686	1,015	307 (47, 567)	0.019
Nervous system disorders*	320–389	1,001	463 (46%)	832	170 (36, 303)	0.027
Cardiovascular disease	390–398 402 404–429 440–448	2,485	1,660 (67%)	2,024	461 (146,777)	0.019
Pneumonia and influenza	480–487	1,480	724 (49%)	1,237	243 (58, 429)	0.025
Emphysema	492	113	80 (71%)	76	38 (20, 56)	0.007
Chronic liver disease and cirrhosis	571	158	31 (20%)	120	38 (11, 65)	0.021
Nephritis, nephritic syndrome, nephrosis	580–589	392	177 (45%)	259	134 (57, 210)	0.011
Effects of heat and light	992	655	347 (53%)	4	651 (641, 662)	<0.001

*Includes: epilepsy, Parkinson's, Alzheimer's

In addition to cardiac, respiratory, and heat effect disorders, admissions for nervous system disorders and kidney disorders were significantly higher than expected. This is determined from computing the excess risk.

(continued)

> **Boxed Example 2** (continued)
>
> $$\text{Excess risk}_{(\text{condition A})} = \text{Observed rate}_{(\text{condition A})} - \text{Expected rate}_{(\text{condition A})}$$
> $$\text{Excess admissions}_{(\text{diagnosis A})} = \text{Observed admissions}_{(\text{diagnosis A})} - \text{Expected admissions}_{(\text{diagnosis A})}$$
> $$\text{Excess admissions}_{(\text{Nervous system disorders})} = 1{,}001 - 832 = 170$$
> $$\text{Excess admissions}_{(\text{Nephritis,nephritic syndrome, nephrosis})} = 392 - 259 = 134$$
>
> **Managerial Epidemiology Implications:** Measuring excess risk, namely the absolute difference between two risk measures, is an important epidemiologic technique to determine for planning surge capacity in health care. In this example, except for emphysema and cardiovascular conditions among the elderly, those susceptible for hospital admission during a heat wave have underlying and comorbid conditions of diabetes, renal diseases, and neurologic diseases. Ensuring staff for a general medical-surgical hospital in-patient population is as important as well as staffing cardiopulmonary specialists during conditions when a persistent high heat index is anticipated within a community.

Q.4. Identify a current environmentally provoked human disease reported in the popular media. Obtain a risk assessment report concerning it. How does this risk assessment pertain to your responsibilities as a health care manager? As a member of the community?

References

Analitis, A., Katsouyanni, K., Biggeri, A., Baccini, B., Forsberg, L., Bisanti, L., Kirchmayer, U., Ballester, F., Cadum, E., Goodman, P.G., Hojs, A., Sunyer, J., Tiittanen, P., and Michelozzi, P., 2008, Effects of cold weather on mortality: results from 15 European cities within the PHEWE Project, *Am. J. Epidemiol.* **168**:1397–1408.

Atlantic Oceanographic and Meteorological Laboratory, 2007, Hurricane: frequently asked questions (August 16, 2008), http://www.aoml.noaa.gov.

Barrett, R.E., Cho, Y.I., Weaver, K.E., Ryu, K., Campbell, R.T., Dolecek, T.A., and Warnecke, R.B., 2008, Neighborhood change and distant metastasis at diagnosis of breast cancer, *Ann. Epidemiol.* **18**:43–47.

Bernard, B.P. (ed.), 1997, Musculoskeletal Disorders and Workplace Factors: A Critical Review of Epidemiologic Evidence for Work-Related Musculoskeletal Disorders of the Neck, Upper Extremity, and Low Back, DHHS (NIOSH) Publication No. 97–141 National Institute of Occupational Safety and Health, Cincinnati, OH.

Blanchard, M.S., Eisen, S.A., Alpern, R., Karlinsky, J., Toomey, R., Reda, D.J., Murphy, F.M., Jackson, L.W., and Kang, H.K., 2006, Chronic multisymptom illness complex in Gulf War I veterans 10 years later, *Am. J. Epidemiol.* **163**:66–75.

Centers for Disease Control and Prevention, 2008, Emergency preparedness and you (August 16, 2008), http://www.bt.cdc.gov/.

Chan, C., Lin, Y., Chen, H., Chang, T., Cheng, T., and Chen, L., 2003, A population-based study on the immediate and prolonged effects of the 1999 Taiwan earthquake on mortality, *Ann. Epidemiol.* **13**:502–508.

Chou, Y., Huang, N., Lee, C., Tsai, S., Chen, L., and Chang, H., 2004, Who is at risk of death in an earthquake? *Epidemiology* **160**:688–695.

Correa P, Haenszel W, and Tannenbaum S., 1982, Epidemiology of gastric carcinoma: review and future prospects, *Natl. Cancer Inst. Monogr.* **62**:129–134.

Daley, W.R., Brown, S., Archer, P., Kruger, E., Jordan, F., Batts, D. and Mallonee, S., 2005, Risk of tornado-related death and injury in Oklahoma, May 3, 1999, *Am. J. Epidemiol.* **161**:1144–1150.

Dominici, F., Peng, R.D., Zeger, S.L., White, R.H., and Samet, J.H., 2007, Particulate air pollution and mortality in the United States: did the risks change from 1987 to 2000? *Am. J. Epidemiol.* **166**:880–888.

Dorn, T., Yzermans, C.J., Guijt, H., and van der Zee, J., 2007, Disaster-related stress as a prospective risk factor for hypertension in parents of adolescent fire victims, *Am. J. Epidemiol.* **165**:410–417.

Feng, S., Tan, H., Benjamin, A., Wen, S., Liu, Z., Zhou, J., Li, S., Yang, T., Zhang, Y., Li, X., and Li, G., 2007, Social support and posttraumatic stress disorder among flood victims in Hunan, China, *Ann. Epidemiol.* **17**:827–833.

Ishigami A., Hajatl S., Kovats R.S., Bisanti L., Rognoni M., Russo M., and Paldy A., 2008, An ecological time-series study of heat-related mortality in three European cities, *Environ. Health* 2008 **7**: 5 doi:10.1186/1476–069X-7-5, http://www.ehjournal.net/content/7/1/5.

Jirtle, R.K., and Skinner, M.K., 2007, Environmental epigenomics and disease susceptibility, *Nat. Rev. Genet.* **8**:252–262.

Johnson, H., Kovats, S., McGregor, G., Stedman, J., Gibbs, M., and Walton, H., 2005, The impact of the 2003 heat wave on daily mortality in England and Wales and the use of rapid weekly mortality estimates, *Euro. Surveill.* **10**:pii = 558, http://www.eurosurveillance.org/ViewArticle.aspx?ArticleID = 558.

Kovats, R.S., and Ebi, K.L., 2006, Heatwaves and public health in Europe, *Euro. J. Pub. Hlth.* **16**:592–599.

Lammerding, A.M., and Paoli, G.M., 1997, Quantitative risk assessment: an emerging tool for emerging foodborne pathogens, *Emerging Infectious Dis.* **3**:483–487.

Lienhardt, C.,2001, From exposure to disease: the role of environmental factors in susceptibility to and development of tuberculosis, *Epidemiol. Rev.* **23**:288–300.

Lin, S., Reibman, J., Bowers, J.A., Hwang, S., Hoerning, A., Gomez, M.I., and Fitzgerald, E.F., 2005, Upper respiratory symptoms and other health effects among residents living near the World Trade Center site after September 11, 2001, *Am. J. Epidemiol.* **162**:499–507.

Meng, Y., Wilhelm, M., Rull, R.P., English, P., Nathan, S., and Ritz, B., 2008, Are frequent asthma symptoms among low-income individuals related to heavy traffic near homes, vulnerabilities, or both? *Ann. Epidemiol.* **18**:343–350.

Morris, P.D., 1995, Lifetime excess risk of death from lung cancer for a U.S. female never-smoker exposed to environmental tobacco smoke, *Environ. Res.* **68**:3–9.

National Center for Injury Prevention and Control, 2007, *In a Moment's Notice: Surge Capacity for Terrorist Bombings*, Centers for Disease Control, Atlanta, GA.

National Oceanic and Atmospheric Administration, 2008, Tsunami (August 16, 2008), http://www.noaa.gov.

Needleman, H., 2004, Lead poisoning, *Ann. Rev. Med.* **55**:209–222.

Nelson, N.J., 2006, Migrant studies aid the search for factors linked to breast cancer risk, J. Natl. Cancer Inst. **98**:436–438.

Peel, J.L., Tolbert, P.E., Klein, M., Metzger, K.B., Flanders, W.D., Todd, K., Mulholland, J.A., Ryan, P.B., and Frumkin, H., 2005, Ambient air pollution and respiratory emergency department visits, *Epidemiology* **16**:164–174.

Prüss-Üstün, A., 2006, *Preventing Disease Through Healthy Environments: Towards an Estimate of the Environmental Burden of Disease*, World Health Organization Press, Geneva, Switzerland.

Ramirez, M., and Peek-Asa, C., 2005, Epidemiology of traumatic injuries from earthquakes, *Epidemiol. Rev.* **27**:47–55.

Rentz, E.D., Marshall, S.W., Loomis, D., Casteel, C., Martin, S.L., and Gibbs, D.A., 2007, Effect of deployment on the occurrence of child maltreatment in military and nonmilitary families, *Am. J. Epidemiol.* **165**:1199–1206.

Schildcrout, J.S., Sheppard, K., Lumley, T., Slaughter, J.C., Koenig, J.Q., and Shapiro, G.G., 2006, Ambient air pollution and asthma exacerbations in children: an eight-city analysis, *Am. J. Epidemiol.* **164**:505–517.

Schneiderman, A.I., Braver, E.R., and Kan, H.K., 2008, Understanding sequelae of injury mechanisms and mild traumatic brain injury incurred during the conflicts in Iraq and Afghanistan: persistent postconcussive symptoms and posttraumatic stress disorder, *Am. J. Epidemiol.* **167**: 1446–1452.

Schober, S.E., Zhang, C., Brody, D.J., and Marano, C., 2008, Disparities in secondhand smoke exposure—United States, 1988–1994 and 1999–2004, *MMWR* **57**:744–747.

Semenza, J.C., McCullough, J.E., Flanders, W.D., McGeehin, M.A., and Lumpkin, J.R., 1999, Excess hospital admissions during the July 1995 heat wave in Chicago, *Am. J. Prev. Med.* **16**:269–277.

Shultz, J.M., Russell, J., and Espinel, Z., 2005, Epidemiology of tropical cyclones: the dynamics of disaster, disease, and development, *Epidemiol. Rev.* **27**:21–35.

Sommer, A., and Mosley, W.H., 1972, East Bengal cyclone of November, 1970: epidemiological approach to disaster assessment, *Lancet* **299**:1029–1036.

Steenland, K., 1999, Risk assessment for heart disease and workplace ETS exposure among nonsmokers, *Environ. Health Perspect.* **107**(Suppl. 6):859–863.

U.S. Department of Health and Human Services, 2000, *Healthy People 2010: Understanding and Improving Health*, 2nd ed., US Government Printing Office, Washington, DC.

Wellenius, G.A., Bateson, T.F., Mittleman, M.A., and Schwartz, J., 2005, Particulate air pollution and the rate of hospitalization for congestive heart failure, *Am. J. Epidemiol.* **161**:1030–1036.

Zablotska, L.B., Bogdanova, T.I., Ron, E., Epstein, O.V., Robbins, J., Likhtarev, I.A., Hatch, M., Markov, V.V., Bouville, A.C., Olijnyk, V.A., et al., 2008, A cohort study of thyroid cancer and other thyroid diseases after the Chornobyl accident: dose-response analysis of thyroid follicular adenomas detected during first screening in Ukraine (1998–2000), *Am. J. Epidemiol.* **167**:305–312.

Chapter 9
Delivering Health Care with Quality: Epidemiological Considerations

Learning Outcomes

After completing this chapter, you will be able to:

1. Evaluate indicators for assessing the quality of health care services in terms of their appropriateness, advantages, and limitations.
2. Identify a process targeted for quality improvement and propose methods for monitoring its ongoing effectiveness.
3. Outline a study design for determining if a new intervention can reduce the incidence of an adverse event in a population of hospitalized patients.

Keyterms Confidence interval • Quality indicator • Risk adjustment • Sentinel event • Variation

Introduction

The notion that evaluating the process of caring for a patient should extend beyond accreditation specifically to address a dimension considered as "quality of care" was put forth by Donabedian as early as 1968. However, concern over the lack of "consistent, high quality medical care to all people" was brought to national attention by the Institute of Medicine's (2001) report, "Crossing the Quality Chasm." This sparked interest in quality management as an organizational strategy although the practice of total quality management was adopted by some organizations a decade earlier (Counte et al., 1995, 1992; Glandon et al., 1993). Organizations were slow to adopt quality management strategies, largely because of the significant information requirements to assess the multiple domains thought to comprise "quality" in the populations they served. At the federal level, quality principles have also espoused, but from a different perspective. One of the two overarching national health goals cited in *Healthy People 2010* is "Goal 1: Increase Quality and Years of Healthy Life" (USDHHS, 2000). The premise is that through access to quality care across all components of the

D.M. Oleske (ed.), *Epidemiology and the Delivery of Health Care Services: Method and Applications,*
DOI 10.1007/978-1-4419-0164-4_9, © Springer Science+Business Media, LLC 2009

continuum of care, health disparities will be reduced and the quality and years of healthy life for all Americans will be realized. Access to health care is one indicator used to measure progress toward this goal along with other epidemiological measurements such as avoidable hospitalizations and proportion of persons appropriately counseled about health behaviors. Regardless of private or public pursuit of quality in the delivery of health care, the goals of quality management are parallel to that of epidemiology in that both seek to improve the health of populations. This chapter explores the epidemiological concepts to assess quality, identify opportunities for improvement, and to examine the impact of change on organizational performance and health outcomes.

Interrelationship Among Health Care Quality, Quality Management, and Epidemiology

The Institute of Medicine defines quality as "the degree to which health services for individuals and populations increase the likelihood of desired health outcomes and are consistent with current professional knowledge" (Institute of Medicine, 1990). Quality of care is technically an abstract term and cannot be measured directly. It is a multidimensional construct and should ideally be measured as such. However, unidimensional indicators are typically used to measure quality and these are based upon the condition or process being evaluated. The practice of quality management practice is based upon the principles of continuous quality improvement (CQI) and involves continuous planning, control, and improvement (Palmer et al., 1991). The planning process requires measurement of the quality phenomena, the identification of risk factors which could potentially reduce quality, and the planning of strategies for continuous improvement in performance. Quality control represents the management processes selected to enable compliance with standards of performance and the methods to routinely reassess the level of compliance. The improvement philosophy of quality management targets the implementation of strategies for raising the bar in performance, not focusing on the deficiencies that need correction. The ultimate goal of quality management is to improve the health of a population through identifying unwanted variation, instituting control strategies aimed at risk factors that affect the quality of care, and providing interventions that positively influence customer (patient) assessments of the quality of their care and their health outcomes. Quality management seeks to improve the performance of both providers and the organization. Thus, individual competence is important as well as organizational infrastructure and both are key to the successful implementation of quality initiatives. The more extensive that quality management is embraced, the more likely the organization or providers are to exhibit high performance on quality indicators (Wang et al., 2006; Weiner et al., 2006). Quality management is not intended to directly produce revenue per se. But according to Weber et al. (2001), "it can be a protective maneuver for organizations in that clinical risks are minimized and cost-control opportunities become apparent." Moreover, a secondary financial benefit can be derived according to these authors suggesting that customer satisfaction is influenced by quality. In the context of health care quality, epidemiology is utilized to measure performance and performance improvement initiatives in the delivery of health care services across the continuum of care. Epidemiology provides the foundations for the measurement, monitoring, and analysis of the delivery of the quality of health care by a provider, organization, or insurer.

Performance According to Standards, Guidelines, and Other Management Strategies

The current practice of quality management has as its foundations quality assurance. Quality assurance is the systematic implementation and functioning of an organization or provider according to appropriate levels of performance for its processes in the delivery of some product, and in the context of this chapter, that product being health care services. Quality assurance programs were the health care industry's first step toward continuous process improvement initiatives. Quality assurance and quality improvement programs emanate from standards regardless of their origin and they serve to formulate, implement and evaluate guidelines, and other management strategies. And, all these initiatives have their origins in epidemiologic data or measures. To ensure that health care that performance levels are achieved and processes are under control, the organization must comply with laws, standards, guidelines from professional organizations, and other mandates. These also serve as the basis for the particular quality measurement strategies and improvement initiatives undertaken by an organization.

Performance According to Standards

According to Weber et al. (2001), "a standard is a statement that defines the performance level, processes, and structures that must be in place to assure quality of care." Process performance is designated by laws, regulations, mandates, or by standards put forth by regulatory, accrediting bodies, payors, or other organizations and hence they may be "required" or voluntary. Some examples are provided here.

The Illinois Hospital Report Card Act (P.A. 93–563, eff. 1–1–04) requires extensive hospital reporting to consumers on unit RN staffing levels, records of staff orientation and training, and hospital reports of nursing hours per patient day, average daily hours worked of nursing, average daily census, infection-related measures for the facility for selected procedures, nursing vacancy, and turnover rates. Evidence of compliance with the rules of this Act is necessary for continued licensure. Licensure and accreditation are necessary for reimbursement from most payors. The reporting requirements associated with this Act are extensive and computerized systems, such as an electronic health record will facilitate reporting. Although laws and regulations may require quality performance standards other than related to reporting, they do not necessarily specify the types of quality improvement projects that must be undertaken to achieve compliance with the standards to be allowed to provide health care services.

The Joint Commission on Accreditation of Healthcare Organizations (http://www.jointcommission.org) sets forth performance standards related to the quality of care which impact accreditation status of hospitals, long-term care facilities, behavioral health centers, and ambulatory care facilities. Examples of JCAHO standards are the requirements pertaining to the collection of data and reporting of measures on the quality of clinical performance which represent the organization's management of conditions such as those related to acute myocardial infarction, heart failure, and community-acquired pneumonia. JCAHO as part of its standards for home care also specifies the collection of data on the patient's perception of the quality of care (2009 Standard PI.01.01.01).

The International Organization for Standardization ISO (International Organization for Standardization), a nongovernmental organization that brings together the public and private sectors, enables a consensus on matters of performance that meet both the requirements of business and the broader needs of society. The ISO has developed a family of performance management standard designations (ISO 9000 and ISO 1400) and is increasingly sought by health care organizations. To receive ISO 9000 designation, an organization must demonstrate certain principles including: customer focus, leadership, involvement of people, use of process approaches, system approach to management, continual improvement, factual approach to decision making, and mutually beneficial supplier relationships. ISO 14000 is awarded to those organizations which demonstrate continuous improvement in its environmental performance to reduce its harmful effects on the environment as in the case of health care organizations, the safe disposal of medical wastes as an example (http://www.iso.ch/iso/iso_catalogue/management_standards/iso_9000_iso_14000.htm, January 3, 2009).

Magnet status designation by the American Nurses' Credentialing Center (ANCC) represents excellence in nursing care based upon standards of nursing practice and nursing sensitive quality indicators. The ANCC is also example of an organization which "achieved ISO 9001:2000 certification for professional services rendered in the administration of the Magnet Recognition Program® for excellence in health care organizations and the Accreditation Program for excellence in continuing nursing education (http://www.nursecredentialing.org/Magnet.aspx, January 3, 2009)."

Clinical Practice Guidelines

The purpose of a clinical practice guideline (CPG) is to assure conformity of performance with a care delivery process that subject matter experts in the area have put forth as the "standard of care." A CPG from a quality perspective is intended to reduce unwanted variation in the delivery of health care. CPGs are a type of evidence-based practice except that practice operation parameters (e.g., timing of intervention) operationalize the evidence in a manner consistent with organizational policies and procedures and the governing laws of the geographic area of the health care organization. The National Guideline Clearinghouse (2000) maintains a data-base of CPGs which contains many nationally recognized standards of care. CPGs in the database meet the following criteria: (1) describe the process involved in the development along with other pertinent information to assist in decision-making; (2) be focused on a specific set of clinical circumstances; (3) be produced under the auspices of a relevant professional association, government agency, health care organi-zation or health plan; (4) be based on a comprehensive, verifiable literature search and review, and summarization of evidence published in peer-reviewed journals; and (5) be current (developed, reviewed or revised within last 5 years). Some specialty professional organizations have developed practice guidelines with the most notable by the American Academy of Pediatrics (AAP) and the American College of Obstetrics and Gynecology, *Guidelines for Perinatal Care*, 6th ed. (AAP, Elk Grove Village, IL, 2007). CPG can also be developed by expert consensus within an organi-zation or group practice setting such as by clinics focusing on reproductive medicine for local particularly when there is no consensus in the profession regarding the standard of care (Gleicher et al., 2000). A subtype of the CPG is a clinical pathway (see Boxed Example 2). A clinical pathway (also sometimes referred to as a critical pathway) is the template which provides clear criteria on track and measurement of a patient's progress regarding milestones aimed at achieving the desired clinical outcome(s). The distinguishing feature of a clinical pathway is that it provides clini-cal management information in terms of the specific sequencing and timing of actions by a health care provider to achieve patient goals. Specialty professional organizations are an important source of clinical pathways. For example, the American Academy of Physical Medicine and Rehabilitation (http://www.aapmr. org/hpl/clinpath.htm, January 3, 2009) provides a wide range of clinical pathways from those pertaining to diagnosis and treatment or a procedure. Neither CPGs nor the clinical pathways are intended to replace professional judgment and hence varia-tion is allowed, but should be documented. According to Weber et al. (2001), critical success factors for implementing a CPG include: "physician commitment; a multi-disciplinary team of caregivers leading the effort, dissemination, and use of data [from the CPG]; and, computerized information systems support." Compliance in using the CPG can be reinforced through the use of standing orders on areas of multidisciplinary consensus and computerized decision-support prompts at keep time points as reminders. Because of the complexity of some guidelines, training on the use of the guidelines is also critical for compliance and may require a higher level of training such as the use of a nurse practitioner to assess and initiate a patient on the CPG (Wisnivesky et al., 2008). CPGs may be useful in reducing disparities in health outcomes from treatment but must include factors pertaining to race and ethnicity that may impact the outcome must be incorporated. For example, a tobacco cessation pharmacotherapy CPG may not be utilized in a low income population without benefit coverage of the recipients Medicaid plan (Gilles et al., 2008). To optimize the effectiveness of a CPG, it should be periodically reevaluated and refined as necessary. An epidemiologic longitudinal design can be used for this purpose and identify gapsin the overall care by race, gender, and age (Peterson et al., 2008). CPGs are most effective when feedback is given to the users regarding the clinical outcomes achieved (Grover et al., 2001) (Boxed Example 1).

Boxed Example 1 Evaluating the Effectiveness of a Clinical Pathway

Problem: Clinical pathways, based upon evidence and consensus for the diagnosis and/or management of a condition, are thought to reduce the variation in the delivery of care, both in terms of the quantity and types services delivered as well as the timing of the use resources. Physicians may not put a patient on a pathway for reasons including not knowing the criteria for patient enrollment, too much paperwork for enrollment, and opposition to the philosophy of a standard care protocol for all patients with a certain condition.

Methods: A retrospective cohort study of 22,196 records of patients hospitalized for pneumonia, 5,219 of whom were on a pneumonia clinical pathway (PCP) as determined from a nonrevenue charge code reflecting a physician's order for the pathway on the hospital's computer system. A clinical decision-support software electronically assigned a severity level to each patient based upon presentation, comorbidities, chronic diseases, age, race, sex, socioeconomic status, and smoking.

Data:

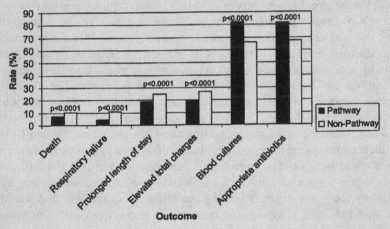

Source: Hauck et al. (2004). Reprinted from *Annals of Epidemiology*, Vol. 14, with permission from Elsevier

Odds ratios and 95% confidence intervals of patients on pneumonia clinical pathway relative to patients on nonpathway care for four outcomes stratified by severity score (Source: Hauck et al., 2004)

Severity score	Mortality OR (95% CI)	Prolonged HLOS[a]OR (95% CI)	Blood culture OR (95% CI)	Respiratory OR (95% CI)	Appropriate antibiotic use OR (95% CI)
1	0.37 (0.20–0.70)	0.34 (0.22–0.54)	2.33 (1.36–4.00)	0.20 (0.12–0.33)	2.08 (1.45–2.99)
2	0.47 (0.32–0.69)	0.65 (0.53–0.80)	2.62 (1.67–4.09)	0.30 (0.19–0.45)	2.30 (1.45–3.64)
3	0.67 (0.51–0.89)	0.91 (0.70–1.17)	2.64 (1.74–4.03)	0.33 (0.24–0.45)	2.29 (1.46–3.58)
4	0.91 (0.67–1.24)	0.73 (0.59–0.90)	2.41 (1.60–3.63)	0.49 (0.35–0.69)	2.10 (1.54–2.85)
5	0.82 (0.69–0.97)	0.80 (0.63–1.02)	2.14 (1.36–3.36)	0.44 (0.33–0.61)	1.85 (1.44–2.36)
Total	0.68 (0.60–0.78)	0.70 (0.59–0.84)	2.38 (1.55–3.65)	0.38 (0.30–0.48)	2.13 (1.55–2.93)

OR odds ratio; *CI* confidence interval

[a] Prolonged HLOS = Hospital length of stay, >75th percentile of 8 days

> **Boxed Example 1** (continued)
>
> **Managerial Epidemiology Interpretation:** *The clinical pathway resulted in* favorable patient outcomes, and administrative and process measures. These outcomes were consistent, in general, across all severity levels. Over 80% of PCP patients received antibiotics according to the guidelines. Patients on PCP were over two times more likely, overall, to have a blood culture performed and have appropriate antibiotics administered. Since patients were more likely to receive a blood culture in the PCP group, this represented better medical management, quicker hospital discharge, and lower mortality. Starting a clinical pathway upon hospital admission for all severity levels of pneumonia patients is supports quality and cost-effective care.

Utilization Management

Utilization management (UM) is the prospective and retrospective review of the episode of care regarding its appropriate progress in a pathway, placement in the health care system during an episode of care, and/or the duration of the care episode. Retrospective UM would review whether or not a hospital admission from an emergency department (ED) was appropriate. If the admission was found to be inappropriate, the development of admissions criteria for that particular case or the training of ED staff regarding the case circumstances would be an UM function. UM might also be in contact after the admission with hospital administration regarding better screening of patient insurance regarding criteria for hospital admission. Prospective monitoring may include the follow-up of a patient regarding length of stay in an intensive care unit, notifying the patient, family, and attending physicians when reimbursed days are close to being met. Prospectively, alternatives to ICU care while remaining within quality guidelines may also be suggested by UM and as such the process aids in ensuring the appropriateness of care. As longer lengths of hospital stay are associated with an increased likelihood of hospital-acquired infection, this is another example of how UM can serve as important function in delivering health care with quality. In evaluating lengths of stay UM personnel use quality practices in benchmarking hospital stays using decision-support systems based upon hospital data for similar cases or relative to normative information from proprietary sources Interqual (Mitus, 2008).

Clinical Research Protocols

Increasingly, the enrollment of a patient onto a phase III clinical trials is accepted as a quality of care practice. The National Institutes of Health defines a Phase III clinical trial as follows:

...a broad-based, prospective study, including community and other population-based trials, usually involving several hundred or more people, to compare an experimental intervention with a standard or control or compare existing treatments. It often aims to provide evidence for changing policy or standard of care. It includes pharmacologic, non-pharmacologic, and behavioral interventions for disease prevention, prophylaxis, diagnosis, or therapy http://grants.nih.gov/grants/glossary.htm#C (January 9, 2009).

The enrollment of a patient is viewed as a quality initiative because both the "standard of care" and the experimental intervention are simultaneously delivered according to strict and prospectively monitored circumstances. Clinical research protocols provide a strict set of criteria for entry to precisely identify the diagnostic condition under investigation, rigorously define the treatment regimen or procedure (including exceptions), and timing of follow-up with measurements along the time period in all study groups. Institutional Review Boards (see chapter "Ethics and Managerial Epidemiology Practice") and Data Safety Monitoring Boards (DSMB) also monitor the results of large clinical trials. The DSMB is comprised of physicians, statisticians, and patient advocates, a majority of whom are not connected with the trial who review the data periodically (at least annually to ascertain treatment outcome and any unexpected or severe adverse reactions).

Clinical trials often employment measurements of outcomes not only related to the biological condition under study, but also to subjective (e.g., quality of life) and economic indicators of success. Additionally, clinical trials may utilize (in the case of those sponsored by the National Institutes of Health) an external monitoring board. There are many large formal long-standing cooperative groups overseeing large clinical trials such as those aimed at various subsets of cancers conducted by the Eastern Cooperative Oncology Group (ECOG, http://www.ecog.org) and large independent clinical trials focused on a particular intervention for a defined period of time, such as many of those supported by the National Institutes of Health (e.g., Antihypertensive and Lipid-Lowering Treatment to Prevent Heart Attack Trial, ALLHAT).

A current registry of federally and privately supported clinical trials conducted worldwide can be found at: http://clinicaltrials.gov/. Registered clinical trials are not only limited to evaluation of therapies, but also are used to examine the quality of processes and are not limited to medical clinical trials. The Structured Early Labor Assessment and Care by Nurses Trial Group (Hodnett et al., 2008) is a randomized clinical trial of complex nursing and midwivery intervention aimed at improving birth outcomes.

Case Management

Case management according to the Commission for Case Manager Certification (CCMC) is "a collaborative process that assesses, plans, implements, coordinates, monitors, and evaluates the options and services required to meet an individual's health needs, using communication and available resources to promote quality, cost-effective outcomes (http://www.ccmcertification.org/index.html, January 3, 2009).

Case management processes are focused on enhancing the performance of particular units or organizations to effectively and efficiently addressing the needs of specific patient populations such as managing the care of a client with an occupational injury or disability and returning that individual to the work setting or an optimum level of function. There are different models of case management, but those based upon clinical pathways to direct patient care are intended to have as goals not only the financial outcomes of length of stay and resource consumption, but also to manage clinical outcomes of morbidity and mortality.

Risk Management

The purpose of risk management is to provide support to health care providers by managing potential or actual liability situations. The risk management process involves the analysis of facts in an untoward event, assisting clinicians in communicating the appropriate information to the patient and family, and guidance in documenting the circumstances relating to the event in an objective manner (Rubeor, 2003). Risk management offices may maintain databases representing areas of risk in an organization, such patterns of incident reports, filed claims, settled claims, and patient satisfaction reports according to physician, physician characteristics, and service category (e.g., neurosurgery, obstetrics, etc.). The analysis of these data may provide areas for proactive interventions. One of the most important aspects of risk management is the promotion of a complete and accurate record of the patient encounter in the organization. Kolber and Lucado (2005) assert that the quality of "documentation is as important as the quality of the care that is delivered to patients, since medical records are legal documents and serve as valuable evidence as to what transpired between patients and the healthcare providers." In formulating risk management strategies pertaining to documentation, the organization should have policies and procedures related to basic charting rules apply including alterations, procedures for including informed consent, and any experimental protocols the patient is undergoing, how incident reports are contained within the record, and how the release of information is handled to be the Health Insurance Portability and Accountability Act of 1996 (HIPAA) Privacy Rule compliant, procedures for documentation of telephone conversations, and more recently protocols for electronic communication (through emails). Although structured as a database, the same principles apply to an electronic health records, but in addition, the storage and transmission of the electronic information is subject to different protocols for transmission (see chapter "Ethics and Managerial Epidemiology Practice"). Quality documentation is also a reminder of the legal obligation all health care providers have in relationship to patient care. Such is the case regarding the relationship between consistent documentation and care related to measured quality indicators such as the documentation related to wound care and how the documentation needs to be a reflection of the organization's current practices, policies, and procedures otherwise legal issues could arise both related to the documentation and potential quality issue. Thus, principle of risk management is also fundamental to managerial epidemiological practice, namely, sound decisions cannot be made unless the data are of high quality.

Benchmarking

Benchmarking is a quality management initiative undertaken to see if the organization is performing within acceptable parameters, usually established and displayed a percentile. A percentile is the value of the percentage distribution equal to or below the given value. Scored data can be computationally transformed to a percentile value to facilitate the interpretation. For example, a mean patient satisfaction score of 4.9 (out of 5.0 being the highest) may be transformed to a more meaningful interpretation if it were to be determined that the value of 4.9 is equivalent to the 99th percentile of favorable satisfaction. The transformed data are then displayed typically in terms of quartiles with the 50th percentile as the median value and the 75th percentile representing the upper quartile and the 25th percentile containing the lower end of the distribution. These quartiles provide performance thresholds that could be targeted for quality improvement. If a hospital is only at a 50th percentile, there is ample room for improvement as this hospital's performance is no better than half of the hospitals compared. Benchmarking can be done for internal organizational purposes, but increasingly this information is available to the public through government agencies, private organizations, and proprietary sources. Hospital Compare (http://www.hospitalcompare.hhs.gov) and Nursing Home Compare (http://www.medicare.gov/NHCompare/home.asp) benchmark databases maintained by the Centers for Medicare and Medicaid are examples. Benchmarking is a practice not unique to US health care. The United Kingdom's National Health Service benchmarks hospitals according to geographic area, type, and patient volume and relative to various quality improvement project results (http://www.nhsbenchmarking.nhs.uk). Organizations self-identifying performance at less than the desired threshold should examine the high performing organizations for best practices in service delivery, realignment of structure for process improvement, or other strategies.

Boxed Example 2 Benchmarking the Quality of Nursing Home Care

Problem: Residents of nursing homes are a vulnerable population. Poor care results in poor quality of life for these residents and an economic burden on society for treatment of complications related to adverse events.

Data: Data from the Minimal Data Set collected for the Center for Medicare and Medicaid Services linked with the Online Survey and Certification and Reporting System (OSCAR), and other related links to data systems provide the basis for

---

(continued)

Boxed Example 2 (continued)

Nursing Home Compare. Data for one quality indicator, percent of high-risk long-stay residents who have pressure sores. Pressure sores are usually caused by constant pressure on one part of the skin because of lack of patient movement, incontinence, and poor nutrition. They may take a long time to heal. The indicator reflects the percentage of short-stay residents who have developed pressure sores, or who had pressure sores that did not get better between their 5-day and 14-day assessments in the nursing home. Lower percentages are better.

Results: The following graph benchmarks one skilled care facility relative to others in the state and nation. It illustrates that the performance of the facility in managing this condition was better than others in both the state and the nation.

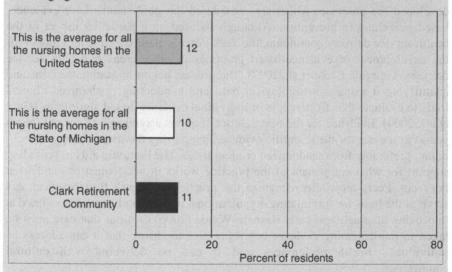

Present of high-risk long-stay residents who have pressure sore.
Source: www.medicare.gov/NHCompare/home.asp, Date Last Updated: April 1, 2009

Managerial Epidemiology Interpretation: The prevalence of pressure sores is one measure of the residents' physical condition. To the consumer this is one source of information that shows how well the nursing home is caring for its residents. Managers of skilled care facilities recognizing increased consumerism via the Internet should give particular attention to this and other publicly available indicators of the quality of care. For this indicator, the nursing home prevalence of pressure sores is lower than both the state and national averages. The goal should be zero percent prevalence of pressure sores. The facility manager should institute increased efforts aimed at preventing pressure sores in all residents including instituting protocols for frequent turning, assessing and improving nutrition, and attention to proper and clean padding on boney prominences.

Best Practices

The use of best practices is a technique or methodology that is perceived to be an innovation and intended to improve the quality and effectiveness of health care delivery. To be a best practice, the users must consistently find that the innovation improves the effectiveness of health care delivery according to some preestablished criterion. Although clinical experience with a large number of patients with a specific condition or the experience of an organization with a specialized challenge (staff security in managing mental health wards) can help shape a best practice, they are best when they are evidence-based (Cowman and Bowers, 2008; Todd and James, 2008). Evidence-based health care is an important quality initiative as it intends to standardize care based upon the best, current clinical evidence. The U.S. Preventive Services Task Force, an independent panel, has developed the processes which are considered the gold standard for evidence-based guidelines in prevention. Although focused on a particular aspect of the health service delivery continuum, the Task Force's methods serve as a model for the development of evidence-based practices in other areas of health service delivery (Guirguis-Blake et al., 2007). The process begins by stating the issue and quantifying it using epidemiological data and conducting randomized clinical trials to evaluate the effectiveness of individual evidence-based algorithms (Gary et al., 2004). Evidence for the best practice requires a synthesis of current (last 5 years) as a basis for the scientific evidence supporting the methodology or technique, preferably from randomized clinical trials. The literature aids in providing support for what component of the practice works in what situations and what does not. Peers must also recognize the practice as "best." Best practices can serve as the basis for formulating organizational policies and procedures aimed at improving the quality of care. Hasnain-Wynia (2006) cautions that care must be taken in implementing evidence-based practice to ensure that it can address an individual's health preferences and it can be delivered with cultural competence.

Measuring Quality Epidemiologically

Epidemiologic measures are well suited to measuring quality to achieve standards or guidelines owing to the fact that quality is fundamentally a population-based construct. The focus, however, is to identify, assess, and prioritize quality concerns or quality improvements in populations receiving health care. Epidemiologic measures of health care quality may be derived from administrative databases (claims files, surveillance systems) or from epidemiologic studies. They can be developed for all phases of the levels of health care, prevention, screening, treatment, rehabilitation, and even palliative care. Quality of care measures can be global, disease specific and even reflect disciplinary-based care (e.g., nursing sensitive indicators). Within each care delivery type, epidemiologic measures can also be used to assess the structure, processes, and outcomes of care according to the framework of the classic Donabedian (1988) model of the evaluation of the quality of care. Examples of epidemiologic measures according to this model are displayed in Table 1. Epidemiologic measures can also be used to assess the quality of care for a specific phase within the delivery of care (e.g., prevalence of pregnant women having prenatal care within the first trimester), an episode of care (e.g., hospitalization for a preventable condition), or a process of care (e.g., compliance with a practice guideline by a provider) or delivery setting.

Table 1 Examples of epidemiologic measures using the Donabedian framework for assessing quality of care (Adapted from: Weber et al., 2001)

Structure measures
- Number of patients per RN
- Number of patients per licensed personnel
- Percentage of contract nursing personnel
- Number of patients per case manager
- Percentage of board certified physicians
- Number of practice guidelines
- Interdisciplinary practice committee

Process measures
- Percentage of pregnant women receiving prenatal care in the first trimester
- Childhood immunization completion rate by recommended vaccine type
- Mammography rate in past 2 years among women aged 40+ years
- Percent of diabetics receiving insulin or oral hypoglycemic and who had an eye exam in past year
- Beta-blocker prescription filled for those after myocardial infarction with no evidence of contraindication
- Percentage of patients screened for nutrition admitted to a hospital or ambulatory clinic setting
- Percentage of patients assessed for pain upon admission to the hospital or ambulatory clinic setting
- Percentage of short-stay residents in skilled nursing care or rehabilitation services following a hospital stay given influenza vaccination during the flu season
- Percent of residents as extended or permanent residents who were physically restrained

Outcome measures
- Mortality rates:
  1. In-hospital death rates by clinical service area (e.g., neonatal intensive care unit), procedure, or diagnosis
- Incidence rates:
  1. Hospital-acquired infection rates
  2. Adverse incidence rate (fall injury rates, medication error rates)
- Survival rates:
  1. Cancer patient survival rate by anatomic site and stage
  2. Patient and graft survival rate by transplant procedure type
- Other rates:
  1. Percentage of postoperative patients experiencing pain control
  2. Patient satisfaction rates with services provided and the patient care environment

The level of measurement used in a quality assessment will determine which analytic and statistical methods are selected for analysis. The most common measures used in quality assessment are: the determination of sentinel events, rate measures, and measures of variability.

Sentinel events are occurrences of such significance in terms of mortality or potential for mortality that the occurrence of one of these requires thorough review of the circumstances related to its occurrence by the health care organization and its leadership. The Joint Commission for Accreditation of Healthcare Organizations defines sentinel events for hospitals. The identification of a sentinel even requires a determination of its type, setting of occurrence, source of the event, event outcomes, and method of the organizations response to preventing further occurrence of the event. Displayed in Table 2 are the most common sentinel events occurring in hospitals.

Rate measures can be used in assessing the process or outcome of care in terms of what is the magnitude of the processes or outcomes achieved (or not achieved). Rate measures used can be static measures (average population at risk denominator) or based upon a person-years denominator (e.g., survival rates). Prevalence measures are used to evaluate processes involved in care delivery, such as the prevalence of patients under glycemic control at the recommended target level for

Table 2 Healthcare sentinel events monitored (Source: Joint Commission for the Accreditation of Healthcare Organizations, 2005, 2007 available at http://www.jcaho.org)[a]

Type of sentinel event	2005	2007
Wrong-site surgery	12.8	13.0
Patient suicide	13.1	12.4
Medication error	10.1	9.3
Delay in treatment	7.6	7.5
Patient fall	5.3	5.8
Patient death/injury in restraints	3.9	3.7
Assault/rape/homicide	3.4	3.7
Perinatal death/loss of function	3.1	3.0
Transfusion error	2.6	2.3
Infection-related event	1.9	2.1
Anesthesia-related event	1.6	1.7
Medical equipment-related	1.6	1.7
Patient elopement	1.9	1.6
Fire	1.8	1.5
Maternal death	1.4	1.5
Ventilator death/injury	1.2	1.0
Infant abduction/wrong family	0.6	0.7
Utility systems-related event	0.5	0.5
Unintended retention of foreign body	0.4	2.9
Other	12.6	12.5

[a]Settings measured: general hospital, psychiatric hospital, behavioral health facility, emergency department, long-term care facility, ambulatory care, home care, clinical laboratory, health care network, office-based surgery

HBA(1c) of <7.5% (McKinney et al., 2008). Outcome rate measures of quality include: in-patient mortality rates, readmission rates, and morbidity rates (e.g., rates of complications). The Agency for Healthcare Research and Quality (AHRQ) has proposed 26 rate measures as "inpatient quality indicators" from hospital administrative data. According to AHRQ (2006), quality indicators "reflect the quality of care inside hospitals and include inpatient mortality for certain procedures and medical conditions; utilization of procedures for which there are questions of overuse, underuse, and misuse…" (Table 3). AHRQ has also developed a set of "prevention quality indicators" which represent conditions present upon admission to a hospital for which good outpatient care or early intervention can prevent the need for hospitalization, complications, or worsening of disease (see http://www.quality-indicators.ahrq.gov/pqi_overview.htm). Because most of the care in hospitals is

Table 3 Inpatient quality indicators (Source: Agency for Healthcare Research and Quality, 2006)

Mortality rates for medical conditions
- Acute myocardial infarction (AMI)
- AMI, without transfer cases
- Congestive heart failure
- Stroke
- Gastrointestinal hemorrhage
- Hip fracture
- Pneumonia

Mortality rates for surgical procedures
- Esophageal resection
- Pancreatic resection
- Abdominal aortic aneurysm repair
- Coronary artery bypass graft
- Percutaneous transluminal coronary angioplasty
- Carotid endarterectomy
- Craniotomy
- Hip replacement

Hospital-level procedure utilization rates
- Cesarean section delivery
- Primary cesarean delivery
- Vaginal Birth After Cesarean (VBAC), uncomplicated[a]
- VBAC, all[a]
- Laparoscopic cholecystectomy
- Incidental appendectomy in the elderly
- Bi-lateral cardiac catheterization

Area-level utilization rates
- Coronary artery bypass graft
- Percutaneous transluminal coronary angioplasty
- Hysterectomy
- Laminectomy or spinal fusion

[a]Higher rates are more favorable

provided by nursing, the National Quality Forum (NQF, 2004) developed a set of indicators representing the quality of nursing care termed "Nursing-Sensitive Care Indicators." There are 15 measures, seven of which are epidemiologically based: (1) pressure ulcer prevalence, (2) falls prevalence, (3) falls with injuries, (4) restraint prevalence, (5) urinary catheter-associated urinary tract infection for intensive care unit (ICU) patients, (6) central line catheter-associated blood stream infection rate for ICU and high-risk nursing patients (HRN), and (7) ventilator-associated pneumonia for ICU and HRN patients. The denominators for these rate measures are either in terms of number of inpatients or person-time units of exposure (e.g., central line-days for ICU patients). Quarterly reporting is recommended by NCF for the first three listed measures. Rate measures are also used in quality assessment to compare the performance of one organizational unit (e.g., a hospital) to some benchmark rate (e.g., all hospitals in a state) after computing confidence intervals (usually 95%) for the point estimates of the rates compared. A confidence interval represents the band of values around the estimate rates in which with a certain level of certainty the true value is expected to lie. Large differences between rates can be easily detected. Detecting small differences requires larger sample sizes. The meaning of small significant differences in large samples may yield a Type I error. Hence, the level of Type I error should be a prior established and typically at $\alpha = 0.05$ and with cautious interpretation. Rules for obtaining the size of the sample compared are specified by the agency requesting the rate information for benchmarking. The duration of the period for which the rate is computed is a function of the particular type of rate. For example, a 30-day period to assess mortality may be preferred over a more narrow time period for some conditions. However, the longer the time period for constructing a rate measure for a postdischarge condition (e.g., readmission, mortality, etc.), the less likely the event is related to the original care episode. Burt et al. (2008) define an emergency department admission within 7 days of a hospital discharge for patients older than 30 days as an important measure to focus on when improving inpatient care quality. Boxed Example 2 illustrates the use of the prevalence rate of cardiac disease to gauge the appropriateness of trends in cardiac procedure rates.

Variability in rates is an important exists regarding the delivery of health care because of the incidence, prevalence, and severity diseases in a community and its demographic composition. Controlling unwanted variation is the goal, but defining unwanted or unnecessary variation is a bigger challenge. Utilization rate measures, such as hospitalization rates, procedure rates, are used to assess variability. Unwanted variability exists when variability in the utilization of health care cannot be explained by the disease patterns or the demographics of a community and it is important to determine the source of the variability. Tseng et al. (2005) identified that seasonal factors may contribute to variation health care utilization. The sinusoidal pattern of monthly hemoglobin A_{1c}, a marker of glycemic control with peaks March through April suggest seasonal physiologic or behavioral responses, may trigger adverse hemoglobin A_{1c} levels followed by increased hospitalization or mortality. The examination of variability begins with a precise definition of the disease of health problem. Numerator counts are commonly collected from claims data. Next, the cohort of individuals receiving services needs to be defined. It is not appropriate to use the hospital population for the denominator as patients may utilize multiple hospitals within a defined geographic area. Unwanted or excess variability is evaluated graphically and/or statistically. A statistical test of the variance (*F*-test) comparing the variance of two or more rates is one method of assessing variability.

Risk adjustment according to Blumenthal et al. (2005) is "a series of techniques that account for the health status of patients when predicting or explaining costs of health care for defined populations or for evaluating retrospectively the performance of providers who care for them." Risk adjustment is often applied when comparing rate measures to account for differences in patient populations served by different organizations or programs. The major types of risk adjustment strategies consider: (1) client demographic characteristics only, (2) client demographic characteristics plus provider and characteristics to adjust for ascertainment and selection bias by the provider (e.g., acceptance of a transfer from a skilled care facility, hospital teaching status, etc.), and (3) client demographic and clinical characteristics (comorbidities existing prior to admission, identified during care episode). While rate standardization described in chapter "Descriptive Epidemiological Methods" is intended to compare disease rates in communities by accounting for age, gender, and race, risk adjustment may also consider other variables depending upon the intent of the risk adjustment. When populations are compared with respect to treatment outcomes, among organizations, provides, x health plans, current comorbidities, past medical history of the patients served, and provider characteristics are included. Risk adjustment may also include other factors, depending upon the patient population such as the inclusion of physical or cognitive abilities when assessing the quality of care for rehabilitation patients (Iezzoni, 2004). Factors in addition to demographic characteristics are used in risk adjustment as they can affect the outcomes and hence the interpretation of the quality of care provided independent of the processes of care. Information from Diagnostic Related Group (DRG) Number or ICD-9-CM code on administrative records of the patient encounter typically provides the clinical data for risk adjustment for comparing outcomes of treated populations. As compared with rates standardization an arithmetic weighting for adjustment, risk adjustment is typically a two-step procedure with a multiple linear regression providing a predicted or expected outcome given the set of characteristics added to the model. The observed rate (O) is compared with the expected rate (E) derived from the regression model such that the significance of O/E = 1 (no difference between the observed rate and the expected rate) is computed as follows:

z-score=([O-E]/SE)where SE is the standard error calculated as $[p_i(1-p_i)]^{1/2}/N$

and N is the number of patients in which the ith patient has an estimated probability p_i of developing the outcome. If O = E, there is no difference in outcomes from what would be expected. If O > E, the outcomes are greater than expected and if the measure is of adverse events, the ratio is unfavorable. If O < E, and O measures unfavorable events, then the ratio is favorable. Figure 1 illustrates improvement in

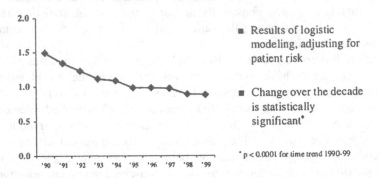

Fig. 1 Observed vs. expected adjusted risk of death from coronary bypass grafting (CABG) surgery (Source: Grover et al., 2001). Reproduced from Gover, F.L., et al., 2001, *Annals of Surgery* 234: with permission of Lippincott Williams & Wilkins (http://lww.com)

outcomes related to procedures as the O/E ratio declines over time after the intro-duction of a quality improvement practice, specifically a decreased adjusted risk of surgical death following coronary artery bypass grafting. Details on other risk adjustment strategies can be found elsewhere (Pope et al., 2004).

In addition to risk adjustment for clinical variables to compare outcomes of care, there is a need to risk adjust population responses that are not related to treatment outcomes. This is the case of comparing perceptions of the quality of care. Variation in the perceptions of the quality of care is influenced by many factors including those of the respondent and features of the delivery system or health plan providing service (Gillies et al., 2006; O'Malley et al., 2005). Variables proposed for risk adjustment of patient ratings of the quality of care include age, gender general health status, mental health status, education, race, Spanish language, and help in completing a questionnaire (O'Malley et al., 2005). Regardless of populations compared, some form of "risk adjustment" is an essential component of data that are reported publicly.

Quality Improvement Tools and Techniques

Despite the availability of quality measures and various standards, guidelines and other quality practices, critical incidents occur and success in achieving compliance by providers or health care organizations may vary because of organizational resources available to address matters of quality (Olson et al., 2008). Epidemiologic methods identify and prioritize opportunities for quality improvement. Quality improvement tools are then used to guide in the development of specific interventions aimed at isolating the root cause(s) of a problem for which additional epidemiologic data or an epidemiologic study may be required. To be most effective, the quality improvement tools and techniques utilized should involve a team approach. Those most commonly used in health care are described below (Boxed Example 3).

Boxed Example 3 Detecting Overutilization Rates of Cardiac Procedures

Problem: Utilization of cardiac interventional procedures and invasive testing has increased dramatically over time. It is not known if the prevalence of cardiac disease has increased, if previously underserved populations now have access to care, or financial reasons account for the trend.

Methods and Data: Cross-sectional examination of physician and supplier Medicare claims in the numerator and Social Security Administration demographic data in the denominator. CPT codes defined procedures and ICD-9-CM codes defined acute myocardial infarction (AMI) as a proxy measure of underlying coronary artery disease prevalence. Annual procedure utilization rates were age, race, and gender directly standardized to a standard population based upon the 2001 population distribution.

Results:

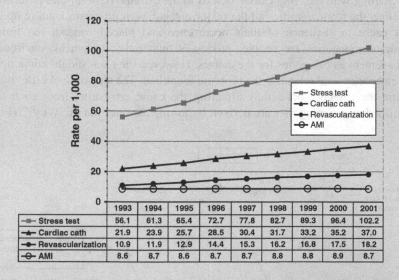

	1993	1994	1995	1996	1997	1998	1999	2000	2001
Stress test	56.1	61.3	65.4	72.7	77.8	82.7	89.3	96.4	102.2
Cardiac cath	21.9	23.9	25.7	28.5	30.4	31.7	33.2	35.2	37.0
Revascularization	10.9	11.9	12.9	14.4	15.3	16.2	16.8	17.5	18.2
AMI	8.6	8.7	8.6	8.7	8.7	8.8	8.8	8.9	8.7

Trends in population-based rates of hospitalization for acute myocardial infarction (AMI), diagnostic testing, and revascularization, adjusted for age, gender, and race, Medicare, 1993–2001. Cath indicates catheterization.
Source: Lucas et al., 2006. Reproduced with permission from the American Heart Association

---

(continued)

Boxed Example 3 (continued)

Managerial Epidemiology Interpretation: The utilization rates, because they were adjusted, reveal that the increases over time were not explained by changes in gender, age, or race, nor AMI prevalence. The study is ecological meaning that the utilization rates and the AMI prevalence rate were correlated from two different samples and not necessarily the AMI rate among persons having the procedure(s). Considering the risk and cost of some of the cardiac procedures, managers of health plans may work with partner physicians to develop protocols for targeting population subgroups, possibly based upon degree of symptoms who could benefit most from the interventions.

Cause-and-Effect Diagram

A cause-and-effect (or "fishbone" or Ishikawa) diagram pictorially represents all the steps in the processes that could be potential causes of a problem. The Ishikawa refinement of this type of diagram is that it cues those constructing the diagram to addressing sets of causes, the specific categories of which depend upon the industry. Starting with the "root cause" placed to the extreme right (or end-point) on the timeline, the team identifies all the major categories of processes leading up to the root cause in sequence of their occurrence and placed beneath the timeline. Common categories are people, processes, materials, equipment, environment, management as categories for the causes. However, the team should come up with the categories used related to the problem identified. The steps or tasks (or "bones") within the category potentially affecting the cause emanating from each of the identified major categories are derived by asking the question of "Why?" (Fig. 2).

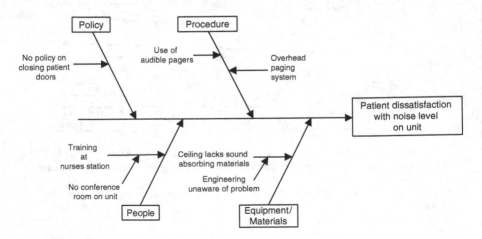

Fig. 2 Cause-and-effect diagram

The team then identifies improvement opportunities associated with the root cause using the diagram as a visual basis for developing teamwork in solving a problem. The diagram also serves to stimulate teamwork in implementing a solution across units within an organization as seldom the causes of a problem are restricted to one department.

Flowchart

Based upon an analysis of performance and the examination of root causes of a problem, the process should be reevaluated by the team. There may be too many hand-offs (leading to quality gaps), the sequencing of processes may be inappropriate, inefficient, or redundant. The flowchart provides a graphical representation of the steps in a process with analysis of the process pictorially by organizing shapes to represent unique actions associated with the process. For example, if a high prevalence of uncontrolled pain was found in a hospital unit, the process may be revised by constructing a flowchart of the "ideal process" to ensure that every patient upon admission has a pain assessment, the score of the assessment is recorded from which a decision is made regarding pain medication administration. Subsequent to the decision, documentation and monitoring continue until discharge of the patient (Fig. 3). The team can then return to a quality improvement model (e.g., PDCA cycle) to evaluate the process to utilizing a graphical or statistical quality control tool to determine if the desired level of performance has been achieved.

Root Cause Analysis

Root Cause Analysis (RCA) is an analysis of the pathway that represents how an event occurred and the "what" and "why" it happened. Rooney and Vanden Heuvel (2004) propose four steps in the process: (1) data collection, (2) causal factor charting, (3) root cause identification, and (4) recommendation generation and implementation. The data collection focuses on the causes that management and staff potentially have control over. Participation of as many individuals as possible in ordering the path leading up to the event is encouraged. Causal charting is similar to a flow chart but in addition superimposes questions warranting additional data needs. The RCA maps all the causal factors using a decision diagram to understand the reasoning that led up to the causal factor. Finally, a summary table according with the following columns: a general description of each causal factor, pathways that led to the factors, and recommendations for each of the root causes identified. The RCA analysis may also be formed as a matrix with the rows addressing the questions, "What is the event?" The RCA analysis is typically used when the quality matter under investigation is a sentinel event.

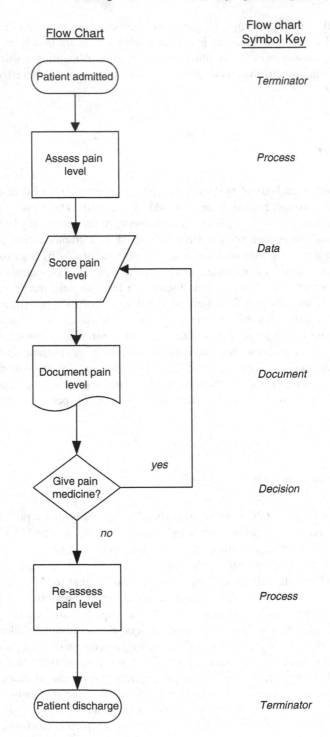

Fig. 3 Flowchart of the process of pain assessment and control

Graphical and Statistical Quality Control Tools

When the process targeted for quality improvement has been identified and refined or otherwise modified, it is necessarily to evaluate ongoing variation in the processes and outcomes of the processes. Graphical and statistical quality control tools are used for this purpose. The goal is to achieve statistical control. These tools aid in gauging if control is achieved.

Check Sheet

A check sheet is the simplest quality control tool as it is a method of recording the raw data from historical sources or for documenting observations. It is typically formatted such that values from the observations or abstractions are put in cells oriented by rows and columns (Fig. 4). A check sheet is intended to facilitate the compilation of data efficiently and accurately. The check sheet should be clear, have all the information required for the assessment readily visible to the recorder, and easy to use. It can be used to count discrete events or record continuous variables (e.g., pain intensity score). The collector of the data should be knowledgeable about the events being recorded and be unbiased in their recording (e.g., not recording a missed pain assessment). The data collected on a check sheet can be for any aspect of quality assessment, structure, process, or outcome. Data compiled from a check sheet can provide an early sign of some major trends or obvious gaps. Subsequent

Project: Pain Control	Dates of Recording: 1/1/09 – 1/7/09			Shift: All			
	Name of Recorder: Ali B. Careful						
Location: PACU	Date of Observation						
	1/1	1/2	1/3	1/4	1/5	1/6	1/7
Number of patients on unit	22	19	22	20	21	20	15
Task per patient							
Pain assessments documented upon admission	20	19	21	20	21	20	15
Pain intensity scores documented on admission	19	15	17	15	16	15	10
Pain medications administered	20	18	21	20	21	20	14
Pain medications administered according to pain intensity algorithm	19	16	21	15	17	14	11
Pain levels re-assessed	18	15	19	15	15	16	10

Fig. 4 Check sheet for quality management project: improving pain control in postsurgical patients

to the recording for the study period, data from the check sheet should be combined over study periods and samples. The check sheet facilitates the formation of graphs or assessments using more advanced statistical quality control tools.

Histogram

A histogram is a graph of which summarizes data collected over time. The frequency of levels (or values) of a variable is represented on the y-axis and the variable representing the process measure on the x-axis (Fig. 5). It aids in visualizing the central tendency (process too high, too low, within expectations), shape (normal, skewed), and dispersion of values (maximum, minimum). The median is contained in the bar representing the peak of the distribution. In the case of Fig. 6, the median primary care provider turnover rate (an indicator of the quality indicator of the continuity of care) was 7.1%. A turnover rate of 10% or higher has been found to be associated with a lower proportion of managed care members satisfaction (Plomondon et al., 2007). The positively skewed distribution in this figure thus indicates there is much room for improvement in decreasing the primary care turnover rate.

Pareto Chart

When problems are identified, the visual representation their relative magnitude aids in incentivizing improvement. A Pareto chart (or bar chart) is a frequency

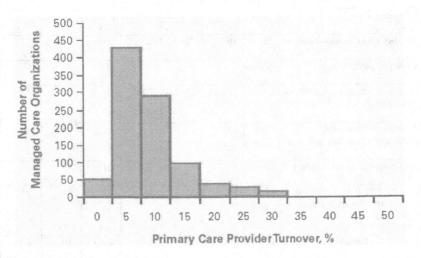

Fig. 5 Histogram of primary care provider turnover rates (Source: Plomondon et al., 2007. Reprinted with permission from the *Am. J. Manag. Care*........)

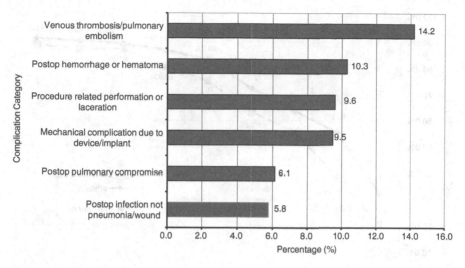

Fig. 6 Pareto chart of hospital inpatient most common specific procedure complications (Source: Hohmann, S.F. (2009). Data from University Health System Consortium. UHC Clinical Data Base/Resource Manager, reproduced with permission of the University Health System Consortium, Oak Brook, IL)

distribution of categorical data displayed in descending rank order. The data selected for the chart are collected at a defined period of time in consideration of when process changes may occur. The data for the Pareto chart in Fig. 6 were collected from hospital discharge abstracts and compiled via special software developed by the University Health System Consortium (UHC Complication Profiler) to identify not only which patients are at risk for particular procedures, but also algorithms for complications based upon ICD-9-CM diagnosis or procedure codes or Diagnostic Related Group (DRG) Numbers. This Pareto chart helps to identify surgical processes which could be improved and provides baseline data for comparing intervention results. Boxed Example 2 illustrates a Pareto chart used in benchmarking a single health care facility relative to others.

Run Chart

A run chart is a line graph used for monitoring process measures in real time over a defined period of time, typically before and after an intervention, to visualize performance change. The outcome (performance measure) is plotted on the x-axis and a time variable, scaled at regular intervals, is plotted on the y-axis. Data for each time point (30 recommended) are gathered on a regular and consistent basis, plotted in chronological order and shared and reviewed soon thereafter with the team. The run chart gives a visual display of overall performance. The run chart in Fig. 7 shows an increasing drug eluting stent utilization rate. This run chart reflects

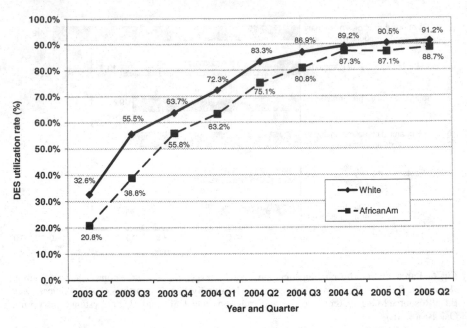

Fig. 7 Run chart of drug-eluting stent (DES) utilization rate, Whites versus African Americans, by Quarter, 2003 Quarter 2 to 2005 Quarter 2, University Health System Consortium Hospitals. Source: Hohmann, S.F. (2009). Data from University Health System Consortium: UHC Clinical Data Base/Resource Manager. Reproduced with permission of the University Health System Consortium, Oak Brook, IL

continuous improvement in performance with both races over time benefiting from the new technology.

Control Chart

A control chart is a form of statistical process control used to monitor, control, and identify significant variation within a process with the goals of continuous improvement and reduction in variation. The control chart consists of three lines: a central line (a measure of central tendency), an upper control limit, and a lower control limit. The straight line representing a measure of central tendency is based upon historical data, a grand measure of central tendency computed from all samples collected during the monitoring phase, or some other normative value established by a standard of practice or an organizational benchmark and is bounded by control limits. Similarly, the upper and lower confidence limits are computed from the same data as that used to compute the measure of central tendency and can be set at one, two, or three (most commonly) times the standard deviation (Fig. 8). Data points representing values derived from random samples of the process or outcome under study are then plotted for each time interval on the chart. A process is said to be under control when all the values from the samples fall within the designated control limits.

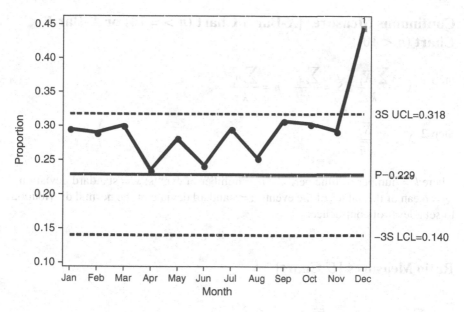

Fig. 8 Control chart

The formulae for constructing the measures of central tendency and confidence intervals for a control chart depend on the level of measurement (e.g., interval, rate, etc.), the variability of the sample size measured over time, and the existence of a preestablished objective standard that would establish the center line. Formulae for calculating common control charts are below:

Rate (or Proportion) Measures [P Chart]

Step 1: $x_i = n_i \cdot P_i$ $\quad \overline{P} = \dfrac{\sum x_i}{\sum n_i} \quad \overline{n} = \dfrac{\sum n_i}{k}$

Step 2: $\sigma_{\overline{P}} = \sqrt{\dfrac{(\overline{P} \cdot (1 - \overline{P}))}{\overline{n}}}$

Step 3: $\overline{P} \pm z \cdot \sigma_{\overline{P}}$

where $k=$ number of time periods; $n_i =$ total number in the denominator ("population at risk"); $P=$ rate = events/population at risk × factor of 10 (or calculate as a proportion); $\sigma_p =$ standard deviation of the rate; $z=$ standard deviate of the normal distribution to set the level of confidence (95% or 99%)

Continuous Measures [X-Bar S Chart ($n > = 10$) or X-Bar R Chart ($n < 10$)]

Step 1 $\bar{\bar{X}} = \dfrac{\sum \bar{X}_i}{k}$ $\bar{S} = \dfrac{\sum s_i}{k}$ $\bar{n} = \dfrac{\sum n_i}{k}$

Step 2 $\bar{X} \pm z \cdot \dfrac{\bar{S}}{\sqrt{\bar{n}}}$

where k = number of time periods; n_i = number of events; s_i = standard deviation $\bar{x}_i$ = mean of the values of the events; z = standard deviate of the normal distribution to set a level of confidence.

Ratio Measures [U Chart]

$$\bar{U} = \frac{\sum x_i}{\sum n_i} \qquad \sigma_u = \frac{\sqrt{\bar{U}}}{\sqrt{n}} \qquad UCL = \bar{U} + 3\sigma_u \qquad LCL = \bar{U} - 3\sigma_u$$

where $\bar{U}$ = mean ratio; X_i = number of events, e.g., number of adverse drug reactions; n_i = number of units of measurement, e.g., 1,000 patient day increments; σ_u = standard deviation; UCL = upper confidence limit; LCL = lower confidence limit.

There are two types of variation of concern in health care and identified through a control chart, special variation and common cause variation. Unexpected or unnatural variation is called special cause variation. Special cause variation is identified when sample points lie outside the confidence (or control) limit. This situation warrants an investigation regarding the cause with the purpose of eliminating the circumstances in the process that gave rise to the variation. Special variation, then, becomes the focus of quality improvement efforts. Special variation may be due to employees, unusual circumstances, or events (e.g., epidemic of pneumonia in the community giving rise to an increase in ED admissions resulting in an increase in average waiting time to see a physician). Common cause variation is natural and expected or inherent. If common cause variation is identified, process redesign is the best method of control. Recalculation of the confidence limits may be indicated if a change in process has resulted in a major shift in the measure of central tendency. If control charts are compared subsequent to process redesign, the charts should use the same scale for both the x-axis and y-axis.

Sampling

Ideally, a census of all patients should be monitored with the quality control tools. A census eliminates any doubts in determining performance that sampling error is not a consideration. Time and resource constraints may render this as not feasible, but this is less of a consideration if the organization utilized electronic health records. Sampling is an acceptable alternative under certain conditions and if used, the sample must be through a random process. There are two common random sampling methods, simple random sampling and systematic random sampling. A simple random sample is obtained when every n observation has an equal chance of being selected from population N. This sample can be selected using a table of random numbers, a spreadsheet software (as is available with Microsoft Excel), or computer statistical software package. A systematic random sample selects records from a population N to obtain n size sample where $j = N/n$ is the sampling interval and k is a random start between 1 and j such that records continue to be selected as k, $k + j$, $k + 2j$, $k + 3j$...until the desired sample size is reached. Regardless of the sampling method chosen, the sample selected must also be large enough to ensure that the parameter estimated (e.g., mean, proportion) yields an acceptable error range (e.g., within a ±3% error). Typically, the sample size is also a function of the number of records available. When information about the quality of care obtained from population surveys (e.g., employee or patient satisfaction), the response rate is an important consideration in determining the size of the sample needed. Over sampling is advised in these circumstances to account for nonparticipation. The amount of over sampling should be in proportion with the combined estimated rate of refusals and of those who are not able to be contacted so as to ensure an adequate sample size for final analysis. For further details concerning statistically computing the sample size required for study, the reader should consult Levy and Lemeshow (2008). Sampling details may also be put forth by a particular accrediting body regarding in what circumstances sampling is allowed, what circumstances 100% of the records are required for quality performance review, and the time frame for the sample (e.g., a specific date, monthly, etc.). For example, monthly random sampling of 20% when patient volume is 50–99 is required by the Joint Commission for Accreditation of Healthcare Organization for use in Disease Specific Care (DSC) certified program for stroke (http://www.jointcommission.org).

Systematic Improvement

To be effective, quality management and improvement must be systematic, employing the scientific method, and continuous. Epidemiologic studies can aid in evaluating programmatic efforts aimed at quality improvement (see chapter "Epidemiological Study Designs for Evaluating Health Services, Programs, and Systems," Fig. 1). However, in practice a gap in quality identified through epidemiological descriptive measure may arise. Response to the gap may require immediate attention such that arising from multiple complaints to a nurse manager by patients and family members of uncontrolled pain during an evening shift. A model used for a more immediate evaluation is the plan-do-check-act (PDCA) cycle (Fig. 9). The steps in the PDCA cycle according to Weber et al. (2001) are:

Performance Improvement Process

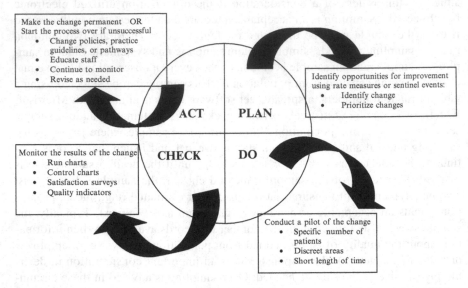

Fig. 9 Plan-do-check-act model of performance improvement process (Adapted from: Weber et al., 2001)

- Plan. To plan a change or fix a problem, plans should be formulated based upon epidemiological or other data, and input from team members.
- Do. Team members implement the plan intended to change the process, usually as a pilot or on a small scale initially.
- Check. The team observes and otherwise evaluates the results of the change. The data systems used in the planning phase can be used to determine the plan that was effective. Quality improvement tools such as control charts can also aid in this step.
- Act. If the desired change is observed (e.g., process under control, the prevalence of controlled pain increased), then the intervention would be implemented on a larger scale. If the desired change is not observed, readjustments to the intervention are made or it is abandoned and the cycle is repeated.

PDCA utilizes the quality tools and techniques previously described to evaluate new or existing quality management strategies. Gordon et al. (2008) used the PDCA framework after identifying the average 24-h pain intensity score in patients was tracking upward and uncovered during a Joint Commission accreditation survey. In addition to the pain-intensity data, the planning cycle found low compliance to clinical pathways and prompted a review of the evidence in the literature regarding pain management strategies. The Do phase launched a new policy and the Check phase involved continuous chart audits including prevalence of pain reassessment. The Act phase involved 23 inpatient units and the ED and consisted of clinical rounds regarding the new policy and pain intervention reassessment with the final result of achieving the target prevalence of compliance (>90%). Torkki et al. (2006) utilize the PDCA cycle to improve the efficiency of urgent surgery in a trauma center with the objective of improving quality of care. In doing so, the utilization rates of the operating room was maximized and also improved efficiency by reducing overtime needs.

Summary

The quality improvement process must be ongoing within an organization. There are a number of different quality indicators and specific tools used to assess and monitor quality depending upon the goals of the performance measured. As with any epidemiological study, the information obtained from quality assessment is only as useful as the quality of the data. The health care manager should ensure the infrastructure to support the accuracy of data and the timeliness of its retrieval such that quality is a continuous process and provides meaningful information to improve the quality of patient care. And, that information must be meaningful to all stakeholders in health care, providers, insurers, and consumers. An engaged dialog among all stakeholders is essential for CQI in health care. And, lastly, the increasing public disclosure of information related to health care will likely be the main driver of quality in a resource constrained environment.

Discussion Questions

Q.1. Disparities in mortality rates among ethnic/racial groups may emerge in part because of differences in the quality of care received. Propose clinical epidemiological measures that a health plan can use to determine if disparities exist among its members by ethnicity and race regarding care for diabetes, breast and cervical cancer, and prenatal care [Hint: see National Committee for Quality Assurance, http://www.ncqa.org]. Assuming disparities exist, propose target(s) goals for each measure for reducing the disparities and quality improvement(s) plans to achieve each of those targets.

Q.2. It is hypothesized that physician-perceived quality of care impacts quality outcomes of patients enrolled in a managed care plan. Design a survey form which could be used in a longitudinal study to evaluate if outcomes of diabetes care improve in relation to physician perceptions of the structure and processes in a managed care plan to deliver care for these types of patients. Propose methods to evaluate that your survey form will have properties to ensure its validity over time (Hint: See Wholey et al., 2003).

Q.3. The Braden Scale is a measure to assess a patient's risk for a pressure ulcer. A score of 18 predicts the risk of a pressure ulcer with 70% sensitivity and 77% specificity. The receiver-operator characteristic (ROC) curve for Whites is

0.75 and 0.82 for Blacks (Bergstrom and Braden, 2002). Would the Braden Scale be useful in predicting risk of a pressure ulcer as a measure of the quality of nursing care in a long-term care facility? What additional information is required to determine the validity and reliability of this Scale?

Q.4.   Propose an epidemiological indicator which could be used to measure the quality of care provided by a health care organization. Discuss the advantages and limitations of the indicator that you selected.

References

Agency for Healthcare Research and Quality (AHRQ) (February, 2006). Inpatient Quality Indicators Overview. AHRQ Quality Indicators. Agency for Healthcare Research and Quality, Rockville, MD (January 11, 2009), http://www.qualityindicators.ahrq.gov/iqi_overview.htm.

Burt, C.W., McCaig, L.F., and Simon, A.E., 2008, Emergency department visits by persons recently discharged from U.S. hospitals, *National Center for Health Statistics Reports*, No. 6, NCHS, Hyattsville, MD.

Bergstrom, N., and Braden, B.J., 2002, Predictive validity of the Braden Scale among Black and White subjects, *Nurs. Res.* **51**:398–403.

Blumenthal, D., Weissman, J.S., Wachterman, M., Weil, E., Stafford, R.S., Perrin, J.M., Ferris, T.G., Kuhlthau, K., Kaushal, R., and Iezzoni, L.I., 2005, The who, what, and why of risk adjustment: a technology on the cusp of adoption, *J. Health Polit. Policy Law* **30**:453–473.

Cowman, S., and Bowers, L., 2008, Safety and security in acute admission psychiatric wards in Ireland and London: a comparative study, *J. Clin. Nurs.* **18**:1346–1353.

Counte, M.A., Glandon, G.L., Oleske, D.M., and Hill, J.P., 1995, Improving hospital performance: issues in assessing the impact of TQM activities, *Hosp Health Serv. Adm.* **40**:80–94.

Counte, M.A., Glandon, G.L., Oleske, D.M., and Hill, J.P., 1992, Total quality management in a health care organization: how are employees affected? *Hosp. Health Serv. Adm.* **37**:503–518.

Donabedian, A., 1968, The evaluation of medical care programs, *Bull. N.Y. Acad. Med.* **44**:117–124.

Donabedian, A., 1988, The quality of care: how can it be assessed? *J.A.M.A.* **260**:1743–1748.

Gary, T.L., Batts-Turner, M., Bone, L.R., Yeh, H.C., Wang, N.Y., Hill-Briggs, F., Levine, D.M., Powe, N.R., Hill, M.N., Saudek, C., McGuire, M., and Brancati, F.L., 2004, A randomized controlled trial of the effects of nurse case manager and community health worker team interventions in urban African-Americans with type 2 diabetes, *Control Clin. Trials* **25**:53–66.

Gilles, M.E., Strayer, L.J., Leischow, R., Feng, C., Menke, J.M., and Sechrest, L., 2008, Awareness and implementation of tobacco dependence treatment guidelines in Arizona: Healthcare Systems Survey 2000, *Health Res Policy Syst.* **6**:13, ISSN:1478–4505.

Gillies, R.R., Chenok, K.E., Shortell, S.M., Pawlson, G., and Wimbush, J.J., 2006, The impact of health plan delivery system organization on clinical quality and patient satisfaction, *HSR: Health Serv. Res.* **41**:1181–1199.

Glandon, G.L., Counte, M.A., Oleske, D.M., and Hill, J.P., 1993, Assessing your TQM program's impact, *Strateg. Healthc. Excell.* **6**:7–12.

Gleicher, N., Oleske, D.M., Tur-Kaspa, I., Vidali, A., and Karande, V., 2000, Reducing the risk of high-order multiple pregnancy after ovarian stimulation with gonadotropins, *New Engl J. Med.* **343**:2–7.

Gordon, D.B., Rees, S.M., McCausland, M.P., Pellino, T.A., Sanford-Ring, S., Smith-Helmenstine, J., and Danis, D.M., 2008, Improving reassessment and documentation of pain management, *Jt. Com. J. Qual. Patient Safety* **34**:509–517

Grover, F.L., Shroyer, A.L.W., Hammermeister, K., Edwards, F.H., Ferguson, Jr., T.B., Dziuban, Jr., S.W., Cleveland, Jr., J.C., Clark, R.E., and McDonald, G., 2001, A decade's experience with quality improvement in cardiac surgery using the Veterans Affairs and Society of Thoracic Surgeons national databases, *Ann. Surg.* **234**:464–474.

Guirguis-Blake, J., Calonge, N., Miller, T., Siu, A., Teutsch, S., and Whitlock, E., for the U.S. Preventive Services Task Force, 2007, Current processes of the U.S. Preventive Services Task Force: refining evidence-based recommendation development, *Ann. Intern. Med.* **147**:117–122.

Hasnain-Wynia, R., 2006, Is evidence-based medicine patient-centered and is patient-centered care evidence-based? *HSR: Health Serv. Res.* **41**:1–8.

Hauck, L.D., Adler, L.M., and Mulla, Z.D., 2004, Clinical pathway care improves outcomes among patients hospitalized for community-acquired pneumonia, *Ann. Epidemiol.* **14**:669–675.

Hodnett, E.D., Stremler, R., Willan, A.R., Weston, J.A., Lowe, N.K., Simpson, K.R., Fraser, W.D., Gafni, and the SELAN (Structured Early Labour Assessment and Care by Nurses) Trial Group, 2008, Effect on birth outcomes of a formalised approach to care in hospital labour assessment units: international, randomized controlled trial, *B.M.J.* **337**:a1021 doi:10.1136/bmj.a1021.

Iezzoni, L.I., 2004, Risk adjusting rehabilitation outcomes: an overview of methodologic issues, *Am. J. Phys. Med. Rehabil.* **83**:316–326.

Institute of Medicine, 1990, *Medicare: A Strategy for Quality Assurance* (K.N. Lohr, ed.), National Academy Press, Washington, DC.

Institute of Medicine, 2001, *Crossing the Quality Chasm: A New Health System for the 21st Century*, National Academy Press, Washington, DC.

Kolber, M., and Lucado, A.M., 2005, Risk management strategies in physical therapy: documentation to avoid malpractice, *Int. J. Health Care Qual. Assur. Inc. Leadersh. Health Serv.* **18**:123–130.

Levy, P.S., and Lemeshow, S., 2008, *Sampling of Populations: Methods and Applications*, Wiley, Hoboken, NJ.

Lucas, F.L., DeLorenzo, M.A., Siewers, A.E., and Wennberg, D.E., 2006, Temporal trends in the utilization of diagnostic testing and treatments for cardiovascular disease in the United States, 1993–2001, *Circulation* **113**:374–379.

McKinney, P.A., Feltbower, R.G., Stephenson, C.R., Reynolds, C., and the Yorkshire Paediatric Diabetes Special Interest Group, 2008, Children and young people with diabetes in Yorkshire: a population-based clinical audit of patient data 2005/2006, *Diabet. Med.* **25**:1276–1282.

Mitus, A.J., 2008, The birth of InterQual: evidence-based decision support criteria that helped change healthcare, *Prof. Case Manage.* **13**:228–233.

National Guideline Clearinghouse™, 2000, *Fact Sheet*. AHRQ Publication No. 00–0047, http://www.ahrq.gov/clinic/ngcfact.htm (January 3, 2008), Agency for Healthcare Research and Quality Rockville, MD.

National Quality Forum (NQF), 2004, National Voluntary Consensus Standards for Nursing-Sensitive Care: An Initial Performance Measure Set, NQF, Washington, DC.

Olson, J.R., Belohlav, J.A., Cook, L.S., and Hays, J.M., 2008, Examining quality improvement programs: the case of Minnesota hospitals, *Health Serv. Res.* **43**:1787–1806.

O'Malley, A.J., Zaslavsky, A.M., Elliott, M.N., Zaborski, L., and Cleary, P.D., 2005, Case-mix adjustment of the CAHPS® Hospital Survey, *HSR: Health Serv. Res.* **40**:2162–2181.

Palmer, R., Donbedian, A., and Povar, G., 1991, *Striving for Quality in Health Care: An Inquiry into Policy and Practice*, Health Administration Press, Ann Arbor, MI.

Peterson, E.D., Shah, B.R., Parsons, L., Pollack, V.C., Jr., French W.J., Canto, J.G., and Gibson, C.M., and Rogers, W.J., 2008, Trends in quality of care for patients with acute myocardial infarction in the National Registry of Myocardial Infarction from 1990 to 2006, *Am. Heart J.* **156**:1045–1055.

Plomondon, M.E, Magid, D.J., Steiner, J.F., MaWhinney, S., Gifford, B.D., Shih, S.C., Grunwald, G.K., and Rumsfeld, J.S., 2007, Primary care provider turnover and quality in managed care organizations, *Am. J. Manage. Care* **13**:465–472.

Pope, G.C., Kautter, J., Ellis, R.P., Ash, A.S., Ayanian, J.Z., Iezzoni, L.I., Ingber, M.J., Levy, J.M., and Robst, J., 2004, Risk adjustment of Medicare capitation payments using the CMS-HCC model, *Health Care Fin. Rev.* **25**:119–141.

Rooney, J.J., and Vanden Heuvel, L.N., 2004, Root cause analysis for beginners, *Quality Prog.* July:45–53.

Rubeor, K., 2003, The role of risk management in maternal-child health, *J. Perinat. Neonatal Nurs.* **17**:94–100.

Todd, A., and James, C.A., 2008, Apomorphine nodules in Parkinson's disease: best practice considerations, *Br. J. Community Nurs.* **13**:457–463.

Torkki, P.M., Alho, A.I., Peltokorpi, A.V., Torkki, M.I., and Kallio, P.E., 2006, Managing urgent surgery as a process: Case study of a trauma center, *Int. J. Tech. Assessment Health Care* **22**:255–260.

Tseng, C., Brimacombe, M., Xie, M., Rajan, M., Wang, H., Kolassa, J., Crystal, S., Chen, T., Pogach, L., and Safford, M., 2005, Seasonal patterns in monthly hemoglobin A1c values, *Am. J. Epidemiol.* **161**:565–574.

U.S. Department of Health and Human Services (USDHHS), 2000, *Healthy People 2010*, 2nd ed., With Understanding and Improving Health and Objectives for Improving Health. 2 vols. U.S. Government Printing Office, Washington, DC.

Wall, R.J., Ely, E.W., Elasy, T.A., Dittus, R.S., Foss, J., Wilkerson, K.S., and Speroff, T., 2005, Using real time process measurements to reduce catheter related bloodstream infections in the intensive care unit, *Qual. Safe Health Care* **14**:295–302.

Wang, M.C., Hyun, J.K., Harrison, M., Shortell, S.M., and Fraser, I., 2006, Redesigning health systems for quality: lessons from emerging practices, *Jt. Comm. J. Qual. Patient Saf.* **32**:599–611.

Weber, D.R., Neikirk H.J., and Hargreaves, M., 2001, Epidemiology and health care quality management, in *Epidemiology and the Delivery of Health Care Services: Methods and Applications* (D.M. Oleske, ed.), Kluwer/Plenum, New York.

Weiner, B.J., Alexander, J.A., Shortell, S.M., Baker, L.C., Becker, M., and Geppert, J.J., 2006, Quality improvement implementation and hospital performance on quality indicators, *HSR: Health Serv. Res.* **41**:307–334.

Wisnivesky, J.P., Lorenzo, J., Lyn-Cook, R., Newman, T., Aponte, A., Kiefer, E., and Halm, E.A., 2008, Barriers to adherence to asthma management guidelines among inner-city primary care providers, *Ann. Allergy Asthma Immunol.* **101**:264–270.

Wholey, D.R., Finch, M., Christianson, J.B., Knutson, D., Rockwood, T., and Warrick, L., 2003, Evaluating health plan quality 3: survey measurement properties, *Am. J. Managed Care* **9**:S76–SP87.

Chapter 10
Advancing Patient Safety Through the Practice of Managerial Epidemiology

Learning Outcomes

After completing this chapter, you will be able to:

1. Differentiate between medical error and patient safety.
2. Interpret a patient safety indicator.
3. Cite the advances and disadvantages of patient safety indicators according to source of data for the indicator.
4. Identify risk factors for patient safety.
5. Design a system based upon epidemiologic principles to promote patient safety in a health care organization.

Keyterms Health care error • High reliability organization • Patient safety • Patient safety indicator • Patient safety organization

Concern over patient safety arose as an urgent problem with the report, "To Err is Human: Building a Safer Health System," by the Institute of Medicine (IOM) (2000) in which tens of thousands of deaths occurred annually in the USA because of preventable errors in the delivery of their health care. What is patient safety? Patient safety is one component of the larger construct, quality of health care (IOM, 2000). The IOM defines patient safety as freedom from injuries or harm to patients from care that is intended to help them. This means that patients must be protected from harm in any form, accidental injury, adverse events, preventable complications or diseases, or hospital-acquired infections (HAIs), during the process of care. The IOM raised a national consciousness of the hazards of the health care industry by reporting on the thousands of medical errors, both of commission (doing the correct thing wrong) as well as omission (failing to do the correct thing) that occur in hospitals across the nation, many of which are preventable. With the availability of computerized databases providing the backbone of point-of-service delivery information collection and dissemination, epidemiological characterization of the extent of patient safety events is not only possible but also serves to confirm the need for continued attention to this problem. Romano et al. (2003) found 1.12 million patient safety events occurring in 1.07 million hospitalizations at nonfederal

D.M. Oleske (ed.), *Epidemiology and the Delivery of Health Care Services:*
Method and Applications,
DOI 10.1007/978-1-4419-0164-4_10, © Springer Science+Business Media, LLC 2009

acute care facilities in 2000. Of concern, the authors observed an increase between 1995 and 2000 in the incidence of postoperative and nursing-related patient safety indicators, specifically for respiratory failure (31% increase), infection due to medical care (14%), decubitus ulcer (19%), septicemia (41%), and thromboembolism (42%). As with the epidemiology of any health problem, the risk of occurrence of a patient safety indicator exhibits variation by age, gender, and race. Additionally, since this health problem is linked to the service delivery, variation is also observed by geographic location and hospital type. Higher rates are observed with increasing age, among blacks, and at urban teaching hospitals (Romano et al., 2003) (Table 1 of chapter "Delivering Health Care with Quality: Epidemiological Considerations"). Patient safety events can also contribute to excess length of hospital stay, hospital charges, and mortality. The greatest excess in all of these areas results from postoperative sepsis. However, the highest rate of patient safety events has been found for obstetrical trauma, vaginal birth with instrumentation (Zhan and Miller, 2003).

Patient safety is also a global public health concern, particularly related to procedures and HAIs. The volume of major surgery worldwide is large estimated to be 234.2 million in 2004 and high even among poor nations where collectively the volume was 8.1 million or 295 (SE 53) per 100,000 population per year (Weiser et al., 2008). The potential for high risk of death and complications associated with major surgery is high, particularly in nations which cannot devote adequate resources to surgical care. Similarly, in countries with limited resources, the incidence rates of device-associated infection rates in intensive care units (ICU) are three to five times higher than those reported from North American, Western European, and Australian ICU's (Rosenthal et al., 2008). The World Health Organization (2008a) also estimates that at any given time 1.4 million persons are suffering from a HAI and that as many as 70% of injections given by needles or syringes are not properly sterilized resulting in 1.3 million deaths annually largely from bloodborne diseases such as Hepatitis B, Hepatitis C, and HIV infection. With the projected increase in the global population to 6.9 billion in 2010 (United Nations, January 4, 2009, http://esa.un.org/unpp/), these numbers of adverse events compromising patient safety, without appropriate and extensive control strategies, will continue to rise.

Epidemiologic principles can be used to promote patient safety in populations in any nation or community through the prevention, control, elimination of health care errors or reduction of risk factors for potential harm. From a management perspective, epidemiology also aids in establishing safety priorities for areas in which preventive actions should be taken at an early stage. This chapter will present issues in classifying and measuring health care error and its relationship to patient safety. Also considered are approaches to preventing and controlling health care error and promoting patient safety initiatives from an epidemiologic perspective.

A Conceptual Framework of Health Care Error

In order to classify and measure health care error, it is necessary to have a systems perspective of the context of the circumstances in which it occurred. Because the presence or absence of a safe environment is a function of the system, the Reason (2000)

Table 1 Rates of potential safety events by age and sex, US nonfederal acute care hospitals, 2000 (Source: Romano et al. (2003). Copyrighted and published by Project HOPE/*Health Affairs* as Romano, P.S., Geppert, J.J., Davies, S., Miller, M.R., Elixhauser, A., and McDonald, K.M., A national profile of patient safety in U.S. hospitals, *Health Affairs*, 22(2), 154-166, March/April, 2003. The published article is archived and available online at www.healthaffairs.org.

Patient safety indicator	Sex	Age group (years)					
		>1	1–17	18–39	40–64	65–74	75+
Anesthesia reactions	M	0.121%	0.056%	0.047%	0.043%	0.056%	0.062%
and complications	F	0.077	0.072	0.048	0.059	0.075	0.064
Death in low-mortality	M	0.006	0.033	0.049	0.076	0.202	0.511
DRGs	F	0.005	0.021	0.009	0.041	0.139	0.377
Decubitus ulcer	M	0.082	0.289	0.651	1.272	2.134	3.620
	F	0.169	0.212	0.292	1.224	2.188	3.648
Failure to rescue	M	8.235	4.912	10.143	15.271	18.766	23.142
	F	7.317	4.699	6.839	13.367	16.380	20.279
Foreign body left during	M	0.000	0.011	0.006	0.010	0.011	0.007
procedure	F	0.004	0.005	0.008	0.012	0.008	0.006
Iatrogenic pneumothorax	M	0.031	0.028	0.040	0.057	0.086	0.107
	F	0.031	0.024	0.015	0.073	0.106	0.121
Infection due	M	0.181	0.122	0.200	0.279	0.289	0.215
to medical care	F	0.199	0.073	0.071	0.251	0.282	0.175
Postop hip fracture	M	0.000	0.000	0.010	0.027	0.053	0.235
	F	0.000	0.000	0.002	0.015	0.082	0.438
Postop hemorrhage/	M	0.271	0.114	0.134	0.207	0.254	0.297
hematoma	F	0.284	0.089	0.172	0.182	0.203	0.223
Postop physiologic or	M	0.055	0.063	0.099	0.120	0.119	0.138
metabolic derangement	F	0.109	0.059	0.029	0.060	0.092	0.097
Postop respiratory	M	0.460	0.316	0.227	0.397	0.502	0.823
failure	F	0.402	0.266	0.115	0.209	0.445	0.592
Postop thromboembolism	M	0.218	0.152	0.585	0.872	1.045	1.324
	F	0.132	0.135	0.393	0.725	1.192	1.495
Postop septicemia	M	2.070	0.907	1.106	1.178	1.232	1.719
	F	2.071	0.674	0.715	0.839	0.934	1.077
Postop abdominopelvic	M	0.029	0.061	0.126	0.332	0.525	0.500
wound dehiscence	F	0.070	0.068	0.040	0.083	0.210	0.216
Accidental puncture	M	0.097	0.066	0.162	0.312	0.347	0.261
or laceration	F	0.040	0.082	0.427	0.505	0.414	0.261
Birth trauma	M	0.752					
	F	0.577					
Obstetric trauma – vaginal with instrumentation	F		23.062	24.537	22.499		
Obstetric trauma – vaginal without instrumentation	F		10.957	8.600	6.205		
Obstetric trauma–cesarean	F		0.323	0.591	0.831		

Note: DRG is diagnosis-related group. Cerain indicators apply only to certain age of sex strata. If an indicator does not apply to a particular stratum, the corresponding cell is blank organizational accident is most applicable to a health care setting. The significance of this model is that it shifts the emphasis in error management from the person approach to a systems approach emphasizing instead the conditions under which individuals work and building a scheme of defenses around these to reduce the likelihood of error. The model considers the following elements: the context within which an accident occurred, the chain of events that led to the adverse outcomes, the actions of those involved, and the conditions in which the staff were working. If the series of defenses, barriers, and safeguards of a system allows alignment of a series of holes (analogous to a model of layers of Swiss cheese) by which the hazard can pass through, an error will occur.

A systems approach for conceptualizing its occurrence of error is important and should not in itself be the endpoint for promotion of patient safety. This model used for conceptualizing error promotes an understanding of the systems approach required for guidance in proactively developing corrective measures from which lessons can be learned in promoting patient safety.

Classifying Health Care Error

In order to understand to promote patient safety from a management epidemiology perspective, it is necessary to understand to define and classify error. For purposes of this chapter, error arising from the delivery of health care shall be referred to as "health care error" or "error" unless otherwise indicated. Health care error ("error") is an unintended situation caused by a defect in the delivery of care. An error can be an act of commission (doing the wrong thing), omission (not doing the correct thing), or execution (doing the right thing incorrectly, sometimes referred to as a "slip"). There are many different approaches to classifying error. Errors can be classified in terms of severity relative to harm or injury (e.g., near miss, sentinel event), graded (1–4, from probable to certain), or in terms of legal implications (e.g., negligence). Human factors errors can be classified in terms of skill-based, rule-based, or knowledge-based in an attempt to distinguish levels of human behaviors in terms of cognitive complexity (Walsh and Beatty, 2002). Skill-level errors, the most basic level, typically, are a result of movement control inadequacies; rule-based errors emerge from deficiencies in memory to apply or recall the correct rule derived from prior training (e.g., inaccurate recall of the correct procedure for Foley catheter insertion); knowledge-based errors occur with incomplete or incorrect knowledge of a situation often because of resource or system limitations (e.g., history and physical not on patient chart upon entering the operating room). Errors can also be classified on the basis of interventions, namely is a drug or therapeutic intervention required for a counteracting effect of the error, or a withdrawal of the drug to prevent an adverse event. Errors can be classified on the basis of care delivery process: failure to identify patient, failure to diagnose, failure to screen, or failure to follow-up. Errors are sometimes classified according to an outcome measure taxonomy (e.g., medical injury, adverse event, iatrogenic illness, or complication). This latter

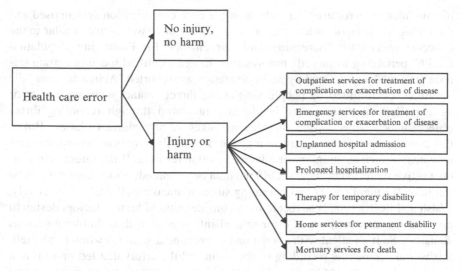

Fig. 1 Classifying health care error in terms of health services outcomes

classification may not be the best as health care error may not necessarily result in an adverse outcome (Fig. 1). There are a number of organizations developing error classification systems including the Joint Commission on Accreditation of Healthcare Organizations (JCAHO)(Chang et al., 2005), the National Coordinating Council for Medication Error Reporting and Prevention (http://www.nccmerp.org), the World Health Organization (2003) as well as professional groups formulating schemes for specialty areas such as ambulatory care (Pace et al., 2005). The selection of an error classification system for managerial epidemiologic practice depends upon the intended goal of the patient safety initiative and the strategy for the measurement of error.

Measuring Health Care Error

After health care error is classified, the next step is its measurement as it relates to patient safety. The origin of the concern for measuring error as a proxy of patient safety has as its origins a public policy issue emerged in response to the malpractice crisis which began to surface in the 1970s (Loeb and O'Leary, 2004). Similar to a mortality rate serving as a proxy measure of health (i.e., lower mortality rates in a population are a proxy measure of a "healthier" population), the absence of health care error is often viewed as a proxy of a safe environment or care process. Safe patient care from an organizational point of view has derived from an on-going system of event reporting, such as the reporting of error, linked to transactional and transformational interactions (Behal, 2004). The particular measurement of error used depends upon the error classification system used and the timing of the error collection, namely, actively or passively and similar to the concepts in chapter "Screening and Surveillance for Promoting Population Health" pertaining to surveillance systems. Errors identified meeting certain criteria classified and defined by an organization are reported. Active failures "the unsafe acts committed by people who are in direct contact with the patient or system (Reason, 2000)" may be directly measured through recording direct observations as slips, lapses, fumbles, mistakes, or procedural violation. But in this context, an error measurement may not necessarily have been recorded unless an outcome such as an injury or adverse reaction resulted. If the intent is to conduct active surveillance, how should the data be measured? Video cameras can be put into all patient rooms and operating suites to measure clinical error actively. Walsh and Beatty (2002) advocate for a consideration of human factors design to promote the measurement of error-related information with technology such as signaling. So if a patient with a wrist band transponder went off when he/she fell, this would compel the recording of the event and the errors that led up to it in a more timely manner. Measuring error in real time may also be possible through recording a simultaneous series of high-risk events occurring, graphic monitors representing multidimensional plots of interrelationships among parameters instead of linear (e.g., lab values, vital signs, drug combinations administered) may be able to identify unanticipated trends such as impending shock or dizziness prior to a fall. This type of measurement system may be particularly important for areas such as emergency departments the pace of which may contribute to a highly likelihood of adverse events. However, this would only solve the measurement problem for immediate-time errors and not those with latent time occurrences (e.g., wound infection). The latent errors are those which occur as a result of decisions, designs, and management style (Reason, 2000). These types of errors are difficult to identify, much less measure, but can be captured through traditional epidemiologic methods such as telephone surveillance (follow-up) of patients at high risk for events such as those undergoing surgical procedures in which unconscious sedation was involved.

The measurement of health care error is also subject to measurement error as error is often are not directly observable unless the harm occurs and is highly visible (e.g., cardiac arrest from infusion of undiluted potassium). Since most health care error is determined from review of a patient's medical record or data compiled from it, the error may be undocumented intentionally or unintentionally. Error may be also confounded with treatment side effects and may not be readily discernable clinically. Regardless of the error targeted, the measurement should also have a high reliability and validity to allow for determining accurate trend and subpopulation analyses, possess low false negativity, be clinically meaningful, and lead to improvements in health care. The more difficult errors to measure are those related to errors of judgment. Use of clinical pathways and practice guidelines as templates of care may help detect these types of errors. Judgment errors, and perhaps even all errors, will require multidimensional metrics to measure them accurately.

Potential Barriers to Error Measurement and Interventions to Improve Error Measurement

Walsh and Beatty (2002) provide a comprehensive summary of the barriers to reporting. These include: lack of value regarding the utility of the reporting process, fear of recrimination, workload demands, not a priority in tasks, and lack of understanding as to what should be reported. In order to address these barriers, the strategy must focus on optimizing human performance relative to improving patient monitoring. As stated previously, it is important to determine which category of error is the objective of the control strategy. From this, the barriers to error measurement can be addressed. For example, if the human factors error attributable to a skill-based error, the reporting can be improved if nursing staff can identify all the tasks associated with various high-risk procedures such as listing all the steps involved in urinary catheterization. Next is to understand the series of actions determined by rule-based behaviors that can cause errors. So if the blood pressure machine is reading zero, but the patient is breathing, the nurse needs to determine what is wrong. Lastly, reporting of error derived from the knowledge-based behaviors are those such as a wrong nursing diagnosis can be facilitated by nurses using coding schemes for nursing diagnoses similar to that of the International Classification of Disease system of coding diagnoses and symptoms. Such a coding scheme is now being developed by the National Quality Forum (NQF) and the Agency for Healthcare Research and Quality (AHRQ) (http://www.qualityforum.org/projects/ongoing/CommonFormats/index.asp, January 1, 2009) and marks the transition of the use of the term "error" to patient safety event.

In addition to the barriers cited above, there are a number of other barriers to accurate measurement of error related more to the methodological aspects. First, because certain errors are not directly observable (e.g., knowledge error) or infrequent case ascertainment may be low and the desirable measurement properties of high validity and reliability may not be able to ever be achieved. Also, computer applications that are designed to detect error (e.g., pharmacy information systems to detect medication error) are not designed to detect human or organization errors linked to them. Duplicate reporting of errors has not been resolved especially for those systems where errors are reported via free text.

The biggest challenge in reporting will be related to communication of the error. Individuals at all levels of the organization may be hesitant to report not knowing the format in which data will be communicated. Thus, balancing the public's (patient and family included) right to know with the level of confidentiality required to have a blameless environment to promote full disclosure and reporting of errors.

Ideally, the best tool for promoting error measurement would be a system that continuously monitors errors and error rates and links them to patient safety measures. With more timely and accurate reporting of error, more rapidly implemented corrective action preventing or decreasing the incidence of these would be expected. However, what is not resolved, even in the literature, is whether or not the reduction in error truly does lead to improved patient safety. This is because the rate of error is typically low or rare (Sugrue et al., 2008). A sufficient sample size for analysis of the impact of an intervention upon error at the hospital level may not be possible. Sample size considerations provide support for statewide reporting systems for medical errors and other adverse events. The Georgia Partnership for Health and Accountability (http://www.gha.org/patientsafety/event_reporting/index.asp#demo) is a model system for web-based reporting of errors and demonstrating how the use of this information can be used to improve safety. It is only through such statewide systems that error data can be compiled in a way such as to yield any meaningful analysis which will lead to corrective solutions. Boxed Examples 1 illustrates how a statewide error reporting system can guide a health care manager in devising error prevention strategies and evaluating their effectiveness.

Boxed Example 1 Interpreting Data from a Statewide Medical Error Reporting System to Improve Patient Safety

Problem: Medical errors are infrequent events. Data compiled across health service delivery settings and populations provide more meaningful and valid indications of areas which need attention for improving patient safety.

Methods and Data: By Executive Order 05–10 on January 11, 2005, Governor Daniels, Jr. of Indiana required the Indiana State Department of Health to develop and implement a medical error reporting system. The reporting system rules required hospitals, ambulatory surgery centers, abortion clinics, and birthing centers to report medical errors. Twenty-seven reportable events were identified in the following categories: surgical events, product or device events, patient protection events, care management events, environmental events, and criminal event. Noncompliance with reporting requirements was enforced with actions ranging from an issue of a letter of correction to a civil monetary penalty in an amount not to exceed ten thousand dollars.

Results: The following were the top four reported medical error events in Indiana in 2007

Medical error event	Number reported
Stage 3 or 4 pressure ulcers acquired after hospital admission	27
Retention of foreign object in patient after surgery in hospital and ambulatory surgery centers	24
Surgery performed on the wrong body part in hospital and ambulatory surgery centers	23
Death or serious disability associated with medication error among inpatient discharges and outpatient visits	8

(continued)

Boxed Example 1 (continued)

Data category	Definition	Total number reported
Inpatient discharges	Admitted to hospital as an inpatient; excludes hospice, skilled nursing facility, and observation patients	785,731
Outpatient visits	Visit for emergency services, outpatient surgery, occupational therapy, rehabilitation, cardiac diagnostic, treatment procedures, psychiatric, or social services	3,281,604
Procedures, hospital	ICD-9 procedures coded 01.00–86.99 inclusive in the principal procedure field as reported by hospital for either inpatient discharges or outpatient visits	1,217,474
Procedures, ambulatory	Any procedures reported by an ambulatory surgery center on State Form 49933, ASC Utilization Report	584,939

Source: Indiana State Department of Health (2008) http://www.in.gov/isdh

Managerial Epidemiology Interpretation: The health care manager must know and be required to report any reportable event defined by the Health Department rules that occur within the facility. The information submitted does not allow for identifying a patient, facility employee, or health care professional, but reporting does require the category of event, the facility where the reportable event occurred, and the quarter and calendar year within which the event occurred. The determination if the event is reportable by the facility is performed by the health care facility's quality assessment and improvement program. This program ensures that the reporting is accurate and timely and that appropriate action is taken to correcting the problem. Correcting the problem begins with an analysis of the data using a root cause analysis or other technique. However, the preferred managerial epidemiologic practice would be to review the compiled data of the reports of all hospitals and ambulatory facilities, particularly of peer institutions to compute the rates of the various 27 required reporting categories to determine the facility's level of risk in each. Based upon the computation of the rates, the health care manager would then target where her facility ranks in medical error rates and consider targeting proactive measures relative to the ones with the highest rates. From the above table, the calculated medical error rates for the State of Indiana overall are the following: 3.4 stage 3 or 4 pressure ulcers per 100,000 hospital discharges; 1.3 retention of foreign object in patient after surgery per 100,000 procedures in hospitals and ambulatory centers; 1.3 surgeries on wrong body part per 100,000 procedures in hospital and ambulatory surgery centers; and 2.7 deaths or serious disability associated with medication error per 1,000,000 inpatient discharges and outpatient visits. Knowing the high frequency of advanced stage pressure ulcers as a leading cause of medical error, managerial epidemiologic practice would give this priority attention by reducing risk factors associated with this condition, including assuring adequate nursing staffing ratios per patient, strict adherence to turning and hygiene protocols, and nutritional assessment and support.

Conceptual Framework for Patient Safety

Patient safety may be conceptualized according to the classic Donabedian model of evaluating health care in terms of structural indicators, process indicators, and outcome indicators. Structural measures would include measures of an organization's safety culture (Sorra et al., 2008; Vogus, 2007), ergonomic hazards in the environment (e.g., fall hazards), and staff–patient ratios. Process measures would include the use of policies and procedures to minimize risk (e.g., fall risk assessment by nursing upon admission). Similar to the quality model, outcome measures of safety may be represented as rate measures (e.g., patient safety indicators) or sentinel events which are "an unexpected occurrence involving death or serious physical or psychological injury or the risk thereof" (The Joint Commission for the Accreditation of Healthcare Organizations, 2007) (e.g., fire associated with oxygen therapy).

Patient Safety Indicators

The accurate classification and measurement of health care error provides the basis for the development of patient safety indicators. The occurrence of an error is the first indication that there is a gap in safety, be it at the structural or process level. Patient safety indicators are built upon complications or error situations known to increase the risk of patient harm or death that are achievable within the health care team's ability to decrease the risk of those adverse outcomes. Similar to the concept of an incidence rate measure, patient safety indicators are general measures of the rate of potentially preventable adverse events that when controlled or prevented reduce a patient's risk of harm. As such, patient safety indicators are outcome measures. Common epidemiologically based patient safety indicators are displayed in Table 1. The selection of an indicator for measuring patient safety depends upon:

- Provider control of the event
- Validity and reliability of the measure
- Specificity and sensitivity of the measure
- Likelihood of preventability
- Generalizability of measure across all health care settings, population subgroups, and health conditions

Patient safety indicators are commonly constructed from administrative databases, the most common of which are billing claims databases, insurance eligibility files, and risk management databases. An organization's Quality Office or Risk Management Office may also be compiling its own information regarding potential indicators such as complaints filed or malpractice suits filed or settled. The AHRQ has developed and made available to the public a software tool to enable capturing and calculating selected patient safety indicators from administrative data coded with ICD-9-CM codes (http://qualityindicators.ahrq.gov/psi_download.htm, January 3, 2009).

The limitations of the use of administrative databases in computing patient safety indicators include: the possibility of inaccuracy of the event (as it is often in the secondary diagnosis field and may not necessarily be used for billing purposes), that the critical incident may have occurred long before it can be detected and interventions implemented, that some clinical information on administrative databases may not be able to be differentiated from preexisting conditions (i.e., prior to the episode of care) or from complications or side effects associated with a particular therapy. Another limitation is related to sample size. The Centers for Medicare and Medicaid Services now require hospitals to add an indicator to determine if certain conditions were present on admission. The use of a date stamp or some other value added to each ICD-CM-9 code in a secondary diagnosis field of a patient's record can be used to satisfy this requirement. Patient safety measures may be presented as crude measures (total number of events in a population at risk times a factor of ten) or as adjusted risk measures. The methodology for risk adjustment of any one patient safety indicator is still being refined. Risk adjustment variables may be confounded by their correlation with measures of quality (e.g., RN staffing levels). Thus, patient safety indicators may be best interpreted according to stratified levels of common structural measures such as hospital type (critical access, teaching, urban, rural) or volume (patient discharge volume, procedure volume).

The limitation of patient safety indicators is also a function of the frequency of the event. Safety events are potentially infrequent rendering some rate indicators of limited value in making decisions in changing processes at less than the organizational unit of analysis. Pooling of safety indicator data across organizations and combining them with data from employment files, more precise information about the impact of some structural features organizational subunits (e.g., medical-surgical units) can be identified. The California Nursing Outcomes Coalition (CalNOC) maintains a database from 252 units from 108 hospitals such that structural variables such as nurse-patient staffing ratios can be examined in relationship to various patient safety indicators (Bolton et al., 2007). Boxed Example 2 presents an example of how patient safety indicators are constructed as epidemiologic measures (Table 2).

Boxed Example 2 Impact of Adding a Present on Admission (POA) Modifier on an ICD-9-CM Code to Improve the Accuracy of a Patient Safety Indicator

Problem: The most widely used patient safety indicators rely on administrative data. The computation of rates from this data source may be biased as the ICD-9-CM codes may not necessary differentiate between complications and preexisting or conditions present upon admission.

(continued)

Boxed Example 2 (continued)

Methods and Data: Coronary artery by-pass graft (CABG) surgery data (ICD-9-CM codes 36.10 – 36.19 and 36.2) from the 1998 to 2000 California State Inpatient Database were used. Each ICD-9-CM code is modified by a POA code. All 30 fields of a patient's diagnoses codes were examined. A record was excluded if the patient's age was less than 18 years, missing gender, or missing discharge status or in hospitals for which greater than 10% of the POA codes were missing or whose percent of ICD-9-CM codes coded as POA of ICD-9-CM was outside of the 95% confidence interval for the CABG patients in the data set (0.67, 0.91). The final data set consisted of 82,063 patients from 111 hospitals.

Results:

	No. of events		Risk pool		1-PPV	Observed rates per 1,000 discharges at risk	
Impact of the POA indicator on observed rates of adverse events							
Patient safety indicators	No POA	POA	No POA	POA		No POA	POA
Decubitus ulcer	228	135	49,463	49,463	0.41	4.61*	2.73*
Failure to rescue	403	324	3,298	2,095	0.20	122.2*	154.7*
Infection due to medical care	374	349	72,954	72,954	0.07	5.13	4.78
Postop hemorrhage or hematoma	524	455	82,046	82,046	0.13	6.39*	5.55*
Postop physiologic and metabolic derangement	191	153	35,003	35,003	0.20	5.46*	4.37*
Postop embolism or DVT	512	343	82,040	82,040	0.33	6.24*	4.18*
Postop sepsis	247	207	30,054	30,054	0.16	8.22**	6.89**
Accidental puncture or laceration	961	848	82,050	82,050	0.12	11.71*	10.34*

DVT deep venous thrombosis, *POA* present-on-admission indicator, *PPV* positive predictive value, *obs* observed, *postop* postoperative
*p-value ≤ 0.05
**p-value = 0.06
Source: Glance et al. (2008)

Managerial Epidemiology Interpretation: Among the CABG population, the patient safety indicator, failure to rescue, had the highest rate. The CABG patient population was at greatest safety risk for failure to rescue. The rate not adjusted for POA underestimated the magnitude of this patient safety risk. The patient safety indicators that most accurately predicted an adverse outcome (i.e., had the highest positive predictive value or lowest false positive), in order, were: decubitus ulcer, postop embolism or DVT, failure to rescue, and post-op physiologic and metabolic derangement. The CABG

Boxed Example 2 (continued)

patient population is at risk for a wide variety of patient safety indicators. The health care manager should assure that policies, procedures, and interventions are in place to address these. The introduction of a rapid response team which includes individuals trained in critical care (including a respiratory therapist) who are available on-call 24/7 throughout a hospital may reduce the incidence of failure to rescue cases. It is also important for the hospital to utilize a coding system that has a POA modifier.

Table 2 Examples of epidemiological measures of patient safety

Measure	Numerator	Denominator
Decubitus ulcer[a]	Any secondary diagnosis fields include ICD-CM-9 codes for decubitus ulcer	Patients with length of stay greater than 4 days. Excludes diagnosis of hemiplegia, paraplegia, quadraplegic; patient admitted from a long-term care facility or transferred from an acute care facility
Failure to rescue[a]	Discharge disposition is death and complication of care includes: pneumonia, DVT/PE, sepsis, acute renal failure, shock/cardiac arrest, or GI hemorrhage	Excludes patients older than 75 years and patients admitted from a long-term facility or transferred from an acute care facility[a]
Hospital-acquired infection[a]	Any secondary diagnosis fields include ICD-CM-9 codes for infectious complication due to medical care, vascular device, implant, or graft	Excludes patients with length of stay less than 2 days and any diagnosis code for immunocompromised state or cancer or cancer DRG
Postoperative hemorrhage or hematoma[a]	Any secondary diagnosis fields include ICD-CM-9 codes for postoperative hemorrhage or hematoma who required a drainage procedure or postoperative control of bleeding	Excludes if only a procedure code for postoperative control of bleeding or drainage procedure and no diagnoses codes related to hemorrhage, hematoma, or drainage, or diagnoses occurred prior to the operative procedure
Postoperative physiologic and metabolic derangement[a]	Any secondary diagnosis fields include ICD-CM-9 codes for physiologic and metabolic derangements	Excludes if ICD-9-CM diagnosis codes for chronic renal failure, acute renal failure where dialysis occurs prior to or on the same day as the operative procedure, or a primary diagnosis of diabetes and a secondary diagnosis code of ketoacidosis, hyperosmolarity, or coma
Postoperative PE or DVT[a]	Any secondary diagnosis fields include ICD-CM-9 codes for PE or DVT	Excluded if only a procedure code for interrupting the vena cava or if PE or DVT occurs before or on same day as operative procedure code

(continued)

Table 2   (continued)

Measure	Numerator	Denominator
Postoperative sepsis[a]	Any secondary diagnosis fields include ICD-CM-9 codes for sepsis	Excluded if the length of stay was less than 4 days, if any of the diagnoses fields included immunocompromised state or cancer or DRG of cancer, or the principal diagnosis field was infection
Accidental puncture or laceration[a]	Any secondary diagnosis fields include ICD-CM-9 codes for accidental cut, puncture, perforation, or laceration	Any hospitalized patient regardless of age
Adverse drug event (ADE)[b]	Number of medication errors that caused discomfort or significantly affected a patient's safety or health	Total doses given or omitted
Medication error[b]	Number of doses in error: any discrepancy (unauthorized, extra dose, wrong dose, omission, wrong route, wrong form, wrong technique, wrong time) between the dose ordered and the dose received	Total doses given or omitted

DRG Diagnostic-Related Group number, *DVT* deep vein thrombosis, *PE* pulmonary embolism, *GI* gastrointestinal
[a]The factor of ten by convention is per 1,000 patients or discharges at risk
[b]The factor of ten by convention is per 100 doses given

Prevention of Health Care Error to Promote Patient Safety

The prevention and control of health care error to promote patient safety is predicated on the knowledge of risk factors known to be associated with health care. Using a systems approach, risk factors for patient safety or common sources of health care error may be categorized as pertaining to the organization, technology, or human context. Examples of specific risk factors in each of these categories are found in Table 3.

The Institutional/Organizational Context

In assessing circumstances leading to an event, staffing, policies and procedures (or lack thereof), physical environment, culture, and leadership and manwagement style all are elements of an institution or organization, all which could contribute to error. One of the most important factors in factor that is key to a high reliability organization is team functioning. The team factors identified in aviation by Hamman (2004) which have relevance for their potential contribution to error in the health care setting are:

Table 3 Categories of systems factors affecting patient safety and associated risk factors (Source: Joint Commission on Accreditation of Healthcare Organizations (2008) available at http://www.jointcommission.org)

Category	Risk factors
Institutional/ organization context	• Lack of clarity or absent policies and procedures for patient safety
	• Team dysfunction (e.g., lack of trust or training, adequate number relative to patient volume, improper composition)
	• Physical separation of team members
	• Lack of staff orientation, training, and retraining
Technical context	• Similar packaging of two different products (e.g., vaccine and tuberculin purified protein derivative [PPD])
	• Improper storage of supplies, equipment, or medications
	• Equipment failure (e.g., monitor burnout)
Human context	• Failure to record accurate and complete information
	• Failure to check
	• Inexperience
	• Inattention
	• Fixation (e.g., with a monitor)
	• Haste
	• Distraction
	• Fatigue
	• Failure to follow procedure

- Historical background of team members
- Physical separation of team
- Psychological isolation (e.g., personality differences)
- Regulatory factors (confusion regarding interpretation over policies and procedures)
- Organizational factors (e.g., isolation from administrative oversight, scheduling problems)

Given the systems approach to conceptualizing error, the identification of "organizational" risk factors as exposures or risk factors for patient safety is emerging, particularly for nursing care and organizational subunits. Aiken et al. (2002) found high patient-to-nurse ratios to be associated with high failure-to-rescue rates. ICU, even those from outside the USA are known to be associated with high rates of device-associated HAI (Rosenthal et al., 2008). Staff education or "lack of" also may affect the level of safety practice within an organization.

Technical Context

Technical factors refer to those physical aspects of the process, equipment, techniques. In assessing if the error is due to technical factors, attribution is that which results from physical items such that these either malfunction, are not available when needed, or whose design can lead to a slip (the right thing done incorrectly) or an error. Items selected for use in patient care ideally should be those which are ergonomically designed, namely consider the psychological and physical attributes of the operator, the suitability to the task, and the acceptability of the technical system.

Human Context

Human factors may be a major cause of as many as 87% of all incidents in health care environments (Walsh and Beatty, 2002). Human factors focus on the individual delivering health care include: health characteristics, anthropomorphic features, behavior, learning, or skills relative to how decisions are made or communicated or performance is conducted. In the stressful health care environment, behavioral factors, such as intimidation and hostility by team members, can arise and are potential safety concerns as they can impede communication and delay critical responses. Rosenstein and O'Daniel (2008) found that as many as 77% of health care providers survey observed disruptive behavior in physicians, with the behavior most frequently reported among those physicians in general. Human factors also may or may not affect safety depending upon whether or not the human is confronted with new situations or routine ones. The human context is anything not attributable to organizational or technology contexts. Different health professions may experience difference patterns of human error. Fabrini and Zayas-Castro (2008) report that after surgical technique judgment errors (29.6%), inattention to detail (29.3%), and incomplete understanding (22.7%) were the categories of most common sources of error in an academic surgery department. Boxed Example 3 illustrates the importance of a nurse performing thorough assessment skills upon hospital admission a patient's risk for a decubitus ulcer and the need to communicate that risk despite what could be a stressful environment such as an intensive care unit.

Boxed Example 3 Determining Risk Factors for Pressure Ulcers in Hospitalized Patients

Problem: Persons at risk for pressure ulcers (also known as decubitus ulcers) in service delivery settings are those who are in long-term care facilities, who have long-lengths of hospital stay, and those who are in intensive care units. It is important to determine who is at highest risk at the time of admission to prevent pressure ulcers and/or to prevent the condition from increasing in grade for consist.

Methods and Data: A longitudinal study design of 121 admissions to a cardiac and surgical intensive care unit at a general hospital and to a nephrology intensive care unit at a university hospital between April and October 2006.

(continued)

Boxed Example 3 (continued)

Excluded were individuals less than 18 years. Each patient was assessed upon admission and upon discharge or death or 2 weeks after admission if the patient was still in intensive care. The Braden Scale (Braden and Maklebust, 2005) was used to classify pressure sore risk level. The severity of illness was assessed using Acute Physiology and Chronic Health Evaluation (APACHE II score).

Results:

Characteristics of patients who never developed pressure ulcers vs. patients who developed pressure ulcers after admission (Data from: Shahin et al., 2008)

Characteristic	−DU[a] ($n = 101$)	+New DU ($n = 4$)	+DU at admission ($n = 16$)
Male	59	3	6
Female	42	1	10
Overweight (BMI > 25 kg/m²)	57	1	10
[b]Braden score <14	32	1	9
Braden score 14 – 18	42	3	6
Braden score >18	27	0	1
Unconsciousness	18	1	4
Urinary catheter at admission	70	4	12

[a]*DU* decubitus ulcer
[b]Higher values of the Braden score reflect fewer risk factors

Managerial Epidemiology Interpretation: The identification of patients at high risk for decubitus ulcers at admissions is critical for prevention of DU, an important safety indicator. To determine the risk of developing a DU during hospitalization, the total number of eligible patients is in the denominator. Because a patient who has a DU may develop a second DU, these individuals may also be considered in the denominator. Overall, the incidence rate of DU in this population is 3.3% (4/121×100%). The prevalence rate of DU at admission is 13.2% (16/121×100%). There are 105 patients at risk for developing a first DU at admission and the rate of new DU during the hospital stay among them is 3.8% (4/105×100%). These rate measures can be used for evaluating the effectiveness of future interventions aimed at reducing the risk of DU. The particular rate measure depends upon the goal of the intervention. If the goal is prevention, the incidence rate of new DU would be the preferable baseline value.

Promoting Patient Safety

In order to implement successful strategies aimed at promoting patient safety, the measurement of the error must be accurate, comprehensive, timely, and yield data to produce meaningful analysis of the cause and baseline for evaluation of the

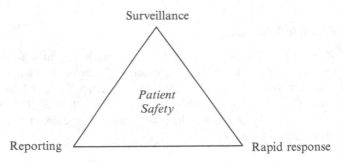

Fig. 2 The epidemiologic triangle for promoting patient safety in health services delivery

effectiveness of interventions. Without proper error identification processes in place, the error may remain occult and rescue measures taken after the occurrence of the error may not be undertaken and corrective systems unlikely. Error needs to be corrected regardless if it does or does not lead to a clinical consequence or adverse health services delivery outcome. The promotion of patient safety, in part, depends upon the control of medical error and identifying associated risk factors. The epidemiologic triangle for promoting patient safety then is dependent upon reporting medical error, surveillance of medical error, and rapid response to medical error (Fig. 2). If any legs of the triangle described below are broken, patient safety is compromised.

Reporting of Medical Error

The essential element for accurate and timely reporting of safety issues is the reporting environment, namely being supported by organizational policy and management action. In this type of environment, information on work processes is continuously collected and corrective action is on-going. Error reporting to ensure a safe environment in this context is viewed as just part of the communications process. Error reporting can be strengthened if it follows these principles: (1) both the public and providers should be able to report, (2) reporting is easy, (3) reporting is confidential, (4) that reporting matters is conveyed, (5) feedback from error reporting systems is given to staff, (6) reporting is linked to learning, and (7) reporting is linked to change processes.

Another element of reporting is the importance of describing the attributes of data for reporting error. Namely, the error should be described and characterized in relation to events that are preventable.

Currently, the impetus for encouraging self-reporting of errors in the form of sentinel events is derived from the JCAHO. JCAHO (2006) encourages the self-reporting of medical errors through its sentinel event policy which includes a major type of medical error, sentinel events that are serious injuries, baby abduction, or accidental deaths. The World Health Organization (WHO, 2005) has issued draft guidelines for the components of an adverse event reporting system. Components include a: classification scheme, statistical methods, learning and accountability, voluntary and confidential processes, and reporting. Other model systems for health care error reporting can be based upon those conditions which are contagious in nature or related to device or technology malfunction. The National Nosocomial Infection Surveillance System collects data on HAIs as part of its responsibility for research and investigation as authorized under Title III, Section 301, Section 304, and Section 306 of the Public Health Service Act (42 USC 241, 242b, 242k, and 242m(d)) (Centers for Disease Control and Prevention, 2005). The NNIS system has been granted a guarantee of confidentiality for the identities of both the patients and the reporting hospitals under Section 308(d) of the Public Health Service Act to analyze, interpret, and publish reports of aggregated data. The NNIS cannot release patient-specific data nor any hospital-specific data without the written consent of the participating hospital. A web-based system assists in reporting hospital in releasing its data to organizations it selects (e.g., state or local health departments and quality improvement organizations). The reliability of NNIS data depends on the assumption that the participating trained infection control professionals use standardized and validated NNIS data collection protocols and have no incentives to over- or underestimate their results in a voluntary, confidential system. However, data quality can be improved in either voluntary or mandatory systems by standard processes (e.g., independent audits and interrater reliability checks). The effectiveness of quality improvement in the NNIS system depends upon participants' trust in the data for comparison across facilities or their use of the data for continuous quality improvement within their facilities. This is a model system for error reporting, but clearly it works for a specific disease entity as long as there are legal protections in place for reporting that leads to quality improvement initiatives.

Recognizing effective error reporting cannot be achieved without legal or regulatory enforcement. For example, a package of legislation is being prepared for submission by the Michigan Health and Safety Coalition to provide mechanisms for the reporting of medical error and near misses. The Michigan Health and Safety Coalition proposed the following key issues for legislative action: (1) the creation of a Michigan Center for Safe Health Care, (2) the establishment and funding of a statewide voluntary, confidential, peer-protected, nonpunitive error reporting system, (3) protecting of patient safety data and reporting without denying patients and families access to information through normal channels when medical errors or unexpected events occur, and (4) change the state's licensing and regulation functions to incorporate culture of safety principles. In the absence of mandated reporting, voluntary reporting of medical error will not be successful unless there are safeguards including against liability and confidentiality of the information and protection from subpoena. A major advancement in this area has been Michigan Public Act 541 of 2008 which provides for the collection and reporting of serious events occurring at hospitals to a qualified hospital patient safety organization (PSO).

Surveillance of Health Care Error

Ideally, a patient safety system should be supported through active surveillance (see chapter "Screening and Surveillance for Promoting Population Health"). This type of system is predicated on the confidentiality of the reporter, the existence of a blameless organizational culture, and quick and easy communication of the reporter (e.g., through an 800 number, web-based reporting, etc.). An electronic prescribing and drug management system offers the potential for a highly effective surveillance for medication error. Equale et al. (2008) report on such a system for physician-initiated drug discontinuation and dose changes with a high specificity (99.7%) and a high positive predictive value (97.3%). The value of this system is that adverse drug reactions are often preceded by drug discontinuation or dose changes and provide an opportunity as an early warning system. The basis for establishing the conditions targeted for surveillance in patient safety emanates from the National Patient Safety Goals established by the JCAHO (Table 4). Barriers to reporting medical error include lack of legal protection, lack of anonymity in reporting, and fear of retribution or punishment. Surveillance is best supported when the organization has a high patient safety culture.

Rapid Response to Health Care Error

The most important action that management can take to improve patient safety based upon epidemiologic principles is to lead the organization to evolving into a "high reliability" organization (HRO). Characteristics of an HRO according to Weick and Sutcliffe (2001) are: (1) preoccupation with failure, (2) reluctance to simplify interpretations, (3) sensitivity to operations, (4) commitment to resilience, and (5) deference to expertise. The promotion of HROs is a strategy other industries have utilized to prevent error. The HRO is more adept at promoting systematic reporting for the

Table 4 National patient safety goals for hospitals

- Improve the accuracy of patient identification
- Improve the effectiveness of communication among caregivers
- Improve the safety of using medications
- Reduce the risk of health care-associated infections
- Accurately and completely reconcile medications across the continuum of care
- Reduce the risk of patient harm resulting from falls
- Reduce the risk of influenza and pneumococcal disease in institutionalized older adults
- Reduce the risks of surgical fires
- Encourage patients' active involvement in their own care as a patient safety strategy
- Prevent health care-associated pressure ulcers
- The organization identifies safety risks inherent in its patient population
- Improve recognition and response to changes in a patient's condition

sake of supporting resilience to respond to hazardous conditions. The purpose of error reporting in these organizations is viewed as part of the culture of eliminating unwanted variability (Reason, 2000). Additionally, the identification of errors in these organizations is a way of promoting training opportunities to recognize and develop system reforms. The key lesson from HROs is that there is redundancy, rules, procedures, extensive training, and migrating decision-making to the center of expertise. The airline industry is a key example of an HRO. The voluntary reporting of error is felt to be fundamental to safety regardless if it occurs at the process or outcome phase. Error reporting in aviation is also encouraged regardless of the severity of the error. Error reporting is facilitated because of the philosophy that errors occur because of faulty system design and that reporting should be on-going because it promotes organizational learning (Wilf-Miron et al., 2002). The operational feature of an HRO which has epidemiologic implications is the expectation of high reporting. High reporting will allow an organizational to take rapid response and learn from the problem at an early stage. The steps in this transformation involve a change in organizational culture, infrastructure support, leadership, and organizational policy changes.

Culture Change

The major strategy for improving the accurate measurement of safety is to promote and organizational culture that according to Hass (2004) moves beyond blame and actually rewards reporting factors which could compromise patient safety. The degree of safety culture within an organization is linked to actions which are associated with medical errors. Specifically, the reporting of medical errors and falls is positively associated with organizations with a high level of safety culture (Vogus and Sutcliffe, 2007). This culture will only be made a reality if all leadership, including nurse leadership, assumes accountability for his/her own role in patient safety as a means of fostering reporting of error. And, this culture of safety will only be achieved if the organization has a patient-centered focus. What constitutes a patient safety culture? The AHRQ (Sorra et al. 2008) surveys US hospitals and to collect information on patient safety culture represented by the following 12 areas:

1. Communication openness
2. Feedback and communication about error
3. Frequency of events reported
4. Handoffs and transitions
5. Management support for patient safety
6. Nonpunitive response to error
7. Organizational learning – continuous improvement
8. Overall perceptions of patient safety
9. Staffing
10. Supervisor/manager expectations and actions promoting safety
11. Teamwork across units
12. Teamwork within units

The results of this survey have been published and can be used by a hospital to benchmark its progress in achieving a patient safety culture (Sorra et al., 2009). Michigan Hospital Association (MHA) Keystone Center for Patient Safety & Quality (2008) supported member collaboration to implement various interventions in participating hospitals aimed at patient safety, but were based upon a comprehensive safety program which integrated "communication, teamwork, and leadership to create and support a 'harm free' patient care culture." Among the successful outcomes associated with the project included a 66% reduction in the rate of central line-associated bloodstream infections over an 18-month period.

Infrastructure Support

In order for error measurement and reporting to achieve a desired level of accuracy, health care managers must provide the infrastructure structure to be compliant with community standards and regulations. Concomitant with implementing a culture of safety, the organization should implement a system of redundancies for identifying error and the conditions that lead up to it (e.g., the slips, near misses, etc.). Next, the categories of error that will be collected by the system need to be determined by the leadership (e.g., medication error, surgical errors, etc.). Once the categories and nomenclature for the errors that will be collected and measured have been identified, the data must be compiled into a reporting system.

The ideal reporting system has the features of being low cost, easy access, potential for anonymity, and rapid analysis. This can be accomplished with a web-based system. Additional features of an error reporting system described by Handler et al. (2000) should include identifying the error as soon as possible and providing a structure within the organization, such as a safety committee to ensure that the data are being reviewed and recommendations acted upon. Error surveillance systems can be active or passive. Passive surveillance identifies the error after it occurs. Active surveillance is the process of attempting to identify the error before it occurs, most commonly through direct observation or through error marker situations. Error marker situations are those requiring the use of reversal agents (e.g., naloxone) or other therapeutics, etc.

Pronovost et al. (2006) describe a system which not only compiles information on the errors themselves but also hazards giving rise to those incidents. These authors advocate the collection of contributing factors such as team factors, patient factors, technology, and work environments.

Following Reason's model, the measurement, collection, and reporting of error data should be based upon the type of error and the defenses that were violated which gave rise to the error.

Promote the adoption of the electronic health record and other decision support applications to address the fragmentation of information about patients and the complexity of their condition. Recognizing that errors are often generated as a result of multisystem failure, up-to-date comprehensive information is necessary. Thus, use of an electronic health record with decision support capabilities and real-time analysis of errors (e.g., Virtual Checklist) provides a seamless approach to error identification. If organizations fully utilized electronic health records, there would be little need for staff to be preoccupied with specific error reporting as expert systems would automatically identify such from the database of inputted information. Safety officers and support personnel are also required infrastructure requirements to collect and monitor error data, ensure the standardization of common procedures in its collection, analyze the data, and disseminate findings.

Training

After implementing an on-going culture of safety and providing the infrastructure for it, on-going training is essential. While formal policies and procedures should certainly be the focus of any training effort, these are typically skill- or rule-based. Training to improve patient safety should also address human factors. The implementation of a training program based upon systemic mindfulness as described by Weick and Sutcliffe (2001) is an example of a strategy aimed at human factors to promote error reporting. The mindfulness approach provides a perspective of viewing every step within a system in terms of its potential for a catastrophic event and learning to interpret causation from ambiguity. And most importantly, error is viewed less punitively in the mindfulness approach being characterized more as a process orientation to each step in the system. Mindfulness training will not only aid in reporting errors related to skill- or rule-based conditions, but this may also greatly aid in the identification of the more difficult knowledge-based errors.

Leadership Initiatives

For an organization to truly engage in a process by which to improve error identification, an examination of the current leadership style is required to determine if the current style supports the cultural change. Leadership accordingly would include the organization's board as well. One approach is to adopt the leadership style of HROs. This leadership style prepares the workforce to have a "collective preoccupation with the possibility of failure (Reason, 2000)." The commitment of executive leadership to promoting a culture of safety in the organization is essential because repairs may need to be at the system level in made in response to errors identified.

With the leadership style and commitment in place, executive leadership actions should follow the following operational elements to promote patient safety offered by Morath (2004):

1. "Declare patient safety urgent and a priority.
2. Accept executive responsibility.
3. Import and apply new knowledge and skills.

4. Establish blameless reporting.
5. Assure accountability.
6. Align external controls.
7. Accelerate change."

The actions associated with these elements must be on-going to be effective.

Organizations Supporting Patient Safety Initiatives

The universal recognition across nations of the need to prevent health care error has led to the formation of a number of organizations dedicated to various aspects of patient safety (Table 4 of chapter "Delivering Health Care with Quality: Epidemiological Considerations"). These organizations propose indicators for patient safety, compile and disseminate data and information to consumers and professionals, a few focus on regulatory aspects, and some support new affiliated organizations or divisions within them in recognition of the specialized attention that patient safety requires. The World Health Organization (WHO, 2008a) has formed the World Alliance for Patient Safety in 2004 with its members dedicated to reducing the risk of health care-associated infection in their health systems. The World Alliance for Safety (WHOs) aims to eliminate or nearly eliminate risks to patient safety with the same intensity as the WHO is committed to eliminating such diseases as polio. Global themes for patient safety adopted by the Alliance include eliminating central line-associated bloodstream infections, promoting clean care as safe care, improving the safety of surgical care, tackling antimicrobial resistance, the development of measurement systems (including nomenclature) for compiling information from disparate sources to analyze and promote the development of best safety practices, and engaging patients through health care literacy projects to partner in safety efforts (WHO, 2008b). Within the National Health Service of the United Kingdom, the National Patient Safety Agency focuses its efforts on patient safety with the emphasis on a rapid response system based upon high reporting (National Health Service Confederation, 2008). The importance of rapid reporting is also recognized in the USA as essential to supporting patient safety initiatives. Support for rapid reporting was one of the stimuli for the enactment of The Patient Safety and Quality Improvement Act of 2005 (Public Law 109–41), signed into law on July 29, 2005. This law provided for the creation of PSOs to collect, aggregate, and analyze confidential information reported by health care providers. The Agency for Healthcare Quality and Research now certifies PSOs. The purpose of this designation is to represent that the PSO-certified organization confer privilege and confidentiality to the information reported with peer review protection. Thus, a PSO, such as the Institute for Safe Medication Practices and the Michigan Health & Hospital Association Patient Safety Organization (MHA PSO), can work with other PSOs and provide analysis of error data because both are federally certified PSOs. Patient safety will become an increasing focus of accrediting bodies and regulations of government agencies, insurers, and employers. The Centers for Medicaid and Medicare Services (CMS) implemented a provision of the Deficit Reduction Act of 2005 (DRA) on October 1, 2007 which began in October 2008 regarding not providing reimbursement for selected patient safety indicators, unless present on admission and these include: catheter-associated urinary tract infections, decubitus ulcers, vascular catheter-associated infection, surgical site infection of the mediastinum after coronary artery bypass graft surgery, and hospital-acquired injuries. Additional ones will be targeted for withhold reimbursement in 2009 including ventilator-associated pneumonia, *Staphylococcus aureus* septicemia, deep vein thrombosis, and pulmonary embolism. The JCAHO has been in the forefront of accrediting bodies in the development of patient safety goals for all service delivery forms, including hospitals, ambulatory care centers, and others. The patient safety goals for hospitals that are represented in Table 5 are representative of the goals for the other health service delivery categories.

Table 5 Organizations supporting patient safety and selected initiatives

Organization/website	Purpose/mission	Selected initiatives
Agency for Healthcare Research and Quality http://www.ahrq.gov	"To improve the quality, safety, efficiency, and effectiveness of health care for all Americans."	Patient safety culture survey database TeamSTEPPS™ evidence-based teamwork system training curriculum
Centers for Medicare and Medicaid Services http://www.cms.gov		
Institute for Healthcare Improvement http://www.ihi.org	"Improving health care"	Improvement tracker allows tracking any of the measures currently available in the Topics area of IHI.org (e.g., surgical site infections) and sharing of information with members
Institute for Safe Medication Practices http://www.ismp.org	"To advance patient safety worldwide by empowering the healthcare community, including consumers to prevent medication errors."	"List of Error-Prone Abbreviations, Symbols, and Dose Designations"
Joint Commission on Accreditation of Healthcare Organizations http://www.jointcommission.org	"To continuously improve the safety and quality of care provided to the public through the provision of health care accreditation and related services that support performance standards."	National patient safety goals

(continued)

Table 5 (continued)

Organization/website	Purpose/mission	Selected initiatives
The Leapfrog Group http://www. leapfroggroup.org	"To trigger giant leaps forward in the safety, quality and affordability of health services by supporting informed healthcare decisions by those who use and pay for health care; and, promoting high-value health care through incentives and rewards."	Leapfrog hospital quality and safety survey data reports for hospitals
National Safety Council http://www.Nsc.org	"To educate and influence people to prevent accidental injury."	Weekly safety tip widget for posting on website
U.S. Food and Drug Administration http://www.fda.org	"… protecting the public health by assuring the safety, efficacy, and security of human and veterinary drugs, biological products, medical devices, our nation's food supply, cosmetics, and products that emit radiation. The FDA is also responsible for advancing the public health by helping to speed innovations that make medicines and foods more effective, safer, and more affordable; and helping the public get the accurate, science-based information they need to use medicines and foods to improve their health."	DailyMed website that provides up-to-date information about FDA approved labels (package inserts) and medication content http://dailymed.nlm. nih.gov/dailymed/ about.cfm
U.S. Department of Veterans Affairs National Center for Patient Safety http:// www.patientsafety.gov	"…to develop and nurture a culture of safety throughout the Veterans Health Administration."	Medical team training Patient safety tips and tools for patients Patient safety assessment tool
World Alliance for Patient Safety http://www.who. int/patientsafety/ worldalliance/en/	"Raises awareness and political commitment to improve the safety of care and facilitates the development of patient safety policy and practice in all WHO Member States."	International Classification for Patient Safety (ICPS)

Summary

The health care consumer, regardless of health delivery setting, has a right to expect that the environment and that the processes of delivering care in it are safe. Since patient safety is an evolving concept, epidemiologic methods will aid in refining its classification for improving the accuracy of its measurement to aid in accuracy identifying patient safety risk factors and to better target their prevention and control. New and emerging laws and regulations will provide the framework for defining safety, but to assess their effectiveness, epidemiologic measures will be essential in continuing to monitor safety practices through the construction of surveillance systems and programs in response to data derived from them. Accurate assessment and documentation, an important practice in epidemiology, will be essential in determining what conditions are present upon admission to a health care setting and who are at risk for safety concerns. These practices will not only improve patient safety in populations receiving health care services but will also have important financial implications to the provider. The managerial epidemiological basis of patient safety also is the consistent identification, reporting, and control of medical error while the research continues to refine those factors which promote patient safety. The challenges that lay ahead are defining and classifying the degree of "exposure" to safety practices within an organization or by a provider in relationship to patient safety outcomes. The paradigm shift that needs to occur in health care management epidemiology practice is to organize health care in terms of the deployment and maintenance of interdisciplinary teams to function in multifunctional systems for providing health care to populations not just individuals as a means of preventing error and promoting patient safety.

Discussion Questions

Q.1. Identify two patient population subgroups served by your health care organization that are high risk for health care errors. What patient safety risk factors do they have? Outline a strategy for preventing these risk factors.

Q.2. Select a patient safety indicator. Discuss the advantages and limitations of this measure.

Q.3. Describe how organizational culture influences the emergence of patient safety risk factors. Propose strategies that a health care manager can use to reduce the prevalence of those risk factors.

Q.4. Select one of the agencies listed in Table 5 whose mission includes promoting patient safety. Determine how that agency can interface with your organization in promoting patient safety.

References

Aiken, L.H., Clarke, S.P., Cheung, R.B., Sloane, D.M., and Silber, J.H., 2006, Educational levels of hospital nurses and surgical patient mortality, *J.A.M.A.* **290**:1617–1623.

Aiken, L.H., Clarke, S.P., Sloane, D.M., Sochalski, J., and Silber, J.H., 2002, Hospital nurse staffing and patient mortality, nurse burnout, and job dissatisfaction, *J.A.M.A.* **288**:1987–1993.

Behal, R., 2004, An organization development framework for transformational change in patient safety: a guide for hospital senior leaders, in *The Patient Safety Handbook* (B.J. Youngberg and M. Hatlie, eds.), pp. 51–65, Jones & Bartlett, Sudbury, MA.

Bolton, L.B., Aydin, C.E., Donaldson, N., Brown, D.S., Sandhu, M., Fridman, M., and Aronow, H.U., 2007, Mandated nurse staffing ratios in California: a comparison of staffing and nursing-sensitive outcomes pre- and postregulation, *Policy, Politics, & Nurs. Practice* **8**:238–250.

Braden, B.J., and Maklebust, J., 2005, Preventing pressure ulcers with the Braden scale: an update on this easy-to-use tool that assesses a patient's risk, *Am. J. Nurs.* **105**:70–72.

Centers for Disease Control and Prevention, 2005, National Nosocomial Infections Surveillance System (NNIS) (April 7, 2007), http://www.cdc.gov/ncidod/dhqp/nnis.html.

Chang, A., Schyve, P.M., Croteau, R.J., O'Leary, D., and Loeb, J.M., 2005, The JCAHO patient safety event taxonomy: a standardized terminology and classification schema for near misses and adverse events, *Int. J. Qual. Health Care* **17**:95–105.

Equale, T., Tamblyn, R., Winslade, N., and Buckeridge, D., 2008, Detection of adverse drug events and other treatment outcomes using an electronic prescribing system, *Drug Saf.* **31**:1005–1116.

Fabri, P.J., and Zayas-Castro, J.L., 2008, Human error, not communication and systems, underlies surgical complications, *Surgery* **144**:557–63.

Glance, L.G., Li, Y., Osler, T.M., Mukamel, D.B., and Dick, A.W., 2008, Impact of date stamping on patient safety measurement in patients undergoing CABG: experience with the AHRQ Patient Safety Indicators, *BMC Health Ser. Res.*, available December 28, 2008 from: http://www.biomedcentral.com/1472–6963/8/176.

Hamman, W.R., 2004, The complexity of team training: what we have learned from aviation and its applications to medicine, *Qual. Saf. Health Care* **13**:i72–i79.

Handler, J.A., Gillam, M., Sanders, A.B., and Klasco, R., 2000, Defining, identifying, and measuring error in emergency medicine, *Acad. Emerg. Med.* **7**:1183–1188.

Hass, D., 2004, Moving beyond blame to create an environment that rewards reporting, in *The Patient Safety Handbook* (B.J. Youngberg and M. Hatlie, eds.), pp. 415 - 422, Jones & Bartlett, Sudbury, MA.

Indiana State Department of Health, 2008, Indiana Medical Error Reporting System (September 28, 2008), http://www.in.gov/isdh.

Institute of Medicine, 2000, *To Err is Human: Building a Safer Health System*, National Academy Press, Washington, DC.

Joint Commission for Accreditation of Healthcare Organizations, 2008, Facts about the Sentinel Event Policy (July 8, 2009), http://www.jointcommission.org/AboutUs/Fact_Sheets/sep_facts.htm.

Loeb, J.M., and O'Leary, D.S., 2004, The fallacy of the body count: why the interest in patient safety and why now? in *The Patient Safety Handbook* (B.J. Youngber and M. Hatlie, eds.), pp. 83–93, Jones & Bartlett, Sudbury, MA.

Michigan Hospital Association Keystone Center for patient Safety & Quality, 2008, Annual Report (December 29, 2008), http://www.mha.org/mha_app/downloads/08%20Keystone%20Annual%20Report.pdf.

Morath, J.M., 2004, The leadership role of the chief operating officer in aligning strategy and operations to create patient safety, in *The Patient Safety Handbook* (B.J. Youngberg and M. Hatlie, M., eds.), Jones & Bartlett, Sudbury, MA.

National Health Service Confederation, 2008, Act on reporting: five actions to improve patient safety reporting, Briefing, Issue 161 (August 17, 2008) http://www.npsa.nhs.uk/patientsafety.

National Patient Safety Foundation, 2003, Our definitions (April 13, 2007), www.npsf.org/html/about_npsf.html.

Pace, W.D., Fernald, D.H., Harris, D.M., Dickinson, L.M., Araya-Guerra, R., Staton, E.W., VanVorst, R., Parnes, B.L., and Main, D.S., 2005, Developing a Taxonomy for Coding Ambulatory Medical Errors: A Report from the ASIPS Collaborative, in *Advances in Patient Safety: From Research to Implementation*. Volume 2. Concepts and Methodology. AHRQ Publication No. 05–0021–2. Agency for Healthcare Research and Quality, Rockville, MD.

Pronovost, P.J., Thompson, D.A., Holzmueller, C.G., Lubomski, L.H., Dorman, T., Dickman, F., Fahey, M., Steinwachs, D.M., Engineer, L., Sexton, J.B., Wu, A.W., and Morlock, L., 2006, Toward learning from patient safety reporting systems, *J. Critical Care* **21**:305–315.

Reason, J., 2000, Human error: models and management, *Br. Med. J.* **320**:768–770.

Romano, P.S., Geppert, J.J., Davies, S., Miller, M.R., Elixhauser, A., McDonald, K.M., 2003, A national profile of patient safety in U.S. hospitals, *Health Affairs* **22**:154–166.

Rosenstein, A.H., and O'Daniel, M., 2008, A survey of the impact of disruptive behaviors and communication defects on patient safety, *Jt. Commission J. Qual. Patient Saf.* **34**:464–471.

Rosenthal, V.D., Maki, D.G., Mehta, A., Alvarez-Moreno, C. Leblebicioglu H., Higuera, F. Cuellar, L.E., Madani, N., Mitrev, Z., Duenas, L., Navoa-Ng, J.A., Garcell, H.G., Raka, L., Hidalgo, R.F., Medeiros, E.A., Kanj, S.S., Abubakar, S., Nercelles, P., Pratesi, R.D., and International Nosocomial Infection Control Consortium Members, 2008, International Nosocomial Infection Control Consortium report, *Am. J. Infect. Control.* **36**:627–637.

Shahin, E.S.M., Dassen, T., and Halfens, R.J.G., 2008, Incidence, prevention and treatment of pressure ulcers in intensive care patients: a longitudinal study, *Int. J. Nurs. Studies.*

Simpson, K.R., 2007, Measuring perinatal patient safety: review of current methods, *J. Obstet., Gynecol. Neonatal Nurs.* **35**:432–442.

Sorra, J., Famolaro, T., Dyer, N., Nelson, D., and Khanna, K., 2008, *Hospital Survey on Patient Safety Culture 2008 Comparative Database Report*, prepared by Westat, Rockville, MD, under contract No. 233–02–0087, Task Order 18, AHRQ Pub. No. 08–0039, Agency for Healthcare Research and Quality, Rockville, MD.

Sorra, J., Famolaro, T., Dyer, N., et al., 2009, *Hospital Survey on Patient Safety Culture 2009 Comparative Database Report*. AHRQ Pub. No. 09-0030, Agency for Healthcare Research and Quality, Rockville, MD.

Sugrue, M., Caldwell, E., D'Amours, S., Crozier, J., Wyllie, P., Flabouris, A., Sheridan, M., and Jalaludin, B., 2008, Time for a change in injury and trauma care delivery: a trauma death review analysis, *ANZ J. Surg.* **78**:949–954.

Vogus, T.J., 2007, The Safety Organizing Scale: development and validation of a behavioral measure of safety culture in hospital nursing units, *Med. Care* **45**:46–54.

Walsh, T., and Beatty, P.C.W. (2002). Human factors error and patient monitoring, *Physiol. Meas.* **23**:R111–R132.

Weick, K.E., and Sutcliffe, K.M., 2001, *Managing the Unexpected. Assuring High Performance in an Age of Complexity*, Jossey-Bass, San Francisco, CA.

Weiser, T.G., Regenbogen, S.E., Thompson, K.D., Haynes, A.B., Lipsitz, S.R., Berry, W.R., and Gawande, A.A., 2008, An estimation of the global volume of surgery: a modeling strategy based on available data, *Lancet* **372**:139–144.

Wilf-Miron, R., Lewenhoff, I., Benyamini, A., and Aviram, A., 2002, From aviation to medicine: applying concepts of aviation safety to risk management in ambulatory care, *Qual. Saf. Health Care* **12**:35–39.

World Health Organization, 2008a, *Patient Safety* (January 4, 2009), http://www.who.int/topics/patient_safety/en/.

World Health Organization, 2008b, *Forward Programme 2008–2009* (January 4, 2009), http://www.who.int/patientsafety/information_centre/reports/Alliance_Forward_Programme_2008.pdf.

World Health Organization, 2005, *WHO Draft Guidelines for Adverse Event Reporting and Learning Systems* (January 19, 2009), http://www.who.int/patientsafety/reporting_and_learning/en.

World Health Organization, 2003, *Towards a Common International Understanding of Patient Safety Concepts and Terms: Taxonomy and Terminology Related to Medical Errors and Systems Failures* (January 19, 2009), http://www.who.int/entity/patientsafety/taxonomy/WHOTaxonomyConsultation Oct2003.pdf

Zhan, C., and Miller, M.R., 2003, Excess length of stay, charges, and mortality attributable to medical injuries during hospitalization, *J.A.M.A.* **290**:1868–1874.

Part III
Spanning Topics

Chapter 11
Epidemiology and the Public Policy Process

Learning Outcomes

After completing this chapter, you will be able to:

1. Apply epidemiologic measures to distinguish among community health problems for receiving priority attention by the policy process.
2. Monitor policy effectiveness in eliminating health care disparities using epidemiologic measures.

Keyterms Health disparity • Health literacy • Public health • Public policy • Stakeholder

Introduction

American governmental public health at the national, state, and local levels has responsibility for assessing population needs, providing assurance for the protection and promotion of health and for developing health policies. The core functions are population-based, grounded in science and epidemiologic and other data, and based on social justice. To serve the public good and protect the health and safety of the people under their jurisdiction, health policy makers are expected to formulate their decisions using current knowledge and evidence as well. For these reasons, public health was chosen as the contextual framework for illustrating the interrelationship between epidemiology and the public policy process.

This chapter includes definitions and descriptions of terms and concepts associated with the policy process. Examples are included that explore and demonstrate the influence of epidemiology on public health policy which affects all levels of health services which is a reason this is considered a spanning topic.

D.M. Oleske (ed.), *Epidemiology and the Delivery of Health Care Services*:
Method and Applications,
DOI 10.1007/978-1-4419-0164-4_11, © Springer Science+Business Media, LLC 2009

Public Health

Understanding the basis for public health is the contextual framework for understanding the interrelationship between public policy and epidemiology. The Institute of Medicine (IOM, 1988) defines the "mission" of public health as fulfilling society's interest in assuring conditions in which people can be healthy with contributions toward this end made by governmental and nongovernmental agencies. The IOM identifies the three core functions of governmental public health: (1) assessment of the health needs of populations including the systematic collection, analysis, and distribution of morbidity, mortality, and disability information; (2) assurance that services to promote and protect the health of the public are provided directly or through others; and (3) development of policy for the protection of health grounded in scientific knowledge and that serves the public interest. Given this perspective, health is regarded as a primary public good in the same manner as employment and participation in the political process which is then specifically supported and advanced by governmental public health. However, in order to achieve its mission and ensure that health is a socially valued goal, public health relies on cooperative efforts of both governmental and not-for-profit agencies, and even industry to achieve goals that are related to the prevention of disease and promotion of health. This intersectoral collaboration to influence health was further emphasized in the Institute of Medicine (2003) report, *The Future of the Public's Health in the 21st Century*, and extended to define a public health system which includes not only governmental health agencies, but also various entities in communities (e.g., schools, religious congregations), public health and health sciences academia, employers, health care delivery systems and organizations, and the media.

The mission is delivered through a framework which defines the essential services of public health which was developed by the Core Public Health Functions Steering Committee in 1994. This Steering Committee included representatives from U.S. Public Health Service agencies and other major public health organizations. The essential services provide a working definition of public health and a guiding framework for the responsibilities of local public health systems. The ten essential public health services are as follows:

Assessment

1. *Monitor* health status to identify and solve community health problems.
2. *Diagnose and investigate* health problems and health hazards in the community.

Policy Development

3. *Inform, educate, and empower* people about health issues.
4. *Mobilize* community partnerships and action to identify and solve health problems.
5. *Develop policies and plans* that support individual and community health efforts.

Assurance

6. *Enforce* laws and regulations that protect health and ensure safety.
7. *Link* people to needed personal health services and assure the provision of health care when otherwise unavailable.

8. *Assure* competent public and personal health care workforce.
9. *Evaluate* effectiveness, accessibility, and quality of personal and population-based health services.
10. *Research* for new insights and innovative solutions to health problems.

The "diagnostic tool" of public health is epidemiology; the "treatment tools" are health behavior change strategies, environmental (sanitarian), and personal health services (e.g., immunization, well-child clinics) (Afifi and Breslow, 1994).

In order to effectively support the core function of policy development, population-based assessments of needs are conducted using epidemiologic and other data. Epidemiology identifies populations at health risk, the causes of health problems, and the development and measurement of interventions for the reduction or elimination of health risks. Epidemiologic methods aid in defining the measurement of the concept of health care disparity, providing the data to identify disparities in populations, and framework for evaluating the methodology which would most appropriately characterize the disparity thereby allowing public health resources to be more effectively targeted. The epidemiologic and other data are then used for engaging the public in participating in the policy development process and decision-making on the allocation of resources.

Public Policy: An Interactive and Iterative Process

Public policy is the development of a governmental response to a societal issue formulated in response to stakeholders, those who share a common interest or commitment, who are themselves intent on finding a solution to the identified problem. The elements of the public policy process are: (1) problem identification (defining the nature of the health care issues and who is affected); (2) formulation (utilizing epidemiological data and studies, expert discussions, testimonials and public opinions, anecdotal reports, and published viewpoints); (3) implementation (the change directed or prescribed by laws, ordinances or municipal regulations, rules of accrediting bodies, and the allocation of resources that follows); and (4) evaluation (assessing the outcomes, the benefits, risks, costs, and progress toward anticipated goal).

The policy process is a reflection of a nation's political belief system, and therefore, in democratic societies, provides opportunity for public participation in the process. When the policy process is interactive and open, input from the public and epidemiological data may be used in any of the elements. In societies where the national political belief system is closed or perceived closed, policy outcomes are more likely to reflect the values and preferences of an official elite. When the policy process limits public input, public support and hence funding for a cause, albeit it one supported with epidemiological data, is likely also to be limited.

The most effective public policies are those that engage and empower communities, disseminate knowledge of the issues, create trust in government consolidate coalitions and belief systems, and garner the support of the economic and financial sectors to support the policy actions. Kotter (1996) provides practical advice for forming a coalition with the first step in "putting together the kind of team that can direct a change is to find the right membership." Toward that end, he suggests that the key characteristics of an effective guiding coalition are: (1) position power or getting the "key players" on board, (2) expertise, (3) credibility, and (4) leaders, a sufficient number "to drive the change process." Community action in support of voluntary policy change has been effective in eliminating environmental tobacco smoking exposure in multiunit housing, smoking policies, and secondhand smoke in rental cars (Matt et al., 2008; Olfene and Harnett-Pettingill, 2008). National coalitions such as the Smokeless States National Tobacco Policy Initiative that spanned 1994–2004 supported by the Robert Wood Johnson Foundation and the American Medical Association are highly effective in achieving policy change throughout the nation. Advocacy, empowerment, and coalitions may be more difficult to achieve in some communities of color, rural areas, Indian country, and blue-collar communities as more intensive grassroots efforts are required and often less resources are available to reach and engage interest and support for advancing a policy. The availability of technology to these groups may facilitate participation to promote policy change and is now being used extensively in the Obama administration for this purpose.

It is evident that there is an increasing use of technology including wireless and the Internet are redefining not only the population, but also who is the "public" in the policy process (formulation, implementation, and evaluation). Public participation in the policy process using these modalities has been dramatically demonstrated in the 2008 Presidential elections. Not only are interest groups formed and nurtured through technologies such as the Internet and text-messaging, but technology enhances communication, collection of data, or the sharing of outcomes with increased effectiveness and efficiency. The American Public Health Association has established a "MegaVote" link for its members to track Congressional voting or to have input in the legislation process by email. The technology associated with the information age brings with it highly interactive opportunities including competitive policy interests like those that surround immunization.

Sharing the science driving health policy in a rapidly changing technological society is just one of many challenges in the policy process in the twenty-first century. Another associated issue related to communication and with the public is the increasing emphasis on health literacy, especially, its role in the elimination of disparities and in decision making. According to the Health Resources and Services Administration (HRSA) of the U.S. Department of Health and Human Services, health literacy is the "degree to which individuals have the capacity to obtain, process, and understand basic health information and services needed to make appropriate health decisions (http://www.hrsa.gov/healthliteracy)." HRSA has identified that health literacy is affected when: (1) health care providers use words that patients don't understand; (2) patients have low educational skills; (3) cultural barriers to health care exist; and (4) the patients have Limited English Proficiency (LEP). These same factors need to be considered when engaging members of a community at large for communication in the policy process.

Changes in policy related to the health system are also highly dependent upon the interaction of politics and policies regarding congruence of goals and direction.

In the USA, health care policy is heavily influenced by the political environment at the state level. This is highly illustrated by the case with Medicaid, whereby states establish the categories of eligibility, coverage, procedures, use different interpretations of quality indicators for reimbursement, and amounts and Medicare for prescription drug coverage (Bellows and Halpin, 2008; Miller and Weissert, 2007). And, as a result, attempting to compare health outcomes of beneficiaries of these programs is difficult. Even the laws governing the reporting transmissible diseases (chapter "The Role of Managerial Epidemiology in Infection Prevention and Control") vary among the states. Regardless, the expectation across all levels of government is that health policies should be based upon scientific data and be able to demonstrate favorable outcomes in the population's health.

The Interrelationship Between Epidemiology and Public Policy

The primary interrelationship between epidemiology and public policy is that both adopt a population-based approach and consider that there are multiple determinants of health, including social, biological, natural and built environments, behavioral, and psychological. Both also recognize that within populations there exists considerable diversity which should be accounted for (epidemiology) and integrated within the mainstream of decision-making (policy) for the benefit of society. Epidemiological data and methods are used in the policy process to:

1. Determine the magnitude, extent, and variability of the health problem regarding who is affected in terms of morbidity, mortality, utilization of health services to assist in the planning process of a policy.
2. Identify risk factors that influence the health of populations, particularly vulnerable population subgroups.
3. Provide data to engage stakeholders in the policy process.
4. Aid in choosing among alternative policies and the allocation of resources within them.
5. Monitor policy effectiveness relative to the rates of persistence, occurrence, or recurrence of health problems or in mortality.

Determining Priority Areas of Concern and Problem Identification for Policy Development Using Descriptive Epidemiologic Data

The identification of priority areas for action by policy initiatives is launched through the use of descriptive epidemiologic data. An abundance of epidemiologic data has identified that the disparities in health among various population subgroups are an example of priority area identified through epidemiologic measures for concern in most every community in the USA as well as globally. Using the ten largest health disparities in the USA among non-Hispanic Blacks relative to other racial/ethnic population subgroups, Keppel (2007) identified the following health problems rated in rank order based upon age-adjusted rates:

1. New cases of gonorrhea (per 100,000 population)
2. New cases of gonorrhea among females aged 15–44 years (per 100,000 female population)
3. Congenital syphilis (per 100,000 live births)
4. New cases of AIDS (per 100,000 population aged ≥13 years)
5. Deaths due to HIV infection (age-adjusted rate per 100,000 standard population)
6. Nonfatal firearm-related injuries (per 100,000 population)
7. New cases of tuberculosis (per 100,000 population)
8. New cases of primary and secondary syphilis (per 100,000 population)
9. Homicides (age-adjusted rate per 100,000 standard population)
10. Drug-induced deaths (age-adjusted rate per 100,000 standard population)

Six of the ten largest condition listed above are related to sexually transmitted diseases, and by default imply that a younger sexually active Blacks has emerged as a population at greatest risk for these disparities. Other descriptive epidemiologic markers of health care disparities are continuing to be evaluated such as the preterm birth differences between black and white infants (Messer et al., 2008).

Disparities may exist for many reasons. But, their identification heightens awareness to identify where disparities exist in the continuum of health care as one means of preventing the disparities. Descriptive epidemiologic data also aid in the formulation of hypothesis to explore reasons for differential in exposures which may account for disparities in health, such as the potential role of unsafe built environments contributing to obesity in African American youth.

Although vital data are important sources for determining the magnitude of the morbidity and mortality of disease, there are many health problems, particularly those related to behavioral disorders for which vital data for policy-decisions are not available. For example, estimates of the incidence and prevalence trends of various forms of addiction (e.g., heroin smoking vs. heroin injectors) by population subgroups are necessary to formulate policies and aid governmental public health in developing prevention strategies and evaluate their effectiveness. Surveillance systems based on treatment centers for such conditions is an important strategy to support policy-decision making (Hickman et al., 2001). However, when utilizing data from these systems, policy makers must be caution as delays in reporting signs or symptoms of conditions may provide underestimates of a condition associated with the potential of social stigma such as HIV/AIDS or injecting drug use.

Using Epidemiologic Studies in Identifying Risk Factors to Guide in the Development of Policies

It is essential that policy decisions which affect the health of populations in the USA as well as in other nations to utilize results derived from epidemiologic studies to identify risk factors. Descriptive epidemiologic studies provide the foundation for identifying risk factors. Epidemiologic rate measures have identified health disparities among various racial and ethnic minorities. These data reveal, for example, that non-Hispanic Blacks who die from HIV disease have approximately 11 times more age-adjusted years of potential life lost before age 75 years per 100,000 population than non-Hispanic Whites; non-Hispanic Blacks had slower progress in reaching 2010 national health objectives for health indicators such as a lower prevalence of prenatal care in the first trimester (75 vs. 89% in Whites) and lower prevalence of influenza vaccination in persons age 65+ years (50 vs. 69% in Whites) (Centers for Disease Control, 2005). Epidemiologic observational studies are also important sources of risk factor information for formulating policy. Longitudinal epidemiologic datasets based upon the collection of individual data are particularly valuable to policy development. Longitudinal studies allow the examination of the impacts upon health effects across sectoral inputs and exposures (e.g., social-economic, economic-environmental) for multiple health problems, provide trended information, and yield data on rates of change in exposure and health problems at the individual level yielding the best estimates of risk factors for particular conditions and health incidence and mortality related to them.

Examples of longitudinal studies important for policy include the Americans Changing Lives Study (Shultz and Wang, 2007), British Cohort Study 1970 (Ferri et al., 2003), The Canadian National Population Health Survey (Orpana et al., 2006), The National Longitudinal Study of Adolescent Health (Yu et al., 2008), and the United States Health and Retirement Survey (Gallo et al., 2006). The Canadian Population Health Study provides information on the rate of change in weight of adults in addition to physical activities. Because significant weight gain (which this study current reveals) is associated with type II diabetes, cardiovascular disease, psychosocial difficulties, and osteoarthritis information about how individuals move from one weight category (gain weight, lose weight, remain stable) to another over time provides valuable data for developing population-based strategies aimed at addressing the growing problem of obesity. The Health and Retirement Survey provides estimates of the impact of loss of employment, particularly immediately before retirement, upon affective symptoms and anxiety, risk factors for cardiovascular and cerebrovascular conditions. Policy makers need to be aware of the health consequences precipitated by job loss to develop programs (e.g., educational retraining stipends) to lessen the likelihood of adverse health outcomes.

Providing Epidemiological Data to Engage Stakeholders in Decision Making

The influence upon policy development arises from many stakeholders. The composition of the stakeholder group depends upon the issue under debate. For example, the debate over concerns over the potency of dioxin and its widespread presence in the environment engaged the public, industry, environmental groups, veterans' groups, and political bodies (Rodricks et al., 2001).

Decision-making factors include the culture of the bodies ascertaining the risk (e.g., some cultures are willing to risk health in favor of advancing economics), the quality of exposure information, confounding factors emerging in the estimates of the risk, the various methods of statistical and study designs used (see also chapter "Descriptive Epidemiological Methods"), how much advocacy exists for the issue and support of a resolution, and the existence of cost analysis, in particular, cost-benefit information. In cost–benefit analysis, epidemiological data provide the benefit information. And, the quality of these data needs to be as closely evaluated for their scientific value as does the definition of the issue considered in policy formulation. The evaluation of tests for genetic testing is an example of the challenges in compiling the growing body of epidemiologic evidence for gene-disease associations (Burke et al., 2002). The determination of policies regarding genetic testing will be complicated by the multifactorial nature of risks associated with many diseases as well as what is the potential for their prevention and treatment. The controversial nature of policies for genetic testing will also engage as stakeholders religious groups, ethicists, health care providers, and insurers.

Another controversial topic emerging is the growing recognition of the social determinants of health care disparities. Wilkinson and Marmot (2003) describe the social determinants of health "perhaps the most complex and challenging" of all known risk factors for health problems. Increasing epidemiologic evidence on the sources of stress such as early life circumstances, social exclusion, working conditions, unemployment, lack of social support, addictive behaviors, lack of access to healthy food, and transportation will bring increasing pressure upon policy and decision-makers to begin to attack the causes of ill health caused by social determinants. Social factors are only one category of risk factors for health disparities. Access to care in consideration of multiple barriers and the potential for substandard quality of care based upon measures of effectiveness, patient safety, timeliness of care, and patient centeredness are other major factors (CDC, 2004). The Center for Disease Control and Prevention's Office of Minority Health, Office of the Director (2005) acknowledges the importance of these other risk factors stating health disparities can only be eliminated with "culturally appropriate public health initiatives, community support, and equitable access to quality health care." As more epidemiological data are available about the causation of disparity, the greater is the probability of its elimination aided by informed policy-making.

The use of epidemiologic data is not only useful in developing policy for the nation and its health services, but also for serving as the foundation for development of US foreign policy. The Institute of Medicine's (2008) recommendations on global health emphasize the importance of "health as a pillar of US foreign policy" as a means of communicating American values and contributing to global economic stability, as well as national security. Epidemiologic data show the shift of the global burden of disease to an increasing rate of chronic conditions and injuries, persistently high child and maternal mortality rates, and the continuing spread of HIV/AIDS. These data will aid in gaining the support of all nations to also commit in partnership to promoting global health.

In the decision-making process phase of policy development, it is essential that all stakeholders have early and continuing interactions regarding the emerging evidence from all sources, data as well as published reports, for framing the issues as well as in the formulation of the policy. The continued disclosure of data concerning provider performance is likely to impact how firms develop policies concerning the selection of health plans for their members. It has also been proposed that these data may also serve to benchmark the effectiveness of health benefits awarded through federal programs (Lansky, 2002).

Epidemiology as an Aid in Choosing Among Alternative Policies

The choice in searching among alternative policies for a health issue should be driven by basing decisions upon the best set of data are available, even though the data may not be as comprehensive as desired. Comparing the strength of the evidence for an intervention in association with known outcomes in terms of odds ratios, relative risks, and their p-values is one method. Another strategy in applying epidemiology to the examination of policy choices can be made in assessing the potential for harm such as analyzing the frequency of false-positives such as the case with prostate-specific antigen (PSA) testing or the optimal timing of screening for colorectal cancer to determine the optimal life-years gained with screening (Lin et al., 2008; Zauber et al., 2008). Cost–benefit or cost-effectiveness analysis is often utilized in choosing among policies whereby epidemiologic data are used in the "benefit" or "effectiveness" component (i.e., the dependent variable) of these equations. Medicare conducts technology assessments utilizing epidemiologic data for making policy choices for coverage levels for a wide range of conditions ranging from the use air-fluidized beds for pressure ulcers to PSA screening for prostate cancer (http://www.cms.hhs.gov/mcd/index_list.asp?list_type=tech). However, sometimes the choice in alternative policies may be driven by a need for further research or the choice may in fact be banned from further consideration. Such is the example of the interest by some stakeholders in advancing a national policy in support of needle exchange programs as a means of combating the spread of HIV infection. In some cultures (e.g., the Netherlands), epidemiological data support these programs as a viable alternative (Vlahov et al., 2001). The political environment will shape whether or not further epidemiological research will be supported or policies will be established regardless of the opinion of other stakeholders.

The concept of "health disparities" is highly controversial and its definition and measurement by epidemiologic methods is essential to the formulation of alternative policies to be considered as a means of reducing differences in health outcomes among population subgroups. The Centers for Disease Control and Prevention (CDC) defines a health disparity as a "[health] difference that occurs by gender, race or ethnicity, education or income, disability, geographic location, or sexual orientation." Hoover et al. (2008) offer the following criteria for ascertaining the existence of a health disparity: "(1) selecting a reference group for the comparison of two or more groups; (2) determining whether a disparity should be measured in absolute or in relative terms; (3) opting to measure health outcomes or health indicators expressed as adverse or favorable events; (4) selecting a method to monitor a disparity over time; and (5) choosing to measure a disparity as a pair-wise comparison between two groups or in terms of a summary measure of disparity among all groups for a particular characteristic." Depending upon the selection of the comparisons, different conclusions may be drawn about the magnitude and direction of health disparities at a point in time and changes over time. Additional considerations are how the "disparity groups" are created. Race and ethnicity are commonly used. However, other measures representing segregation of population subgroups may be included such as degree of isolation or dissimilarity, clustering, and concentration (Messer, 2008).

Disparities can be measured quantitatively in absolute terms (rate differences, numbers affected, between group variances), relative measures (rate ratios), or how far the reference group is the nonreference group is in terms of a 95% confidence interval (Cheng et al., 2008). The quantification of these differences should be examined regardless of cause. Harper et al. (2008) examine four measures of absolute disparity and three measures of relative disparity regarding trends in lung cancer incidence. Based upon their work, they further propose considering which group is most appropriate for the "reference group" in measuring the disparity as well as whether whatever measure of disparity is selected should be weighted by the population sizes considered. In addition to incidence and mortality rates, another common epidemiologic measure used to measure disparities is hospital utilization rates. For example, Wier et al. (2009) found that "patients who were living in the poorest communities were about 8 percent more likely to be admitted through the emergency department (ED) compared to patients living in other communities." The main limitation of utilization rates as a measure of disparities is that information on race, ethnicity, and income are not present on the visit or discharge encounter record and are often imputed and merged from another data source. It is for these reasons that alternative policies, particularly when those are aimed at eliminating or reducing health disparities should be formulated and a suite of epidemiologic indicators be considered in those decisions. Depending upon the measure used to declare that a disparity exists, different levels of policy effectiveness may be observed.

Monitoring Policy Effectiveness

Any policy proposed is considered incomplete unless a plan for evaluating its effectiveness is included. Policy effectiveness can be evaluated descriptively through the examination of rate measures over time. For example, in Canada the impact of primary care reform and other policies for health sector restructuring has been examined through plotting of trends in avoidable hospitalization rates. These data aid in determining if service inequities or population factors influence disparities in health outcomes (Cloutier-Fisher et al., 2006). The application of epidemiologic measures to monitor the policy effectiveness of laws and ordinances upon communities, workplaces, and hospitals, respectively, are displayed in Boxed Examples 1, 2, and 3.

Boxed Example 1 Impact of Alcohol-Related Laws and Motor Vehicle Crashes

Problem: Nearly half of all motor vehicle injuries and fatalities involve alcohol use. Such injuries are costly in terms of direct (hospitalization, rehabilitation) and indirect (higher automobile insurance premiums, wage loss) costs. Many forms of laws exist and with tighter government budgets, promotion of the most effective ones to the public is of importance.

Methods and data: Mortality data were obtained from Fatality Analysis Reporting System motor vehicle crash data from the National Highway Traffic Safety Administration for the period 1980–1997. Population data from the US Census Bureau were used for the denominator. Law lists were compiled from the National Highway Traffic Safety Administration and *Digest of State Alcohol-Related Legislation*. State mortality data were grouped according to type of law.

Results: Adjusted mortality rate ratios for all motor vehicle fatalities calculated using person-years as the denominator for rates, US, 1980–1997(Source: Villaveces et al., 2003)

Alcohol-related law	Adjusted rate ratio	95% confidence interval
Blood alcohol concentration ≤0.08 g/dl per se	0.86	0.83, 0.88
Zero tolerance	0.88	0.86, 0.90
Administrative license revocation	0.95	0.93, 0.98
Sobriety checkpoints	0.99	0.97, 1.01
Mandatory jail term upon first DUI offense	0.95	0.93, 0.98
Primary seat-belt law	0.94	0.92, 0.97
Secondary seat-belt law	1.02	0.99, 1.04

Managerial Epidemiology Interpretation: The law with the greatest impact on the reduction of motor vehicle (MV)-related fatalities was that which established the criteria for driving under the influence as a blood alcohol concentration (BAC) ≤0.08 g/dl per se. This law was associated with a 14% reduction in MV-related deaths $(1 - 0.86 \times 100\%)$. The communication by a health plan manager or an employer benefits manager to their respective population of the specific exposure level cut-off associated of blood alcohol level law may reduce morbidity and health care costs associated with injuries among their respective populations.

Boxed Example 2 Ordinance Impact Upon Workplace Smoking Cessation

Problem: According to the US Surgeon General, no level of secondhand smoke is safe and that protection from exposure can only be accomplished by eliminating smoking from indoor places. Laws and policies are the only means of controlling exposure, but the relative efficacy of the various types is unknown.

Methods: California residents were surveyed regarding the existing of workplace policies on restricting cigarette smoking and responses were compared among counties with different levels of strengths of local ordinances regarding smoke-free areas. The strength of the ordinances was graded by a content analysis of local laws conducted by the American for Nonsmokers' Rights and the California Smoke-Free Cities Project.

Data and Results: Prevalence of smokers who quit smoking within 6 months of the survey according to ordinance strength (Source: Moskowitz et al., 2000)

Ordinance strength	Prevalence of smokers who quit smoking (95% CI)
No ordinance (*referent*)	19.1% (15.4%, 23.4%)
Weak ordinance	24.6% (19.2%, 30.1%)
Moderate ordinance	24.2% (19.7%, 29.3%)
Strong ordinance	26.4% (23.0%, 30.2%)

CI confidence interval

Managerial Epidemiology Interpretation: Public health policy supporting the passage of strong local ordinances to control public exposure to smoking is effective in increasing the prevalence of smokers who quit smoking. The percentage improvement in the population quitting smoking attributable to a strong ordinance was 38% [(26.4 − 19.1%)/19.1%)]. The strength of local ordinances influenced employers' and business' ability to enforce various no smoking policies in the workplace. Healthcare managers should be aware of local ordinances regarding provisions for workplace smoking to ensure that these are adopted as workplace policies.

Epidemiologic study designs can also be used to evaluate policy effectiveness. The advantage of using a specific study design in evaluation is that a comparison (or "control") group provides a comparison at the same time the policy was introduced (Boxed Example 3).

Boxed Example 3 Impact of Smoke-Free Ordinance on Hospitalization

Problem: Second hand smoke as an etiologic factor in lung cancer and cardiovascular is well known. The impact of legislative changes upon protecting the health of the public from second hand smoke is not well established.

Methods and data: A municipal smoke-free ordinance in the city of Pueblo, Colorado took effect on July 1, 2003. Two control sites were selected for comparison: Pueblo County outside the city of Pueblo limits and El Paso County including Colorado Spring. Neither of the control sites had smoke-free laws at the time the study began. Hospitalization data for acute myocardial infarction (AMI) (ICD-9-CM, 410.0 – 410.9) were obtained. Denominators were calculated from U.S. Census Bureau population data for 2006.

Results: The AMI hospitalization rate significantly declined in the City of Pueblo, but not in the two control areas.

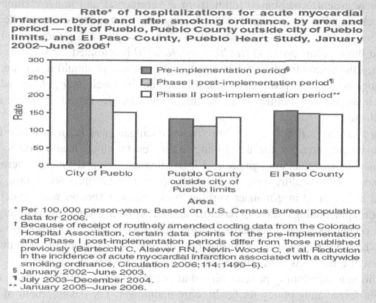

Rate* of hospitalizations for acute myocardial infarction before and after smoking ordinance, by area and period — city of Pueblo, Pueblo County outside city of Pueblo limits, and El Paso County, Pueblo Heart Study, January 2002–June 2006†

* Per 100,000 person-years. Based on U.S. Census Bureau population data for 2006.
† Because of receipt of routinely amended coding data from the Colorado Hospital Association, certain data points for the pre-implementation and Phase I post-implementation periods differ from those published previously (Bartecchi C, Alsever RN, Nevin-Woods C, et al. Reduction in the incidence of acute myocardial infarction associated with a citywide smoking ordinance. Circulation 2006;114:1490–6).
§ January 2002–June 2003.
¶ July 2003–December 2004.
** January 2005–June 2006.

Source: Alsever et al. (2009).

Managerial Epidemiology Implication: Organizations without a smoke-free workplace should consider adopting one, even though local ordinances may not require it. Health benefits of such a policy would extend to potentially reducing acute consequences of second-hand smoke. With an aging health workforce it is imperative to introduce changes in the workplace aimed at prevention and health promotion. Benefits could also be experienced by the employer in the form of reduced lost-workdays and health insurance claims.

A potential limitation of the use of rate measures in monitoring policy effectiveness is that the desired rate of change may have already been occurring by the time the policy was introduced. Similar to obtaining consensus on the health issue itself, stakeholders should likewise be in agreement with the strategies for evaluating the effectiveness of the intervention proposed in the policy.

Examples of Policies Developed Using Epidemiologic Data

A policy document serves to guide in a course of action to government as well as the private sectors. At the national level, for each decade since 1980, public health and public health policy have been guided by national health objectives. Each set of national health objectives has focused on prevention, considered the successes or failures of the previous decade, incorporated new knowledge and technologies, and considered changes in the organization and delivery of public health. Goals and objectives represent broad-based input from governmental and nongovernmental sources including data from national public hearings and electronic responses collected by a federal website. *Healthy People 2010* is an example of a policy document developed through this process. *Healthy People 2010* is intended for the development of health policies for the USA that not only government should reference, but also private and even for-profit firms should consider in developing policies which affect their workforces. Public comments regarding *Healthy People 2020* are now being collected.

Michigan Healthy People 2010 (http://www.michigan.gov) is an example of a policy document intended for developing strategies to guide health policy and improvement in Michigan through the year 2010. It was developed with the overarching philosophy that a healthy economy is best supported by a healthy population. This document is formatted in a manner similar to the national version with objectives based upon epidemiologic data as baseline and target data. Action plans emerging from this policy document included *A Health Status Report* and *A Prescription for Health*, which are intended not only for the Michigan Department of Community Health, but also for all its partnering agencies and stakeholders in Michigan.

In addition to developing policies aimed at health problems, epidemiologic data are used in formulating policy for health care manpower. The development of *The Nursing Agenda for Michigan 2005–2010: Actions to Avert a Crisis* is one such example. This document utilized data pertaining to the aging of the nursing workforce and the general population, recent catastrophic natural disasters and emerging infectious diseases for which a shortage of nurses could impact the health and safety of Michigan citizens. The *Agenda* was developed by the Coalition of Michigan Organizations in Nursing (COMON, 2006) whose members represented 28 Michigan nursing organizations with a constituency of 150,000 nurses. The *Agenda* also received the endorsement of a number of other key (stakeholder) organizations including the Michigan Department of Community Health, Office of the Michigan Chief Nurse Executive, the Michigan Health Council, and the Michigan

Home Health Association. The *Agenda* provides short-range, medium range, and long-range recommendations covering topics such as work environment, work design, nursing education, and scope of nursing practice. A number of the recommended actions also consider the health and safety of the nursing workforce such as alternative approaches to moving/lifting patients and flexible safe working hours staffing.

Summary

Epidemiologic data and studies are essential in formulating policy, as well as evaluating the impacts of policies. It is the obligation of all those who affected by a policy to close the loop and report and communicate to policy makers whether or not they benefited or are harmed by its introduction. To communicate to policy makers in epidemiologic terms is essential to fully address the scope of the impact of the policy in terms of a population and population subgroups not just individuals. Lastly, epidemiology provides the methods for evaluating contributions of the public health and medical care system relative to nonhealth care systems (e.g., housing authorities, public transit systems) in policy formulation and evaluation.

Discussion Questions

Q.1. Communities are increasingly becoming diverse in ethnicity, race, and age. Discuss the challenges in collecting race and ethnic data and the pros and cons of collecting these data for policy decisions. Propose methods for improving the accuracy of collecting race and ethnic data. Would these methods be useful in identifying health disparities? Why or why not? What other information would be important in validating if disparities exist?

Q.2. Select a health issue. Provide or suggest sources of epidemiologic data regarding why it is a concern in terms of its magnitude, mortality and morbidity, and risk to human populations. Identify the stakeholders in the issue. Draft a communication plan appropriate to engage additional stakeholders on the context of the known epidemiologic data on the issues, including its limitations and uncertainties.

Q.3. Based upon the health issue you identified in (2) above, formulate a policy and alternative policies (which include the allocation of resources) to reduce or eliminate the problem, and propose a strategy for monitoring its effectiveness.

Q.4. Given the array of disparities of health problems in the US population, compare and contrast the various epidemiologic measures of determining priorities: age-adjusted rates (including type of standard population use in adjusting rates), years of potential life lost, and age-specific rates. How would your conclusions change, if at all, using the different measures?

References

Afifi, A. and Breslow, I., 1994, The maturing paradigm of public health, *Annu. Rev. Pub. Health* **15**:223–235.

Alsever, R.N., Thomas, W.M., Nevin-Woods, C., Beauvais, R., Dennison, S., Bueno, R., Chang, L., Bartecchi, C.E., Babb, S., Trosclair, A., Engstrom, M., Pechacek, T., and Kaufmann, R., 2009, Reduced hospitalizations for acute myocardial infarction after implementation of a smoke-free ordinance—City of Pueblo, Colorado, 2002–2006. *M.M.W.R* .**51**:1373–1377.

Bellows, N.M., and Halpin, M.A., 2008, Impact of Medicaid reimbursement on mental health quality indicators, *Health Serv. Res.* **43**:582–97.

Burke, W., Atkins, D., Gwinn, M., Guttmacher, A., Haddow, J., Lau, J., Palomaki, G., Press, N., Richards, C.S., Wideroff, L., and Wiesner, G. L., 2002, Genetic test evaluation: information needs of clinicians, policy makers, and the public, *Am. J. Epidemiol.* **156**:311–318.

Centers for Disease Control and Prevention, 2004, Health disparities experienced by racial/ethnic minority populations, *M.M.W.R.* **53**:755.

Centers for Disease Control and Prevention, 2005, Health disparities experienced by black or African Americans – United States, *M.M.W.R.* **54**:1–3.

Cheng, N.F., Han, P.Z., and Gansky, S.A., 2008, Methods and software for estimating health disparities: the case of children's oral health, *Am. J. Epidemiol.* **168**:906–914.

Cloutier-Fisher, D., Penning, M.J., Zheng, C., and Druyts, B.F., 2006, The devil is in the details: trends in avoidable hospitalization rates by geography in British Columbia, 1990–2000, *BMC Health Services Res.* **6**:104.

Coalition of Michigan Organizations of Nursing (COMON), 2006, The Nursing Agenda for Michigan: 2005–2010: Actions to Avert a Crisis (August 16, 2008), http://www.michigancenterfornursing.org.

Ferri, E., Bynner J., and Wadsworth, M. (eds.), 2003, *Changing Britain, Changing Lives: Three Generations at the Turn of the Century*, Institute of Education, University of London, London, UK.

Gallo, W.T., Teng, H.M., Falba, T.A., Kasl, S.V., Krumholz, H.M., and Bradley, E.H., 2006, The impact of late career job loss on myocardial infarction and stroke: a 10 year follow up using the health and retirement survey, *Occup. Environ. Med.* **63**:683–687.

Harper, S., Lynch, J., Meersman, S.C., Breen, N., Davis, W.W., and Reichman, M.E., 2008, An overview of methods for monitoring social disparities in cancer with an example using trends in lung cancer incidence by area-socioeconomic position and race-ethnicity, 1992–2004, *Am. J. Epidemiol.* **167**:889–899.

Hickman, M., Seaman, S., and de Angelis, D., 2001, Estimating the relative incidence of drug use: application of a method for adjusting observed reports of first visits to specialized drug treatment agencies, *Am. J. Epidemiol.* **153**:632–641.

Hoover, K., Bohm, M., and Keppel, K., 2008, Measuring Disparities in the Incidence of Sexually Transmitted Diseases, *Sex Transm. Dis.*

Institute of Medicine (IOM), 1988, *The Future of Public Health*, National Academy Press, Washington, DC.

Institute of Medicine (IOM), 2003, *The Future of the Public's Health in the 21st Century*, National Academy Press, Washington, DC.

Institute of Medicine (IOM), 2008, *The U.S. Commitment to Global Health: Recommendations for the New Administration*, National Academy Press, Washington, DC.

Kotter, J.P., 1996, *Leading Change*, Harvard Business School Press, Boston, MA.

Keppel, K.G., 2007, Ten largest racial and ethnic disparities in the United States base on Healthy People 2010 Objectives, *Am. J. Epidemiol.* **166**:97–103.

Lansky, D., 2002, Improving quality through public disclosure of performance information, *Health Affairs* **21**:52–62.

Lin, K., Lipsitz, R., Miller, T., Janakiraman, S., and U.S. Preventive Services Task Force, 2008, Benefits and harms of prostate-specific antigen screening for prostate cancer: an evidence update for the U.S. Preventive Services Task Force, *Ann. Intern. Med.* **149**:192–199.

Matt, G.E., Quintana, P.J.E., Brewer, A.D., Romero, R., Zkarian, J.M., Guilar, M.G., Chatfield, D.A., and Hovell, M.F., 2008, Smoking policies and secondhand smoke in rental cars, Annual Meeting of the American Public Health Association, No. 3026.

Messer, L.C., 2008, Invited commentary: measuring social disparities in health—what was the question again? *Am. J. Epidemiol.* **167**:900–904.

Messer, L.C., Kaufman, J.S., Mendola, P., and Laraia, B.A., 2008, Black-white preterm birth disparity: a marker of inequality, *Ann. Epidemiol.* **18**:851–858.

Miller, E.A., and Weissert, W.G., 2007, Geography still dictates Rx coverage for many near-poor seniors and disabled persons, *J. Aging Soc. Policy* **19**:77–96.

Moskowitz, J.M., Lin Z., and Hudes, E.S., 2000, The impact of workplace smoking ordinances in California on smoking cessation, *Am. J. Pub. Health* **90**:757–761.

Olfene, A., and Harnett-Pettingill, T., 2008, Smoke-free housing: Eliminating ETS exposure in multi-unit housing through voluntary policy change, Am. Pub. Health Assn. Annual Meeting, No. 3026.

Orpana, H.M., Tremblay, M.S., and Finès, P., 2006, *Trends in Weight Change Among Canadian Adults: Evidence from the 1996/1997 to 2004/2005 National Population Health Survey*, Catalogue no. 82–618-MIE, Health Analysis and Measurement Group Division and Physical Health Measures Division, Statistics Canada, Ottawa, Ontario, Canada.

Rodricks, J.V., Collins, J.J., Farland, W.H., and Tollerud, D.J., 2001, Contrasting roles of epidemiology in dioxin-related policy: lessons learned, *Am. J. Epidemiol.* **154**:S43–49.

Shultz, K.S., and Wang, M., 2007, The influence of specific physical health conditions on retirement decisions, *Int. J. Aging Hum. Dev.* **65**:149–161.

Villaveces, A., Cummings, P., Koepsell, T.D., Rivara, F.P., Lumley, T., and Moffat, J., 2003, Association of alcohol-related laws with death due to motor vehicle and motorcycle crashes in the United States, 1980–1997, *Am. J. Epidemiol.* **157**:131–140.

Vlahov, D., Des Jarlais, D.C., Goosby, E., Hollinger, P.C., Lurie, P.G., Shriver, M.D., and Strathdee, S.A., 2001, Needle exchange programs for the prevention of human immunodeficiency virus infection: epidemiology and policy, *Am. J. Epidemiol.* **154**:S70–S77.

Wier, L., Merrill, C.T., and Elixhauser, A., 2009, *Hospital Stays among People Living in the Poorest Communities*, 2006. HCUP Brief #73, Agency for Healthcare Research and Quality, Rockville, MD.

Wilkinson, R. and Marmot, M. (eds.), 2003, *Social Determinants of Health: The Solid Facts*, 2nd ed., World Health Organization Press, Geneva, Switzerland.

Yu, J.W., Adams, S.H., Burns, J., Brindis, C.D., and Irwin, C.E., Jr., 2008, Use of mental health counseling as adolescents become young adults, *J. Adolescent Health* **43**:268–276.

Zauber, A.G., Lansdorp-Vogelaar, I., Knudsen, A.B., Wilschut, J., van Ballegooijen, M., and Kuntz, K.M., 2008, Evaluating test strategies for colorectal cancer screening: a decision analysis for the U.S. Preventive Services Task Force, *Ann Intern Med.* **149**:659–669.

Chapter 12
Ethics and Managerial Epidemiology Practice

Learning Outcomes

After completing this chapter, you will be able to:

1. Identify potential ethical concerns regarding surveys of health.
2. Design an informed consent form for an observational epidemiologic study.
3. Discuss strategies to increase the security of protected health information.
4. Cite behaviors, positive and negative, which reflect the ethical practice of managerial epidemiology and their implication upon the delivery of health services across the continuum of care.

Keyterms Advanced directives Ethics • HIPAA • Informed consent • Institutional Review Board

Introduction

A profession is an autonomous and self-regulating body which practices a discipline in a competent, learned manner and provides services related to it. A profession also embraces shared core values, obligations, virtues, and defines the level of competence required for its practice. The actions and decisions of a profession impact institutions, other practitioners, and a society. Weed and Coughlin (1999) offer epidemiologists in related context as individuals who "profess to prevent disease in populations through studying the distribution and determinants of disease and applying that knowledge for the public's benefit." Extending that definition to include that the public's benefit is actualized through health services delivery at all levels of prevention and public policy, managerial epidemiology is considered a profession.

Managers who utilize epidemiologic principles regarding the use and distribution of health care resources in populations need to follow ethical guidelines which transect epidemiology, public health, and health care management. Additionally, scientific advances such as genetic screening and gene and stem cell therapy, as well as new health care delivery Paradigms (e.g., financial incentives for certain

D.M. Oleske (ed.), *Epidemiology and the Delivery of Health Care Services*:
Method and Applications,
DOI 10.1007/978-1-4419-0164-4_12, © Springer Science+Business Media, LLC 2009

health-related behaviors, individual or payor), require that ethics be considered in managerial epidemiologic decision-making. Ethics can be defined as the challenges involved in answering questions involving morality, moral disagreements, and conflicting judgments about particular issues. On a broader level, given increases in the population globally and pervasive economic constraints, resource allocation for maintaining a safe level of health in communities of all nations raises growing ethical concerns. Further challenges to allocation of resources are the potential for pandemics and newly emerging diseases (see also chapter "The Role of Managerial Epidemiology in Infection Prevention and Control").

This chapter, therefore, emphasizes concepts related to ethical considerations that would be encountered in the practice of managerial epidemiology. Dilemmas, moral disagreements, and conflicting judgments can occur at every level of the health services delivery continuum, from primary prevention to end-of-life care. The consideration of these challenges in the context of services to populations, not just individuals, heightens the complexity of the ethical concerns and responses to these.

Ethical Elements of Health Care and Health Care Research

Previously, research studies on human subjects have historically been based in academic health centers or government agencies (Heinig et al., 1999). Now human subjects research (commonly called "clinical studies") can be found routinely in almost every aspect of the health services delivery continuum, from experiments of the effectiveness of smoking cessation programs in health maintenance organizations, vaccination trials in nursing homes or other institutionalized population, and even the effectiveness of various forms of end-of-life care.

Research as the fundamental pursuit of new knowledge ideally supports the advancement of health of populations. Randomized clinical trials (see chapter "Epidemiological Study Designs for Evaluating Health Services, Programs, and Systems") provide a unique role in the advancement of the quality of health care through the application of a rigorous structure for evaluation, treatment, and follow-up of study participants. However, research can be harmful for a variety of reasons, including the risks that may be associated with it, known and unknown, ranging from the effects of questioning to the side effects of a new therapy. Research when conducted within an ethical framework is intended to decrease risk and increase the likelihood of a favorable impact upon the health of populations.

The major general principles underlying the ethical conduct of the delivery of health care services and research, including epidemiologic research are: autonomy (respect for individual rights), beneficence (do good), justice (treat fairly, with moral rightness, and in accordance with laws), and nonmaleficence (do no harm). The principles of autonomy and confidentiality are highly linked. To respect a patient's autonomy, the health care provider must also protect the individual's privacy and rights in the decision-making process. These ethical elements are operationalized through informed consent in research as well as in clinical procedures.

Informed Consent

Informed consent is the process whereby a patient or the research subject has the opportunity to make informed decisions, without duress or coercion, about his or health care treatment or research participation. Informed consent is typically obtained in person for the delivery of health care procedures. For some observational research studies, consent may be obtained electronically by having the respondent login to a secure web-based site which displays an electronic version of the consent form and then selecting a choice of consenting to participate or not consenting to participate before proceeding to enter information into a web-based form. In addition to the treatment or research protocol, additional representation of ethical principles in informed consent are the description of the methods for the protection of individual identifiable health data and the identification of risks and amelioration of risks, benefits to the participant and society (in research studies). Research studies consent forms also contains statements regarding the assurance of diversity in the sample (minorities, gender, age), cost considerations for participation, and information describing the circumstances in which an investigator needs to terminate the participant from study or the study, and how results which could impact the health of the participant are communicated. Health care managers have the responsibilities of providing a mechanism and/or policies for oversight of research (e.g., an Institutional Review Board) in any form, including surveys intended for publication to intervention studies are conducted within their organization to ensure that employees or other groups intending to conduct research using the service population, comply with regulations and ethical principles. A written policy on informed consent is a 2008 standard required to be met by the Joint Commission on Accreditation of Health Care Organizations for hospitals (http://www.jointcommission.org).

Informed consent is actually a means of providing structure to resolving ethical dilemmas that may be encountered in the delivery of either health care or clinical research. The essential elements of informed consent based upon the ethical principle that an individual is an autonomous being are: voluntariness, information, understanding, and capacity. Although informed consent is presented herein the context of research, the concept of disclosure is essential in health care as it focuses on the provision of information, be it to the research participant or the patient. All invasive clinical procedures require an informed consent to be completed by the patient. Ethically, the health care provider or the research must disclose the facts that the research participant or patients would consider important in deciding whether to consent or to withhold consent. In the process of administering the consent, the provider (or researcher) must provide the purpose of the consent, the scope of the consent (if applicable), and in the situation of health care, the provider must provide his or her recommendation and disclose if that recommendation is related to a personal interest that may affect his or her judgment, and whether or not those interests are related to the patient's health or anticipated outcomes. In the delivery of health care services, any circumstances requiring the disclosure of information about the patient must be presented in the informed consent process. Circumstances may include the disclosure of information which is required for reporting by law such as HIV, tuberculosis, or other conditions affecting health to organizations such as health departments or the Centers for Disease Control and Prevention.

Standards for the preParation of informed consent forms for participation in research are promulgated through the Office of Human Subjects Research (OHSR). The OHSR operates within the Office of the Deputy Director for Intramural Research (DDIR), National Institutes of Health (NIH). NIH is a federal agency within the US Public Health Service (PHS) of the Department of Health and Human Services (DHHS). Elements of informed consent are displayed in Table 1. Further details concerning informed consent and because laws and regulations concerning the protection of human subjects in research may change over time the reader is also advised to consult the website: http://www.hhs.gov/ohrp/. These same standards provide a framework for informed consent forms used in routine procedures or treatments (e.g., for routine vaccinations) in the health care setting.

It must be pointed out that such standards for informed consent were developed in consideration of Western standards and felt to be another means of also protecting the exploitation of vulnerable or less sophisticated populations and societies. Research conducted or even the delivery of health care in non-Western nations may not necessarily espouse the concept of an individual as a freestanding being who is capable of making decisions independent of the expectations or considerations of others (Loue et al., 1996). The WHO's (1995) *Guidelines for Good Clinical Practice for Trials on Pharmaceutical Projects* offers mechanisms for applying ethical principles when conducting research in cultures and societies that may greatly differ from Western norms. Another organization concerned with the ethics of international clinical research is The International Conference on Harmonisation of Technical Requirements for Registration of Pharmaceuticals for Human Use (ICH). The ICH brings together experts from the pharmaceutical industry in Europe, Japan, and the United States consideration of "maintaining safeguards on quality, safety and efficacy, and regulatory obligations to protect public health (http://www.ich.org)" related to the development and distribution of pharmaceutical agents in humans.

Protection of Health Data

The protection of an individual's health information, for research purposes or for health care services, is governed by the Privacy Rule of the Health Insurance Portability and Accountability Act (HIPAA) (http://www.hhs.gov/ocr/hipaa). There are 18 data elements currently considered protected under rule 45 C.F.R. § 164.514(b) (Table 2) which governs the use and transmission of health information. The participant may consent to the release or viewing of this information through a seParate form or on an informed consent form, depending upon the institutions procedures. Viewing of the information may be in either paper or electronic form. Regardless of the platform, written authorization from the individual whose information is used in a research study is required. In addition to authorization of the

Table 1 Guidelines for Informed consent documents (Source: Office of Human Subjects Research, 2006, available from http://ohsr.od.nih.gov/info/sheet6.html)

I. Conveyance of ethical principles for respect of persons
1. Disclosure of relevant information to prospective subjects about the research
2. Ensure comprehension of the information by participants
3. Assure voluntary agreement

II. Basic elements for written informed consent documents
1. A statement that the study involves research
2. An explanation of the purpose of the research and the expected duration of the subject's participation
3. A description of the procedures to be followed and identification of any procedures that are experimental
4. A description of any foreseeable risks or discomforts to the subject, an estimate of their likelihood, and a description of what steps will be taken to prevent or minimize them
5. A description of any benefits to the subject or to others that may reasonably be expected from the research (Monetary compensation is not a benefit). If compensation or even a token of appreciation for participation will be provided to research subjects or healthy volunteers, the amount and/or items should be stated in the consent document
6. A disclosure of any appropriate alternative procedures or courses of treatment that might be advantageous to the subject
7. A statement describing to what extent records will be kept confidential, including a description of who may have access to research records
8. For research involving more than minimal risk, an explanation and description of any compensation and any medical treatments that are available if research subjects are injured; where further information may be obtained, and whom to contact in the event of a research-related injury
9. An explanation of who to contact for answers to pertinent questions about the research and the research subject's rights (include the Clinical Center's Patient Representative and telephone number)
10. A statement that participation is voluntary and that refusal to participate or discontinuing participation at any time will involve no penalty or loss of benefits to which the subject is otherwise entitled

III. Additional elements
1. If the subject is or may become pregnant, a statement that the particular treatment or procedure may involve risks, which are currently unforeseeable, to the subject or to the embryo or fetus
2. A description of circumstances in which the subject's participation may be terminated by the investigator without the subject's consent
3. Any costs to the subject that may result from participation in the research and who is expected to cover (Travel costs for participation are often customarily provided)
4. What will happen if the subject decides to withdraw from the research and how withdrawal will be handled
5. A statement that the Principal Investigator will notify subjects of any significant new findings during the course of the study that may affect them and influence their willingness to continue participation
6. The approximate number of subjects involved in the study
7. When appropriate, a statement concerning an investigator's potential financial or other conflict of interest in the conduct of the study

324 12 Ethics and Managerial Epidemiology Practice

Table 2 Protected health information (Sources: USDHHS, 2003, *Summary of the HIPAA Privacy Rule* available at http://www.hhs.gov/ocr/privacysummary.pdf and USHDDS, 2003, *Standards for Privacy of Individually Identifiable Health Information* available at http://www.hhs.gov/ocr/hipaa/guidelines/guidanceallsections.pdf)

The following identifiers of the individual or of relatives, employers, or household members of the individual must be removed to achieve the "safe harbor" method of de-identification:

1. Names.
2. All geographic subdivisions smaller than a State, including street address, city, county, precinct, zip code, and their equivalent geocodes, except for the initial three digits of a zip code if according to the current publicly available data from the Bureau of Census: (1) the geographic units formed by combining all zip codes with the same three initial digits contains more than 20,000 people; and (2) the initial three digits of a zip code for all such geographic units containing 20,000 or fewer people is changed to 000.
3. All elements of dates (except year) for dates directly related to the individual, including birth date, admission date, discharge date, date of death; and all ages over 89 and all elements of dates (including year) indicative of such age, except that such ages and elements may be aggregated into a single category of age 90 or older.
4. Telephone numbers.
5. Fax numbers.
6. Electronic mail addresses.
7. Social security numbers.
8. Medical record numbers.
9. Health plan beneficiary numbers.
10. Account numbers.
11. Certificate/license numbers.
12. Vehicle identifiers and serial numbers, including license plate numbers.
13. Device identifiers and serial numbers.
14. Web Universal Resource Locators (URLs).
15. Internet Protocol (IP) address numbers.
16. Biometric identifiers, including finger and voice prints.
17. Full face photographic images and any comparable images.
18. Any other unique identifying number, characteristic, or code, except as permitted for reidentification purposes provided certain conditions are met. In addition to the removal of the above-stated identifiers, the covered entity may not have actual knowledge that the remaining information could be used alone or in combination with any other information to identify an individual who is subject of the information. 45 C.F.R. § 164.514(b).

individual data elements, the use of the information must be specified. These procedures reinforce the ethical obligation of health care professionals from disclosing information about the patient's case to others unless authorization for access has been granted from the patient. Yet, in the course of clinical practice regarding the care of a patient there is often an exchange of information with other health care providers deemed critical to the care. These are justifiable so long as precautions are taken to limit the ability of others to hear or see confidential information (e.g., secure login to patient information by physicians, computerized tracking of who views the information, etc.).

There are two methods used for de-identifying records. One is called the "safe harbor method." This method removes all 18 data elements listed in Table 2 and thus creates a zero change that anyone might be able to identify the patient through a review of the medical record alone and/or with other sources of information. The "little chance" method is a statistical process in which some of the data elements are removed lessening the chances that the patient care be identified through a review of the medical record.

The storage and transmittal of Electronic Protected Health Information (EPHI) is a major concern owing to the portability of such information through electronic means (e.g., email) and devices (e.g., cell phones). The organization should develop a security strategy for the storage and transmittal of EPHI. According to 45 C.F.R. § 164.306(b)(2) of the HIPAA Security Standards security strategies utilized by a health care manager in health care data storage and transactions should consider.

(i)   "The size, complexity and capabilities of the covered entity.
(ii) The covered entity's technical infrastructure, hardware, and software security capabilities.
(iii) The costs of security measures.
(iv) The probability and criticality of potential risks to [EPHI]."

Security training is essential for all staff handling health care information, but it may not be sufficient to prevent security breaches because of individual errors or systems failures. The chances of any change in personnel or IT change (software, hardware) or other organizational discontinuities may also give rise to breaches of confidentiality or integrity of personally identified health information (Collmann and Cooper, 2007). Good information management based upon quality practices (see chapter "Advancing Patient Safety Through the Practice of Managerial Epidemiology") including Failure Mode and Effects Analysis (Cohen et al., 1994) and routine communication on handling health information will help maintain information security.

In addition, the organization needs to determine whether or not the information needs to be accessed off-site or electronically transmitted. If information is transmitted off-site, risk analysis and risk management strategies, policies and procedures for safeguarding the EPHI, and adequate workforce training regarding security awareness and knowledge of the security policies and procedures must be done.

The risk analysis should be based upon who should have access to the information based upon their role within the organization and only those who need to know the EPHI. Policies and procedures should cover access, storage, and transmittal of EPHI across all devices used in the organization, including sanctions for violation of policy. Risk management strategies for all devices and portable systems would include virus-protection and firewall software utilization, password management procedures, session termination protocols, access monitoring, archival backups, secure electronic connections, and use of deletion tools.

Protection of data when manipulated for analysis is also important. Included in this strategy is not to reveal the identity of individual's data either in quantitative or visual form (e.g., photographs). Only grouped data should be presented. Rules should be formulated in advance to ensure that conclusions from grouped data that are small in number could potentially disclose the individuals in a group or stigmatize the group by virtue of the results.

Risks and Benefits

Risk enters in to any study design, treatment, health program, or policy. The ethical consideration in that communication of risk should be transparent, namely, its existence must be acknowledged and the assumptions upon which risk estimates are based as stated. Risks including foreseeable discomforts to the subject should be described in lay terms the likelihood of their occurrence and the measures that will be taken to prevent them or minimize the risks should they occur.

Benefits considered are those which pertain to the individual and society at large. Monetary compensation for study participation, even travel reimbursement or tokens of appreciation for study participation are not considered benefits.

Diversity of Participants

Diversity of participation in human subjects research is particularly important in clinical research. Toward that end, the NIH requires its funded clinical research to include both genders and be diverse in racial and ethnic groups. Researchers are also encouraged to examine differential effects on such groups in the event that results are identified which could impact a standard of care, that population subgroups are differentially affected by the treatment in terms of clinical outcome or response or side effects, or that data are found which could change in health policy.

Cost

From an ethical perspective, the participant must be informed about the costs of participation. Included in the information should be a statement if as a result of participation any injuries or side effects associated with participation will or will not be compensated. Cost may be a major barrier to participation, both direct and indirect costs, in some study designs. Direct costs may include loss of wages for time spent in participation, travel associated with participation. Indirect costs include the need for child and family care and other personal obligations to participate in the study (Brown et al., 2000). Commonly, a clause may be included in an informed consent form that the research is not responsible for the treatment of any adverse consequences associated with study participation. Thus, lack of insurance to cover costs of any adverse effects of participation, and this disproportionately would affect minorities and low income persons. As mentioned earlier, costs enabling enrollment and follow-up in the study are not a benefit of study participation. Compensation may be provided to research subjects even to healthy volunteers, and if it is, the amount should be stated in the consent form.

Confidentiality and Privacy Concerns

Respect for the individual in terms of protecting the confidentiality of their information in research or health care arises regardless of one's ethical framework. The ethical principle of nonmaleficence is invoked such that access to health-related information about an individual should be restricted so as to minimize harm in the event it was disclosed either intentionally or unintentionally. Various laws govern who and in what circumstances health information could be shared or transmitted. For example, laws exist mandating the reporting of abuse, in circumstances where a specific disease such as HIV, of wounds resulting from specified weapons or events, and the monitoring of records by government or accrediting organizations for quality assurance purposes. As referred to above, technological means of protecting confidentiality and privacy exist, but these should not substitute for the ethical behaviors the health care professional should practice in this regard, such as not discussing patient information in public places or in the presence of other patients, health care providers, or friends or family who do not need to know about the circumstances of treatment or diagnosis.

Ethical Factors Affecting Participation in Research Studies and Utilizing Health Care

Numerous factors have been cited in the literature concerning participation in research studies involving an understanding of disease etiology as well as for participation in experimental diagnoses or treatment studies (devices, drugs, and other therapies including behavioral). These same factors also influence not only the patient or member of the community's choice to seek health care, but also the type of health care he/she can access and is willing to accept. It is essential that trust is established, respect for the participant's culture, language, and structural factors (e.g., poverty, tribal affiliation), and privacy and confidentiality are assured (Giuliano et al., 2000; Vega et al., 2007) in the delivery of health care as well as in research. In fact, some of the actions and laws designed to protect human subjects in research and treatment that may in fact affect trust and cost (Ness et al., 2007). Multiple forms (e.g., HIPAA plus informed consent) and complex, lengthy procedures for recruiting and enrolling study participants, even with the intent of protecting privacy, may negatively affect public trust, add cost to study participation and may dissuade individuals from participating in research (Dunlop et al., 2007; Ness et al., 2007). Safeguards of privacy may actually be a barrier to the recruitment of patients through registries (e.g., tumor registries, twin registries) as typically some level of physician interaction is involved. Established physician relationships may not necessarily exist (e.g., the case of a second opinion for cancer) or may involve multiple physicians and variation in policies exists regarding recruitment through registries (Beskow et al., 2006). The balance regarding contacting patients through registries using different strategies without physician involvement such as educating patients in advance regarding the purpose of the research, the procedures to be used, expected benefits to the participant and society, the potential of reasonably foreseeable risks and alternatives to participating in the research still requires further discussion at a policy level.

With the aging of the population, there will be increasing ethical challenges related to the participation in research and related to the delivery as well as the termination of care. Generational differences may result in a patient's wishes and values to be quite different than the values of the family and health care providers. A "value" is the moral certainty of an informant of the "rightness" of his or her course of action or decision. Although the principle of respect for an individual obligates the health care provider to include the patient in decisions regarding health care, the principle of beneficence may require a family member or significant other to act upon the behalf of the patient in life-threatening or end-of-life circumstances, resulting in an ethical conflict. Advance directives, required by many hospitals as part of the admissions process, are a means of resolving this potential ethical conflict. Advance directives are legal documents that convey an individual's decisions about end-of-life care to those who need to make decisions about your treatment in the event of the individual's incapacitation to make those decision (see National Institutes of Health, available October 28, 2008 at http://www.nlm.nih.gov/medlineplus/advancedirectives.html). Cognitive and physical impairments and dependence upon others affect not only participation but limit engagement in treatment. Expression of choice and volunteerism may be feasible in cognitively and impaired individual, but new strategies for their recognition may have to be developed (Loue, 2004).

Ethical Allocation of Resources in Populations

With a changing environment in terms of climate, pollution, and growth of industry, the possibility increases for an environmental disaster. With a growing world population, vast involuntary migrations due to wars and civil conflicts, voluntary migrations for economic pursuit, and international travel, the likelihood of outbreaks of infectious diseases and even pandemics are increased. The increasing global population increases the possibility of more extensive human casualties than would be anticipated even a 100 years ago. The potential for a disaster, natural or man-made, is a call to prompt the development not only of preparedness plans by health care providers, health care organizations, businesses, and government, but the threat of a disaster also provides the impetus for developing an ethical framework for the allocation of resources to protect and preserve the health of communities across a variety of situations. Planning for a disaster such as a pandemic assumes that normal businesses operations and public safety infrastructures will be disrupted and the distribution of essential goods and services including public health will be interrupted or unavailable, and hence an ethical framework for the distribution of resources is essential not only during the event itself, but also for managing the sequellae resulting from it. Influenza pandemics of historical importance are the "Spanish flu" of 1918, the "Asian flu" of 1957, and the "Hong Kong flu" of 1968 (Kilbourne, 2006). Another influenza pandemic is eminent, but the specific strains and predicted time of occurrence are unknown.

Ethical frameworks for planning decision-making in the event of a pandemic have been proposed by a number of groups (Garrett et al., 2008; Kinlaw and Levine, 2007; Thompson et al., 2006; WHO, 2007). The elements of developing an ethical framework for decision-making in the allocation of resources from these authors are summarized below:

- The formation of a working group of experts in the health condition of concern, public health, organizational ethics, and clinical ethicists
- Review of the ethics literature on the condition
- Stakeholder vetting of the framework developed through information, education, and communication
- The development of the ethical framework utilizing and ethical process (accountability, inclusiveness, public engagement, openness, transparency, reasonableness, and responsiveness)
- The development of values that inform the process (duty to provide care, equity or equal access, individual liberty, privacy, proportionality, protection of the public from harm, social and economic stability, reciprocity, solidarity, stewardship, trust, saving the most lives)
- Sponsorship of the framework by key administrators, public and private sectors
- Dissemination of the final ethical framework to key stakeholders
- Development of a resource allocation protocol based upon the ethical framework and values
- Continuous review of the ethical framework for decision-making

In pluralistic societies, values are diverse and continuously changing. Health care managers when practicing with an epidemiologic framework must be aware of their own values and the standards of ethical behavior in the communities in which they practice. Thus, to make informed decisions, there is the need for the continuous reevaluation and revision as necessary the ethical framework, even if anticipating the same disease entity (e.g., influenza) will reoccur to challenge the society's resources. Even the characteristics of a pandemic might change in terms of what if any vaccines are available and if vaccines are available who are most likely to benefit. The reevaluation requires engagement of clinicians, organizations, public health, and stakeholders in each iterative process with the perspective that the goals of population health, the protection of safety and services, and to treat all fairly. However, each of these goals is not necessarily equal with the allocation of resources. For example, in the event of a pandemic, health care workers and public safety personnel and children may be given priority before all other persons. The implementation of this prioritization scheme may result in an ethical dilemma as ethically all persons should be honored with human dignity and it is still open for debate regarding how can this be maintained if priority is given to those with a better chance of survival or of a younger age.

There are a number of other ethical considerations in the allocation of resources, not only in terms of disasters but also in terms of resource allocation for end-of-life care. Allocation decisions for disasters are based upon the nature and scope of the recipients of the services, such as requiring vaccinations in times of epidemics for health workers' for safety and obligation reasons, mandating vaccinations for certain categories of the general population, or for criteria for prioritization of the recipients of resources regardless of their legal status in a country. Situations where mandated vaccinations are required, regardless of circumstances, also raise the ethical concerns in the event vaccine-related injuries or illnesses occur (Mello, 2008). The nature of international cooperation and assistance, both in terms of receiving as well as providing assistance, are also ethical considerations in terms of disasters because the balance of the internal resources for the protection of the public need to be balanced against the protection of the public from outside threats.

The allocation of resources in the treatment setting is optimally a joint decision by the patient and the health care provider. However, for adults living with serious and potentially life- or mind-threatening conditions, family members, partners, and health care providers are often faced with ethical dilemmas regarding the nature of continued treatment. Advance care planning (advanced directives, wills, power of attorney) clarify decision-making in matters of the allocation of resources for continued care. The provision of written information about advance directives in hospitalized patient populations is a standard addressed in the Joint Commission on Accreditation of Healthcare Organizations (http://www.jointcommission.org) for hospitals in 2008. Rates of advance care planning are influenced by potentially modifiable factors such as relationship with primary care physicians, knowledge of the process itself, and the willingness of physicians' to initiate discussion of the topic (Morrison and Meier, 2004).

Managerial Epidemiology Practice to Promote Ethical Conduct

One of the fundamental ways to practice managerial epidemiology with ethical conduct is to know how one's behaviors, decisions, and actions conform to the professions' standards of ethics. Both the American College of Epidemiology (ACE) and the American College of Healthcare Executives (ACHE) have put forth guidelines for practice that are relevant to any individual engaged in the practice of population-based health care management. The guidelines put forth by the ACHE and the ACE represent standards of practice for the practitioners of management epidemiology. The ACE *Ethics Guidelines* (2000) covers: the professional role of epidemiologists including avoiding conflicts of interest and partiality; responsibility in minimizing the risks and protecting the welfare of research participants; providing benefits and assuring equitable distribution of risks to individuals and society; assuring confidentiality, privacy, and appropriate informed consent; maintaining the public trust; communicating ethical requirements to colleagues, employers, and sponsors and confronting unacceptable conduct; and duty to community in reporting results, as public health advocates, and respecting cultural diversity (Table 3). McKeown et al. (2003) describe the ACE *Ethics Guidelines* as addressing the core values and duties of epidemiologists and virtues important to professional practice, and the duties and obligations of epidemiologists and how these are applied in practice. The *ACHE Code of Ethics* (2007) addresses the breadth considering an individual executive's behavior, responsibilities to patients and others served, to the organization, to employees, to community and society, and the duty to report violations of the code to the organization's Ethics Committee (Table 4).

Table 3 American college of epidemiology outline of Ethics guidelines elements (Source: American College of Epidemiology, 2000, available from http://www.acepidemiology2.org/policystmts/EthicsGuide.pdf. Reprinted with permission from ACE, Raleigh, NC)

Part I – Core values, duties, and virtues in epidemiology
  1.1. Definition and discussion of core values
  1.2. Definition and discussion of duties and obligations
  1.3. Definition and discussion of virtues

Part II – Ethics guidelines
  2.1. The professional role of epidemiologists
  2.2. Minimizing risks and protecting the welfare of research participants
  2.3. Providing benefits
  2.4. Ensuring an equitable distribution of risks and benefits
  2.5. Protecting confidentiality and privacy
  2.6. Obtaining the informed consent of participants
    2.6.1. Elements of informed consent
    2.6.2. Avoidance of manipulation or coercion
    2.6.3. Conditions under which informed consent requirements may be waived
  2.7. Submitting proposed studies for ethical review
  2.8. Maintaining public trust
    2.8.1. Adhering to the highest scientific standards
    2.8.2. Involving community representatives in research
  2.9. Avoiding conflicts of interest and partiality
  2.10. Communicating ethical requirements to colleagues, employers, and sponsors and confronting unacceptable conduct
    2.10.1. Communicating ethical requirements
    2.10.2. Confronting unacceptable conduct
  2.11. Obligations to communities
    2.11.1. Reporting results
    2.11.2. Public health advocacy
    2.11.3. Respecting cultural diversity

Part III – Discussion and clarification of guidelines
  3.1. The professional role of epidemiologists
  3.2. Minimizing risks and protecting the welfare of research participants
  3.3. Providing benefits
  3.4. Ensuring an equitable distribution of risks and benefits

(continued)

Table 3 (continued)

3.5. Protecting confidentiality and privacy
   3.5.1. Maintaining confidentiality (unlinked information; Linked information [anonymous, nonnominal, nominal, or nominative])
   3.5.2. Maintaining security
   3.5.3. Certificates of confidentiality
3.6. Obtaining the informed consent of participants
3.7. Submitting proposed studies for ethical review
3.8. Maintaining public trust
3.9. Avoiding conflicts of interest and partiality
3.10. Communicating ethical requirements to colleagues, employers, and sponsors and confronting unacceptable conduct
3.11. Obligations to communities

Table 4 American college of health care executives code of Ethics (Source: American College of Healthcare Executives, 2007, available from: http://www.ache.org/ABT_ACHE/code.cfm. Reprinted with permission from ACHE, Chicago, IL)

PREAMBLE

The purpose of the Code of Ethics of the American College of Healthcare Executives is to serve as a standard of conduct for affiliates. It contains standards of ethical behavior for healthcare executives in their professional relationships. These relationships include colleagues, patients, or others served; members of the healthcare executive's organization and other organizations, the community and society as a whole. The Code of Ethics also incorporates standards of ethical behavior governing individual behavior, particularly when that conduct directly relates to the role and identity of the healthcare executive. The fundamental objectives of the healthcare management profession are to maintain or enhance the overall quality of life, dignity, and well-being of every individual needing healthcare service and to create a more equitable, accessible, effective, and efficient healthcare system. Healthcare executives have an obligation to act in ways that will merit the trust, confidence and respect of healthcare professionals and the general public. Therefore, healthcare executives should lead lives that embody an exemplary system of values and ethics. In fulfilling their commitments and obligations to patients or others served, healthcare executives function as moral advocates and models. Since every management decision affects the health and well-being of both individuals and communities, healthcare executives must carefully evaluate the possible outcomes of their decisions. In organizations that deliver healthcare services, they must work to safeguard and foster the rights, interests, and prerogatives of patients or others served. The role of moral advocate requires that healthcare executives take actions necessary to promote such rights, interests, and prerogatives. Being a model means that decisions and actions will reflect personal integrity and ethical leadership that others will seek to emulate.

I. The health care executive's responsibilities to the profession of health care management
   The healthcare executive shall:
   A. Uphold the *Code of Ethics* and mission of the American College of Healthcare Executives
   B. Conduct professional activities with honesty, integrity, respect, fairness, and good faith in a manner that will reflect well upon the profession
   C. Comply with all laws and regulations pertaining to healthcare management in the jurisdictions in which the healthcare executive is located or conducts professional activities
   D. Maintain competence and proficiency in healthcare management by implementing a personal program of assessment and continuing professional education
   E. Avoid the improper exploitation of professional relationships for personal gain

(continued)

Table 4 (continued)

F. Disclose financial and other conflicts of interest

G. Use this *Code* to further the interests of the profession and not for selfish reasons

H. Respect professional confidences

I. Enhance the dignity and image of the healthcare management profession through positive public information programs

J. Refrain from participating in any activity that demeans the credibility and dignity of the healthcare management profession

II. The health care executive's responsibilities to patients or others served

The health care executive shall, within the scope of his or her authority:

A. Work to ensure the existence of a process to evaluate the quality of care or service rendered

B. Avoid practicing or facilitating discrimination and institute safeguards to prevent discriminatory organizational practices

C. Work to ensure the existence of a process that will advise patients or others served of the rights, opportunities, responsibilities, and risks regarding available healthcare services

D. Work to ensure that there is a process in place to facilitate the resolution of conflicts that may arise when values of patients and their families differ from those of employees and physicians

E. Demonstrate zero tolerance for any abuse of power that compromises patients or others served

F. Work to provide a process that ensures the autonomy and self-determination of patients or others served

G. Work to ensure the existence of procedures that will safeguard the confidentiality and privacy of patients or others served

III. The health care executive's responsibilities to the organization

The health care executive shall, within the scope of his or her authority:

A. Provide healthcare services consistent with available resources, and when there are limited resources, work to ensure the existence of a resource allocation process that considers ethical ramifications

B. Conduct both competitive and cooperative activities in ways that improve community health care services

C. Lead the organization in the use and improvement of standards of management and sound business practices

D. Respect the customs and practices of patients or others served, consistent with the organization's philosophy

E. Be truthful in all forms of professional and organizational communication, and avoid disseminating information that is false, misleading, or deceptive

F. Report negative financial and other information promptly and accurately, and initiate appropriate action

G. Prevent fraud and abuse and aggressive accounting practices that may result in disputable financial reports

H. Create an organizational environment in which both clinical and management mistakes are minimized and, when they do occur, are disclosed and addressed effectively

I. Implement an organizational code of ethics and monitor compliance

J. Provide ethics resources to staff to address organizational and clinical issues

(continued)

Table 4 (continued)

IV. The health care executive's responsibilities to employees

Health care executives have ethical and professional obligations to the employees they manage that encompass but are not limited to:

A. Creating a work environment that promotes ethical conduct by employees

B. Providing a work environment that encourages a free expression of ethical concerns and provides mechanisms for discussing and addressing such concerns

C. Providing a work environment that discourages harassment, sexual, and other; coercion of any kind, especially to perform illegal or unethical acts; and discrimination on the basis of race, ethnicity, creed, gender, sexual orientation, age, or disability

D. Providing a work environment that promotes the proper use of employees' knowledge and skills

E. Providing a safe work environment

F. Establishing appropriate grievance and appeals mechanisms

V. The health care executive's responsibilities to community and society

The health care executive shall:

A. Work to identify and meet the healthcare needs of the community

B. Work to support access to healthcare services for all people

C. Encourage and participate in public dialogue on healthcare policy issues, and advocate solutions that will improve health status and promote quality health care

D. Apply short- and long-term assessments to management decisions affecting both community and society

E. Provide prospective patients and others with adequate and accurate information, enabling them to make enlightened decisions regarding services

VI. The health care executive's responsibility to report violations of the code

An affiliate of ACHE who has reasonable grounds to believe that another affiliate has violated this *Code* has a duty to communicate such facts to the Ethics Committee

Both sets of guidelines are necessary and complement each other. For example, the ACHE executives Ethics Guidelines do not consider research imperatives that are essential in this era of data-driven studies such as quality, safety, and outcomes assessment to improve health care. The ACE Ethics Guidelines do not consider the organizational factors which may influence the conduct of epidemiologic studies, including informed consents and study designs, and dissemination of their results. Additionally, the Public Health Code of Ethics (Table 5) is complementary to both the ACE and the ACHE guidelines as it emphasizes the necessity of the interaction between government and health care professionals and other organizations in ethical considerations as they affect the health of the public.

Espousing principles of social justice is another aspect of ethical managerial epidemiologic practice. Managers should seek to identify disparities in health, injury, disability, disease, or mortality in populations served and attempt to ensure a more equitable distribution of resources and access to care. With more equitable distribution, variation in health care outcomes among population subgroups will be less likely. However, the effectiveness of more equitable distribution also assumes that recipients of care are able to engage or be active and informed participants in the services. Toward that end health care managers need to be involved regardless

Table 5 Public health code of Ethics (Source: Public Health Leadership Society, 2002)

1. Public health should address principally the fundamental causes of disease and requirements for health, aiming to prevent adverse health outcomes.
2. Public health should achieve community health in a way that respects the rights of individuals in the community.
3. Public health policies, programs, and priorities should be developed and evaluated through processes that ensure an opportunity for input from community members.
4. Public health should advocate and work for the empowerment of disenfranchised community members, aiming to ensure that the basic resources and conditions necessary for health are accessible to all.
5. Public health should seek the information needed to implement effective policies and programs that protect and promote health.
6. Public health institutions should provide communities with the information they have that is needed for decisions on policies or programs and should obtain the community's consent for their implementation.
7. Public health institutions should act in a timely manner on the information they have within the resources and the mandate given to them by the public.
8. Public health programs and policies should incorporate a variety of approaches that anticipate and respect diverse values, beliefs, and cultures in the community.
9. Public health programs and policies should be implemented in a manner that most enhances the physical and social environment.
10. Public health institutions should protect the confidentiality of information that can bring harm to an individual or community if made public. Exceptions must be justified on the basis of the high likelihood of significant harm to the individual or others.
11. Public health institutions should ensure the professional competence of their employees.
12. Public health institutions and their employees should engage in collaborations and affiliations in ways that build the public's trust and the institution's effectiveness.

of the level of health prevention they provide leadership in the continuous distribution of information and education to current and potential recipients of health care. The "rightness" or "wrongness" related to any ethical dilemma in the delivery or health care services or research delivered in conjunction with these services can be guided by referring to the ethical guidelines of the three organizations presented herein. Each health care manager practicing within an epidemiologic framework must also strive to act in a moral and responsible manner to the population served regardless of what occurs within an organization (Boxed Example 1).

Boxed Example 1 Increasing Socioeconomic Disparities in Disability Among the Elderly

Problem: Despite the existence of national health insurance for the elderly (Medicare), there are epidemiologic data which indicate there are disparities in old-age disability by race/ethnicity.

Methods and Data: Data from the National Health Interview Survey (NHIS) were used to characterize over time a sample of 8,000 adults 70+ years. To represent the civilian noninstitutional population, SUDAAN software was used to adjust the survey results with appropriate weights. Disability was conceptualized as activities of daily living (ADL) and instrumental activities of daily living (IADL) and measured by two questions. Those responding "yes" to an ADL limitation were asked if the limitation required assistance with the impairment (IADL-type limitations). Logistic regression models adjusting for time, age, gender were performed and included interaction terms as appropriate. The estimated average annual percentage change in disability was calculated from the estimated odds ratio of the model on the trend variable minus 1 and then multiplied by 100.

Results:

Average annual percentage change in disability, logistic models, 1982–2002	
Any disability	
All people	−2.15**
Years of education	
0–8	−0.88**
9–11	−0.84*
12	−1.61**
13–15	−1.67**
16 or more	−2.53**
Family income quartile	
Lowest	−1.38**
Second	−2.65**
Third	−3.06**
Highest	−3.11**

$*p = 0.05, **p = 01$

The [data] show that the average rate of decline in the prevalence of disability of persons 70+ years is −2.15%, exhibiting a significant downward trend. The largest annual rates of decline in disability are among those with the highest educational level (16+ years, −2.53 vs. 0–8 years, −0.88) and family income (highest, −3.11 vs. lowest, −1.38)

Source: Schoeni et al. (2005)

Managerial Epidemiology Interpretation: Although the prevalence of disability is declining among the population 70+ years, health care managers should not assume that the availability of health care insurance will eliminate disparities, even with insurance offered through the government. Promotion of the adoption of personal health behaviors, collaboration with governmental and private agencies to support healthy environments for the elderly, particularly for those of lower income or education may help to eliminate disparities in disability. These actions are an essential component of health care managers' duties, beyond those to the organization, because of their ethical responsibilities as advocates for public health and their responsibilities to the community and society.

Summary

The ethical responsibilities of management epidemiology practice are broad because of the scope of epidemiology and the various definitions of populations served. Because of the continuous new information derived from epidemiologic studies, the ethical constructs of practice need to continuously be revisited for relevance. Involvement in professional organizations which represent the discipline of managerial epidemiology practice is a way to ensure that ethical practice is congruent with professional standards and current research findings. Keeping abreast of the regulations and laws that impact health care research in humans is a responsibility for ensuring that managerial epidemiology is practiced in an ethical manner. Another ethical responsibility is the professional duty to promote ecological integrity, namely being responsible in preserving a balanced relationship of services and the environment. Lastly, consultation and involvement with members of groups affected (or their representatives) by the research or the health services provided should be ongoing. These stakeholders form the community norms and standards of acceptability of risks and benefits for the health care services provided and any related health care research.

Discussion Questions

Q.1. Design an informed consent form for an observational study of the relationship between preventive health behaviors and utilization of physician services for acute care illness, injuries, and general health check-ups (e.g., regular physical exams). How would the informed consent form have to be modified if the population studied were children?

Q.2. Screening and treatment of early stage breast cancer are highly effective in preventing morbidity and mortality from breast cancer (Boxed Example 2). Discuss the ethical implications of allocating health care for the screening and treatment of breast cancer when available resources for a population (manpower, budget, etc.) are limited. (Note: This could apply to any population from those in a managed care plan to a developing nation.)

Q.3. Tobacco usage is a known risk factor for many health-related problems, both to the individual and others, in the case of second-hand smoke. Should epidemiologic studies which ascertain tobacco usage in any form offer tobacco cessation information and/or health care services for tobacco cessation as part of the research protocol?

Q.4. Many childhood infectious diseases are preventable through vaccination. States have mandatory vaccination laws that require children to receive certain vaccines as a condition of school attendance. Although all states provide medical exemptions, many states also allow religious exemptions and some states allow exemptions based upon philosophical grounds. Opponents of any

Boxed Example 2 Breast Health in Limited-Resource Countries

Problem: As the global population ages, chronic conditions such as breast cancer will become more prevalent. Guidelines for breast cancer control and treatment have been developed for national with a high level of resources available, but not in limited-resource countries (LRC). Even within a limited-resource country, the possibility of inequity in access to early detection and treatment exists because of social and economic disparities, such that the poor are the majority of the population and the wealthier are the smaller number. For this reason in LRC, women often present for care only in the late stages of the disease. Better resource allocation for early detection may improve breast health.

Methods: A panel of breast cancer experts and advocates from around the world met to review the published literature in the context of the WHO guidelines and develop consensus principles for breast cancer screening in LRC (Yip et al., 2008). The WHO (2002) guidelines utilized were formed inconsideration of the following levels of services: (1) Basic level: core resources for any health care and can be applied in a single health care interaction; (2) Limited level: resources used to improve outcome in a major way and may involve single or multiple contacts or health care interactions; (3) Enhanced level: resources that make some optional treatments available; (4) Maximal level: resources applied comParable to a country with high-level resources that improve outcome in a minor way compared with the enhanced level. The scheme is incremental such that it assumes that a health care system should first be able to provide the greatest benefit for the largest number of people possible. Next for each service considered the expert panel determined the strengths and weaknesses and resources required. When disagreement existed, stratification of level of resources within a service was then considered.

Results: In LRCs, at the basic level, imaging services would likely not be universally available and thus the primary emphasis would be on obtaining a history and physical exam. Limited level services in terms of mammography should be offered to age groups at higher risk. Enhanced level services would offer mammography every 2 years in women aged 50–69. Maximal level services would include annual mammography screening in women aged 40 and older.

Managerial Epidemiology Interpretation: Where ever possible studies, health care managers should encourage the participation of minorities and economically disadvantaged populations in well-designed and organized clinical trials of cancer screening initiatives. This will not only benefit the participants, but also benefit their societies and add to knowledge regarding potential social and cultural factors that could affect the outcomes of the screening. However, there are substantial barriers to early detection for breast cancer in LRCs including that in some male-dominated societies the fear of neglect or abandonment. The support of public education and awareness particularly in these target populations regarding the value of screening is essential to ensuring the effective deployment of resources needed to promote breast health in LRCs.

form of vaccination, including childhood, argue that the government does not
have the right to override individual autonomy. Provide epidemiological evidence to address the concerns regarding mandatory vaccinations. Assuming
you are in the role of a health care manager: What are your ethical obligations
to the community as a whole with respect to immunizations? To an individual
child within your managed care plan? How do you balance these interests?

References

American College of Epidemiology, 2000, *Ethics Guidelines*, Available at: http://www.acepidemiology2.org/cttes/ethics/

American College of Healthcare Executives, 2007, *ACHE Code of Ethics*, Available at: http://www.ache.org/ABT_ACHE/code.cfm.

Brown, D.R., Fouad, M.N., Basen-Engquist, K., and Tortolero-Luna, G., 2000, Recruitment and retention of minority women in cancer screening, prevention, and treatment trials, *Ann. Epidemiol.* **10**:S13–S21.

Cohen, M.R., Senders, J., and Davis, N.M., 1994, Failure mode and effects analysis: a novel approach to avoiding dangerous medication errors and accidents, *Hosp. Pharm.* **29**:319–330.

Collmann, J. and Cooper, T., 2007, Breaching the security of the Kaiser Permanente internet patient portal: the organizational foundations of information security, *J. Am. Med. Inform. Assoc.* **14**:239–243.

Dunlop, A.L., Graham, T., Leroy, A., Glanz, K., and Dunlop, B., 2007, the impact of HIPAA authorization on willingness to participate in clinical research, *Ann. Epidemiol.* **17**:899–905.

Garrett, J.E., Vawter, D.E., Prehn, A.W., DeBruin, D.A., and Gervais, K.G., 2008, Ethical considerations in pandemic influenza planning, *Minn. Med.* **91**:37–39.

Giuliano, A.R., Mokuau, N., Hughes, C., Tortolero-Luna, G., Risendal, B., Ho, R.C.S., Prewitt, T.E., and McCaskill-Stevens, W.J., 2000, Participation of minorities in cancer research: the influence of structural, cultural, and linguistic factors, *Ann. Epidemiol.* **10**:S22–S34.

Heinig, S.J., Quon, A.S., Meyer, R.E., and Korn, D., 1999, The changing landscape for clinical research, *Acad. Med.* **74**:726–45. Erratum in: *Acad. Med.* **74**:950.

Kilbourne, E.D., 2006, Influenza pandemics of the 20th century, *Emerging Infectious Dis.* **12**:9–13.

Kinlaw, K., and Levine, F. for the Ethics Subcommittee of the Advisory Committee to the Director, Centers for Disease Control and Prevention, 2007, *Ethical Guidelines in Pandemic Influenza*, (October 31, 2008). *http://www.cdc.gov/od/science/phec/panFlu_Ethic_Guidelines.pdf.*

Loue, S., 2004, The participation of cognitively impaired elderly in research, *Care Manag. J.* **5**:245–257.

Loue, S., Okello, D., and Kawuma, M., 1996, Research bioethics in the Ugandan context: a program summary, *J. Law Med. Ethics* **24**:47–53.

McKeown, R.E., Weed, D.L., Kahn, J.P., and Stoto, M.A., 2003, American College of Epidemiology Ethics Guidelines: Foundations and dissemination, *Science and Engineering Ethics* **9**:207–214.

Mello, M.M., 2008, Rationalizing vaccine injury compensation, *Bioethics* **22**:32–42.

Morrison, R.S., and Meier, D.E., 2004, High rates of advance care planning in New York City's elderly population, *Arch. Intern. Med.* **164**:2421–2426.

Ness, R. for the Joint Policy Committee, Societies of Epidemiology, 2007, Influence of the HIPAA privacy rule on health research, *J.A.M.A.* **298**:2164–2170.

Public Health Leadership Society, *2002, Principles of the Ethical Practice of Public Health, Version 2.2.* (October 12, 2008), http://www.apha.org/NR/rdonlyres/1CED3CEA-287E-4185–9CBD-BD405FC60856/0/ethicsbrochure.pdf.

Schoeni, R.F., Martin, L.G., Andreski, P.M., and Freedman, V.A., 2005, Persistent and growing socioeconomic disparities in disability among the elderly: 1982–2002, *Am. J. Pub. Hlth.* **95**:2065–2070.

Thompson, A.K., Faith, K., Gibson, J.L., and Upshur, R.E.G., 2006, Pandemic influenza preparedness: an ethical framework to guide decision-making, *BMS Med. Ethics* **7**:E12.

U.S. Department of Health and Human Services Office for Civil Rights, *Standards for Privacy of Individually Identifiable Health Information*, Available at: http://hhs.gov/ocr/.

Vega, W.A., Karno, M., Alegria, M., Alvidrez, J., Bernal, G., Escamilla, M., Escobar, J., Guarnaccia, P., Jenkins, J., Kopelowicz, A., Lagomasino, I.T., Lewis-Fernandez, R., Marin, H., Lopez, S., and Loue, S., 2007, Research issues for improving treatment of U.S. Hispanics with persistent mental disorders, *Psychiatr. Serv.* **58**:385–394.

Yip, C., Smith, R.A., Anderson, B.O., Miller, A.B., Thomas, D.B., Ang, E., Caffarella, R.S., Corbex, M., Kreps, G.L., and McTiernan, A., on behalf of the Breast Health Global Initiative Early Detection Panel, 2008, Guideline implementation for breast healthcare in low- and middle-income countries: early detection resource allocation, *Cancer Suppl.* **113**:2244–2256.

Weed, D.L., and Coughlin, S.S., 1999, New ethics guidelines for epidemiology: background and rationale, *Ann. Epidemiol.* **9**:277–280.

World Health Organization, 1995, *Guidelines for Good Clinical Practice (GCP) for Trials on Pharmaceutical Products*, WHO Technical Report Series, No. 850, 1995, Annex 3, Geneva, Switzerland.

World Health Organization, 2002, Executive summary. In *National Cancer Control Programmes: Policies and managerial Guidelines*, WHO, Geneva, Switzerland.

World Health Organization, 2007, *Ethical Considerations in Developing a Public Health Response to Pandemic Influenza*, WHO, Geneva, Switzerland.

Index